Innovations in Data Methodologies and Computational Algorithms for Medical Applications

Aryya Gangopadhyay
University of Maryland Baltimore County, USA

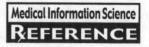

Medical Information Science
REFERENCE

Managing Director: Lindsay Johnston
Senior Editorial Director: Heather A. Probst
Book Production Manager: Sean Woznicki
Development Manager: Joel Gamon
Acquisitions Editor: Erika Gallagher
Typesetter: Jennifer Romanchak
Cover Design: Nick Newcomer, Lisandro Gonzalez

Published in the United States of America by
  Medical Information Science Reference (an imprint of IGI Global)
  701 E. Chocolate Avenue
  Hershey PA 17033
  Tel: 717-533-8845
  Fax: 717-533-8661
  E-mail: cust@igi-global.com
  Web site: http://www.igi-global.com

Library of Congress Cataloging-in-Publication Data

Innovations in data methodologies and computational algorithms for medical applications / Aryya Gangopadhyay, editor.
    p. cm.
  Summary: "This book offers the most cutting edge research in the field of medical applications of technologies, offering insights using case studies and methodologies from around the world"-- Provided by publisher.
  Includes bibliographical references and index.
  ISBN 978-1-4666-0282-3 (hardcover) -- ISBN 978-1-4666-0283-0 (ebook) -- ISBN 978-1-4666-0284-7 (print & perpetual access) 1. Medical informatics. 2. Medical innovations. I. Gangopadhyay, Aryya, 1962-
  R858.I556 2012
  610.72--dc36
                              2011051317

British Cataloguing in Publication Data
A Cataloguing in Publication record for this book is available from the British Library.

Table of Contents

Detailed Table of Contents

Chapter 1

    Yoo Jung An, Fairleigh Dickinson University, USA
    Kuo-chuan Huang, New Jersey Institute of Technology, USA
    Soon Ae Chun, College of Staten Island, USA
    James Geller, New Jersey Institute of Technology, USA

Ontologies, terminologies and vocabularies are popular repositories for collecting the terms used in a domain. It may be expected that in the future more such ontologies will be created for domain experts. However, there is increasing interest in making the language of experts understandable to casual users. For example, cancer patients often research their cases on the Web. The authors consider the problem of objectively evaluating the quality of ontologies (QoO). This article formalizes the notion of naturalness as a component of QoO and quantitatively measures naturalness for well-known ontologies (UMLS, WordNet, OpenCyc) based on their concepts, IS-A relationships and semantic relationships. To compute numeric values characterizing the naturalness of an ontology, this article defines appropriate metrics. As absolute numbers in such a pursuit are often meaningless, we concentrate on using relative naturalness metrics. That allows us to say that a certain ontology is relatively more natural than another one.

Chapter 2

    Shibnath Mukherjee, Yahoo! Research and Development, India
    Aryya Gangopadhyay, University of Maryland Baltimore County, USA
    Zhiyuan Chen, University of Maryland Baltimore County, USA

While data mining has been widely acclaimed as a technology that can bring potential benefits to organizations, such efforts may be negatively impacted by the possibility of discovering sensitive patterns, particularly in patient data. In this article the authors present an approach to identify the optimal set of transactions that, if sanitized, would result in hiding sensitive patterns while reducing the accidental hiding of legitimate patterns and the damage done to the database as much as possible. Their methodology allows the user to adjust their preference on the weights assigned to benefits in terms of the number of restrictive patterns hidden, cost in terms of the number of legitimate patterns hidden, and damage to the database in terms of the difference between marginal frequencies of items for the original and sanitized databases. Most approaches in solving the given problem found in literature are all-heuristic based without formal treatment for optimality. While in a few work, ILP has been used previously as a formal optimization approach, the novelty of this method is the extremely low cost-complexity model in contrast to the others. They implement our methodology in C and C++ and ran several experiments with synthetic data generated with the IBM synthetic data generator. The experiments show excellent results when compared to those in the literature.

Chapter 3

.   *Hongfang Liu, Georgetown University Medical Center, USA*

Manabu Torii, Georgetown University Medical Center, USA

Guixian Xu, Minzu University of China, China

Johannes Goll, The J. Craig Venter Institute, USA

Protein-protein interaction (PPI) networks are essential to understand the fundamental processes governing cell biology. Recently, studying PPI networks becomes possible due to advances in experimental high-throughput genomics and proteomics technologies. Many interactions from such high-throughput studies and most interactions from small-scale studies are reported only in the scientific literature and thus are not accessible in a readily analyzable format. This has led to the birth of manual curation initiatives such as the International Molecular Exchange Consortium (IMEx). The manual curation of PPI knowledge can be accelerated by text mining systems to retrieve PPI-relevant articles (article retrieval) and extract PPI-relevant knowledge (information extraction). In this article, the authors focus on article retrieval and define the task as binary classification where PPI-relevant articles are positives and the others are negatives. In order to build such classifier, an annotated corpus is needed. It is very expensive to obtain an annotated corpus manually but a noisy and imbalanced annotated corpus can be obtained automatically, where a collection of positive documents can be retrieved from existing PPI knowledge bases and a large number of unlabeled documents (most of them are negatives) can be retrieved from PubMed. They compared the performance of several machine learning algorithms by varying the ratio of the number of positives to the number of unlabeled documents and the number of features used.

Chapter 4

Bhaswati Ghosh, Cleveland State University, USA

Partha S. Ghosh, Cleveland Clinic Foundation, USA

Iftikhar U. Sikder, Cleveland State University, USA

Ontology-based disease classification offers a way to rigorously assign disease types and to reuse diagnostic knowledge. However, ontology itself is not sufficient for fully representing the complex knowledge needed in classification schemes which are continuously evolving. This article describes the application of SWRL/OWL-DL to the representation of knowledge intended for proper classification of a complex neurological condition, namely epilepsy. The authors present a rigorous and expandable approach to the ontological classification of epileptic seizures based on the 1981 ILAE classification. It provides a classification knowledge base that can be extended with rules that describe constraints in SWRL. Moreover, by transforming an OWL classification scheme into JESS (rule engine in Java platform) facts and by transforming SWRL constraints into JESS, logical inferences and reasoning provide a mechanism to discover new knowledge and facts. The logic representation of epileptic classification amounts to greater community understanding among practitioners, knowledge reuse and interoperability.

The aim of the study was to determine association between osteoarthritis and metabolic syndrome stratified by age and gender categories. A final sample of 16,149 US residents aged 17 years or older was analyzed using the database National Health and Nutrition Examination Survey (NAHNES III). Variables assessed include age, gender, race, education, poverty income ratio, body mass index, smoking history, metabolic syndrome and its risk components. Continuous and categorical variables were compared in the 2 groups using T and chi-square statistics as appropriate. Multivariate analysis was performed after adjusting for the potential confounders. Five percent subjects self-reported of having osteoarthritis. The prevalence of metabolic syndrome in subjects with osteoarthritis was 40% compared to 21% with no osteoarthritis. Subjects with osteoarthritis were significantly older; were females, non-Hispanic whites, less educated and had high prevalence of diabetes, hypertension and high cholesterol. Age, being female, higher education, being non-Hispanic White, absence of osteoporosis, and body mass index were significant predictors of osteoarthritis. Metabolic syndrome was a risk factor for osteoarthritis in males.

Commercial Web-based Personal-Health Record (PHR) systems can help patients to share their personal health records (PHRs) anytime from anywhere. PHRs are very sensitive data and an inappropriate disclosure may cause serious problems to an individual. Therefore commercial Web-based PHR systems have to ensure that the patient health data is secured using state-of-the-art mechanisms. In current commercial PHR systems, even though patients have the power to define the access control policy on who can access their data, patients have to trust entirely the access-control manager of the commercial PHR system to properly enforce these policies. Therefore patients hesitate to upload their health data to these systems as the data is processed unencrypted on untrusted platforms. Recent proposals on enforcing access control policies exploit the use of encryption techniques to enforce access control policies. In such systems, information is stored in an encrypted form by the third party and there is no need for an access control manager. This implies that data remains confidential even if the database maintained by the third party is compromised. In this paper we propose a new encryption technique called a type-and-identity-based proxy re-encryption scheme which is suitable to be used in the healthcare setting. The proposed scheme allows users (patients) to securely store their PHRs on commercial Web-based PHRs, and securely share their PHRs with other users (doctors).

For health care related research studies the medical records of patients may need to be retrieved from multiple sites with different regulations on the disclosure of health information. Given the sensitive nature of health care information, privacy is a major concern when patients' health care data is used for research purposes. In this paper, the authors propose approaches for integration and querying of health care data from multiple sources in a secure and privacy preserving manner. In particular, the first approach ensures secure data integration based on unique identifiers, and the second one considers data integration based on quasi identifiers, for which a rule-based framework is proposed for cross-linking data records, including secure character matching.

Recent government-led efforts and industry-sponsored privacy initiatives in the healthcare sector have received heightened publicity. The current set of privacy legislation mandates that all parties involved in the delivery of care specify and publish privacy policies regarding the use and disclosure of personal health information. The authors' study of actual healthcare privacy policies indicates that the vague representations in published privacy policies are not strongly correlated with adequate privacy protection for the patient. This phenomenon is not due to a lack of available technology to enforce privacy policies, but rather to the will of the healthcare entities to enforce strong privacy protections and their interpretation of minimum compliance obligations. Using available information systems and data mining techniques, this article describes an infrastructure for privacy protection based on the idea of policy refinement to allow the transition from the current state of perceived to be privacy-preserving systems to actually privacy-preserving systems.

The authors extend their previous work on Ultrasound (US) image lesion detection and segmentation, to classification, proposing a complete end-to-end solution for automatic Ultrasound Computer Aided Detection (US CAD). Carried out is a comprehensive analysis to determine the best classifier-feature set combination that works optimally in US imaging. In particular the use of nineteen features categorised into three groups (shape, texture and edge), ten classifiers and 22 feature selection approaches are used in the analysis. From the overall performance, the classifier RBFNetworks defined by the WEKA pattern recognition tool set, with a feature set comprising of the area to perimeter ratio, solidity, elongation, roundness, standard deviation, two Fourier related and a fractal related texture measures out-performed other combinations of feature-classifiers, with an achievement of predicted Az value of 0.948. Next analyzed is the use of a number of different metrics in performance analysis and provide an insight to future improvements and extension.

Chapter 10

Pimwadee Chaovalit, National Science and Technology Development Agency, Thailand

In the healthcare industry, the ability to monitor patients via biomedical signals assists healthcare professionals in detecting early signs of conditions such as blocked arteries and abnormal heart rhythms. Using data clustering, it is possible to interpret these signals to look for patterns that may indicate emerging or developing conditions. This can be accomplished by basing monitoring systems on a fast clustering algorithm that processes fast-paced streams of raw data effectively. This paper presents a clustering method, POD-Clus, which can be useful in computer-aided diagnosis. The proposed method clusters data streams in linear time and outperforms a competing algorithm in capturing changes of clusters in data streams.

Chapter 11

Xin Li, Georgetown University, USA

In this paper, the authors present a new approach to perform principal component analysis (PCA)-based gene clustering on genomic data distributed in multiple sites (horizontal partitions) with privacy protection. This approach allows data providers to collaborate together to identify gene profiles from a global viewpoint, and at the same time, protect the sensitive genomic data from possible privacy leaks. The authors developed a framework for privacy preserving PCA-based gene clustering, which includes two types of participants such as data providers and a trusted central site. Within this mechanism, distributed horizontal partitions of genomic data can be globally clustered with privacy preservation. Compared to results from centralized scenarios, the result generated from distributed partitions achieves 100% accuracy by using this approach. An experiment on a real genomic data set is conducted, and result shows that the proposed framework produces exactly the same cluster formation as that from the centralized data set.

Chapter 12

Ravinder Singh Malhotra, Sri Guru Ram Das Institute of Medical Sciences
& Research and Center for Public Health Informatics, India
K. S. Ded, Sri Guru Ram Das Institute of Medical Sciences
& Research and Center for Public Health Informatics, India
Arun Gupta, Sri Guru Ram Das Institute of Medical Sciences
& Research and Center for Public Health Informatics, India
Darpan Bansal, Sri Guru Ram Das Institute of Medical Sciences
& Research and Center for Public Health Informatics, India
Harneet Singh, Sri Guru Ram Das Institute of Medical Sciences
& Research and Center for Public Health Informatics, India

Haematemesis and malena are the two most important symptoms of upper gastrointestinal bleeding . The most common cause of upper gastrointestinal bleeding is due to a peptic ulcer. In this paper, the authors research the cause of bleeding. Contrary to previous studies, results favor esophageal varices, e.g., alcoholism or cirrhosis liver post necrotic, as the most common cause of bleeding rather than a peptic ulcer. The authors' study is based on an observational retrospective protocol with records of 50 consecutive patients with GI bleeding, attending the emergency room from February 2007 until September 2009. Results show that the treatment of UGI bleeding has made important progress since the introduction of emergency endoscopy and endoscopic techniques for haemostasis. The application of specific protocols significantly decreases rebleeding and the need for surgery, whereas mortality is still high. The data highlight the decreasing trend of peptic ulcer as the sole cause of bleeding, as shown in previous literature, ascertaining that varices are now the most common variable.

Chapter 13

Computational techniques, such as Simple K, have been used for exploratory analysis in applications ranging from data mining research, machine learning, and computational biology. The medical domain has benefitted from these applications, and in this regard, the authors analyze patterns in individuals of selected age groups linked with the possibility of Metabolic Syndrome (MetS), a disorder affecting approximately 45% of the elderly. The study identifies groups of individuals behaving in two defined categories, that is, those diagnosed with MetS (MetS Positive) and those who are not (MetS Negative), comparing the pattern definition. The paper compares the cluster formation in patterns when using a data reduction technique referred to as Singular Value Decomposition (SVD) versus eliminating its application in clustering. Data reduction techniques like SVD have proved to be very useful in projecting only what is considered to be key relations in the data by suppressing the less important ones. With the existence of high dimensionality, the importance of SVD can be highly effective. By applying two internal measures to validate the cluster quality, findings in this study prove interesting in context to both approaches.

Chlamydia trachomatis (CT) and Neisseria gonorrhoeae (GC) are two common sexually transmitted diseases among women in the United States. Publicly funded programs usually do not have enough money to screen and treat all patients. Therefore, the authors propose a new resource allocation model to assist clinical managers to make decisions on identifying at-risk population groups, as well as selecting a screening and treatment strategy for CT and GC patients under a fixed budget. At the same time, the authors also develop a two-step branch-and-bound algorithm tailor-made for our model. Running on real-life data, the algorithm calculates the optimal solution within a very short time. The new algorithm also improves the accuracy of an approximate solution obtained by Excel Solver. This study has shown that a resource allocation model and algorithm might have a significant impact on real clinical issues.

The rate of people dying from medical errors in hospitals each year is very high. Errors that frequently occur during the course of providing health care are adverse drug events and improper transfusions, surgical injuries and wrong-site surgery, suicides, restraint-related injuries or death, falls, burns, pressure ulcers, and mistaken patient identities. Medical decision support systems play an increasingly important role in medical practice. By assisting physicians in making clinical decisions, medical decision support systems improve the quality of medical care. Two approaches have been investigated for the prediction of medical outcomes: "hours of ventilation" and the "mortality rate" in the adult intensive care unit. The first approach is based on neural networks with the weight-elimination algorithm, and the second is based on genetic programming. Both approaches are compared to commonly used machine learning algorithms. Results show that both algorithms developed score well for the outcomes selected.

In this paper, a set of analyses on the deployment of coronary stents by using a nonlinear finite element method is proposed. The author proposes a convergence test able to select the appropriate mesh dimension and a methodology to perform the simplification of structures composed of cyclically repeated units to reduce the number of degree of freedom and the analysis run time. A systematic study, based on the analysis of seven meshes for each model, is performed, gradually reducing the element dimension. In addition, geometric models are simplified considering symmetries; adequate boundary conditions are applied and verified based on the results obtained from analysis of the whole model.

Hypertension, the leading global risk factor for early mortality, cannot be detected or treated without accurate and practical methods of blood pressure (BP) measurement. Although home BP measurement has considerable popularity among patients, the lack of evidence needed to assure its place in modern clinical practice has hindered its widespread acceptance among physicians. This paper demonstrates that home BP measurement is more accurate than conventional clinic and ambulatory monitoring BP measurement and can be used effectively in clinical practice. On the basis of the data from different studies, it can be concluded that home BP measurement is an improvement over conventional clinic BP measurement. Home monitoring of BP is a convenient, accurate, and widely available option and may become the method of choice when diagnosing and treating hypertension. A paradigm shift is needed in BP measurement as evidence-based medicine suggests that clinic BP measurement should only be used for screening purposes.

Preface

The importance of Information Technology in healthcare cannot be overestimated in today's world. With the rapid development of Information Technology (IT) there is an ever-growing emphasis on the use of IT in the research and practice of healthcare. The research in health information technology has been motivated by several developments, including electronic medical records, emphasis on personalized medicine and research on genomic data, and development of computational techniques for finding patterns, to name a few. Along with these new privacy concerns for electronic medical records and their access to third parties has become an important issue. In this article we discuss some of the recent research on health information technology within the context of the following areas: pattern recognition in medicine, privacy and security issues in healthcare, and clinical decision support.

PATTERN RECOGNITION IN MEDICINE

Pattern recognition algorithms are powerful techniques that can identify hidden patterns in data that can be beneficial for medical diagnosis, treatment management, epidemiological studies, finding longitudinal patterns, information retrieval in medical literature, and integration of different types of data. There is vast potential for applying pattern recognition techniques including algorithms from data mining, machine learning, statistical analysis, and matrix-based methods such as singular value decomposition and spectral analysis in healthcare data. In this section we first provide an overview of some of the common methods that have been developed in the recent literature and then describe a few articles in more details. In our discussion we recognize the overlap between machine learning and data mining methods but differentiate the two fields by the fact that data mining has a more explicit focus on dealing with large databases. Statistical methods are hypothetico-deductive where the main focus is to test and either validate or refute, through rigorous mathematical treatment, a given hypothesis (Hand 1998). Data mining is useful in exploratory data analysis where patterns are found using inductive methods (see Han et al 2006, Tan et al 2006, Dunham 2000 for more details).

Association Rule Mining

Traditionally, data mining methods have been categorized into association rule mining, classification, clustering, and outlier or anomaly detection. Association rules have their roots in market basket analysis where the goal is to find frequently co-occurring items in retail store transactions. Since different transactions (market baskets) typically belong to different customers it is assumed that the transactions are independent of each other. In some applications, such as co-location analyses such assumption is not valid and hence some modifications to the algorithms for association rule mining are needed. Generating association rules using the popular *a-priori* algorithm requires multiple database scans and hence more efficient algorithms such as FP-tree (Han et al 2000) have been proposed. Association rules represent local patterns between items, terms, diseases, patients etc.

Clustering

Clustering is an exploratory technique used in finding homogeneous groups is clustering, which can be useful in finding global characteristics such as the main groupings in datasets. There are several challenges in finding clusters in datasets. Since the goal of clustering is to group similar data points in one group, an appropriate distance measure is needed. The popular distance measure of the Euclidean distance assumes an underlying flat-space geometric representation of the data. Other flat-space geometry measures such Mahalanobis distance (Mahalanobus 1936), Kullback-Leibler distance (Kullback et al 1951), are also used. There are many clustering algorithms, the most popular being the k-means clustering algorithm. However, others such as hierarchical and density-based clustering algorithms are also commonly used. Methods such as k-means and k-medoids tend to discover globular clusters whereas density-based clustering algorithms can discover clusters with arbitrary shapes including those with high aspect ratios.

Dimensionality Reduction

A fundamental challenge in data mining, particularly in clustering, is the high dimensionality of the data. In a high-dimensional space the data gets scattered which makes it difficult to find homogeneous clusters. Dimensionality reduction techniques such as Principal Components Analysis (PCA) (Joliffe 2002) can be used to project the data into a low dimensional subspace as a pre-processing step. The low dimensional subspace is spanned by a set of eigenvectors that correspond to the largest eigenvalues of the covariance matrix of the data. Since the covariance matrix is symmetric the eigenvectors are orthogonal. Hence projecting the original data into the new basis vectors (set of selected eigenvectors) also decorrelates the dimensions. In a recent study (Joshi et al 2010) PCA was applied to glomerural filtration rates of the kidneys for 110 patients tracked over a period of twenty-four months after kidney transplantation with the goal of identifying homogeneous clusters that would explain why some of the transplanted kidneys failed while others did not. The data in the original twenty-four dimensional space did not exhibit any consistent patterns while PCA reduced the dataset to a single dimension. Subsequent analysis showed statistically significant differences between patient clusters with implications such as possible intervention strategies that can be deployed more effective care.

Principal components analysis is a linear transformation of the data that may not preserve nonlinear relationships. Manifold techniques such as multi-dimensional scaling (MDS) (Lee at al 2003), locally linear embedding (LLE) (Saul et al 2003), and ISOMAP (Tenenbaum et al 2000) try to discover low dimensional manifolds for high-dimensional data. However, MDS tries to reconstruct the nonlinear relationships using Euclidean distance and may not be topology preserving. ISOMAP builds a graph using K nearest neighbors and looks for local properties in those neighborhoods. ISOMAP assumes that there are no holes in the data. It is also sensitive to noise. LLE, like ISOMAP also uses nonlinear embedding. However, LLE may not be able to handle high-dimensional data.

Classification

Classification is a supervised technique for pattern recognition where the goal is to classify an instance into one of several discrete pre-defined classes. A classification model is built from a set of existing instances whose class values are already known. A simplified example is to classify a patient into one of two classes (healthy or sick) from a set of observable symptoms. The classification model is created from a training set and its accuracy is estimated using a set of test set. In addition to the overall accuracy other measures of goodness of the classification model are used. Examples of classification algorithms include decision trees, support vector machines, neural networks, and Bayesian classifiers such as the naïve Bayes classifier and Bayesian networks. Examples of classification algorithms in healthcare include Ludwig et al (2010) and Yap et al (2010).

Mining Medical Data Streams

Biomedical signals generated by monitoring devices such as Electrocardiogram (ECG), Electroencephalogram (EEG), and Phonocardiogram (PCG) abound in today's healthcare industry (e.g., Cowley 2006, Lu et al 2005). Systematic analysis of such data can help monitor and detect early signs of critical conditions and possible interventions. However, the data generated by such devices is typically very large and potentially unbounded. For example, an ECG can generate several million data points in a matter of minutes (Chaovalit 2010). Analyzing such data streams is a challenging task that requires efficient algorithms that can detect time-dependent changes efficiently and accurately. Chaovalit (2010) describes an algorithm called POD-Clus for clustering high-speed data streams using a linear time algorithm that can create and update clusters over a period of time. More specifically, the method has the following characteristics: it scans the data only once which is required given the high-speed, high-volume intake of data streams, it creates a compact model (cluster synopsis) of the data and updates it parameters incrementally, it uses a small and fixed amount of memory, it detects outliers, and it can handle cluster evolutions. There are several types of cluster evolutions that are handled by the method: migration of data points from one cluster to another, creation of new clusters either as a result of cluster spilt or mergers, emergence of new clusters, and dissolution of existing clusters. Two algorithms are proposed to handle cases with and without cluster evolutions respectively. If cluster evolution is not expected the algorithm starts with an initial cluster formation, computes the mean and standard deviation (or covariance matrix if the data is multi-dimensional), and updates these measures as new data points are generated. Obviously, the method assumes that the data is follows a Gaussian distribution, which is realistic for large data sets (Thompson et al 1990).

When cluster evolution is expected a number of additional steps are necessary. As new data points arrive, the algorithm checks for outliers that are not within the standard deviations from the centroids of any existing clusters. Outliers may form a new cluster if they are homogeneous. The method monitors the sparsity of the clusters using a threshold and uses a chi-square test to determine if the cluster needs to be split. Clusters can dissolve when a sufficient number of data points migrate to other clusters or groups. Clusters can also be merged when the overlapping region exceeds a predetermined threshold. The method was extensively tested against previous data stream clustering algorithms such as E-Stream (Udommanetanakit et al 2007) as with ground truth validation.

Information Retrieval

The practice of evidence-based medicine requires physicians to retrieve and analyze data from published research, which helps provide the latest treatment to their patients. An example is randomized clinical trials that provide evidence of the effectiveness of drugs on specific patient populations. There is a huge amount of medical information in the form of text documents including research papers in online databases, physician notes, discharge summaries, Web portals, etc. There is a vital need for effective search and retrieval of information from these sources as well as for the organization of these text corpuses into homogeneous groups or clusters. This remains a challenge even with the advanced technology found in today's world. One important characteristic needed for information search and retrieval tools in this context is the ability to remove obsolete documents and narrow the search down to the set of newer documents or respond to queries with specific time windows. These methods should be incremental and dynamic in order to avoid expensive re-computation every time changes are made. A dynamic document clustering method is described in Ramesh (2011) that creates singular value decomposition (SVD) of a term-document matrix (TDM) that contains term weights as products of term and inverse document frequencies normalized by the document size. The document clustering is done using the left singular vectors of the TDM corresponding to the largest eigenvalues. Since only a few singular values are selected a truncated SVD is created consisting of the submatrices corresponding to the original left and right singular vector matrices and the submatrix of the original singular value matrix with only the selected subset of singular values. The challenge is to incrementally update the truncated SVD when new terms and/or documents are added to the existing text corpus. Re-computing the SVD for the entire TDM each time is computationally expensive. However, *fold-in* methods have been suggested for incremental updates of the singular vector matrices of the TDM. A new fold-in method and subsequent clustering are suggested is Ramesh (2011). When new documents arrive, the TDM for the newly added documents is created and the new TDM is projected into the truncated SVD space. In addition to folding-in the method also describes a method called "windowing" that updates the truncated SVD when users select a specific time window for document clustering or retrieval. The method is validated using medical abstracts from Pubmed.

PRIVACY AND SECURITY

The Health Insurance Portability and Accountability Act (HIPAA), enforced by the Office for Civil Rights, is the national standard for security of electronic health information and the protection of identifiable information of patients. With the growing digitization of heath records the issues of patient privacy and security of electronic medical records are becoming increasingly important. In this section we first discuss the privacy issues in healthcare data and then the issues related to security.

Privacy

Research on health information technology requires collection of data from a variety of sources including government agencies, healthcare providers, insurance companies, etc. The sensitive nature of healthcare data and the social and legal implications of the disclosure of such data require that such data be protected against any possible violation of the privacy of individuals. However, it is also important to share such data with researchers to advance the state of the art in medical research. It has been shown that publicly available datasets that remove all identifying information about individuals can be compromised using linkage attacks (Samarati et al 1998). This presents an interesting dichotomy that requires the dual objectives of having to share the data in its original or some perturbed or transformed version such that both data utility and privacy will be preserved. The area of privacy preserving data mining offers solutions to this dichotomy by providing perturbation methods that hide private information while preserving patterns in the data.

The research on privacy preserving data mining can be broadly categorized into the following groups: data anonymization methods, data perturbation methods, cryptographic methods, methods dealing with specialized data types such as genomic data, image data, spatial data and protection of location privacy, incremental methods for privacy preserving data mining, privacy preserving data imputation, and privacy preserving data integration. In this article we will provide an overview of the latest work in this area. Interested readers are referred to books such as Vaidya et al (2006) and Aggarwal et al (2008) for a more detailed treatment of this area. Data perturbation methods distort the data while preserving the underlying data distributions. Additive data perturbation methods were among the first data perturbation methods suggested in the literature. These methods add random noise to the data while preserving the data distributions (Agrawal et al 2001). However, such methods were shown to be vulnerable to attacks based on correlations (Kargupta et al 2003). Subsequently, random projection-based methods were suggested that would reduce the dimensions of the original data my multiplying it with a random matrix (Liu et al 2006). While the work described in Liu et al (2006) provided some privacy there was no provable worst-case privacy guaranty, which was achieved in a subsequent work described in Mukherjee at al (2008). The data perturbation and transformation based approaches suggested throughout the privacy preserving data mining literature have a fundamental problem when it comes to healthcare data in that the data utility is severely compromised in most cases. A more recent research describes a perturbation method for preventing 3D reconstruction of CT axial images used by radiologists for the diagnosis of various diseases such as carotid aneurysm (Chen et al 2011). The method is based on edge detection of individual DICOM slices, creating a map for each slice, and adding random voxels as mask to each slice. The mask is smoothed by making the voxel intensities similar to those of the closest skin surface. The diagnostic information below the skin surface is fully preserved.

Another area of research in privacy preserving data mining focused on secure mining of data with distributed inputs from a number of data owners (sites). This branch of research, also known as secure multi-party computation, typically use cryptographic techniques to securely compute mathematical functions such that all parties can see the final results but not the individual data which is sensitive (see Verkios et al 2004 for a survey). Li (2010, 2011) described a method for privacy preserving clustering for gene expression microarrays on distributed data. Three different data partitioning scenarios were considered: horizontal, where each site has a different set of genes but all sites have the same set of experimental conditions, vertical, where each site has the same set of genes but different experimental conditions, and mixed, where each site has a different set of genes and a different set of experimental conditions. This method also reduces data transmission cost that can be prohibitively large for genomic data. Experimental results showed the feasibility of the approach with high degree of accuracy in PCA and clustering.

Security

Electronic health record systems (EHRs) can provide many benefits such as reducing cost, improving the quality of care, and empowering patients to maintain their own health-related information. The ability to record and maintain health-related information provides patients to have more control over their own information and increases their awareness about their health condition. However, electronic storage of data also brings increasing threats for inappropriate access to such data with devastating consequences. Government agencies across the world (such as HIPAA in the United States) have developed directives to safeguard patient privacy. This necessitates research and development of methods to secure such systems against unauthorized access to data.

While legislations control the privacy and electronic communications of EHRs personal health record systems (PHRs) such as Google Health (Google 2007) and Microsoft Health Vault (Microsoft 2007) are still outside the scope of such legislation (Ibraimi et al 2010). One problem with PHRs is that a patient cannot create fine-grained and dynamic access control policy on their health data where the access is all or nothing. Another concern is that the sensitive health information such as history, drug-use, and sexual orientation are stored in a third-party server without any authority over the access control mechanisms established by the third party host. The major issues related to PHR systems are the ability for patients to provide differential access control and guaranteed security against unauthorized access to such data.

Ibraimi et al (2010) describe a public key encryption method for securing personal health records. Patients might want to share their health information with their primary care physicians that can be achieved using a proxy re-encryption mechanism. Public key encryption schemes create a pair of private and public keys. Anyone can encrypt a message with the public key. However, the private key is needed to decrypt the encrypted data (the cyphertext). The identity-based proxy re-encryption scheme (Green et al 2007) extends public key encryption by allowing the patient (delegator) to create a proxy re-encryption key that can be used by a designated physician (delegatee) to re-encrypt the cyphertext and subsequently decrypt the original data using their own private key. Thus, the delegator does not need to share his/her own private key with anyone else. This scheme is useful is PHR systems because (1) the data is secure in a third party server because it is encrypted, (2) the patient can share his/her data with designated physicians, and (3) the patient can dynamically change access policy with out having to decrypt the data. One potential drawback of the identity-based proxy re-encryption is that the proxy (in this case the physician) can re-encrypt all of the patient data and get access to them. Hence, this mechanism is still all-or-nothing, which does not let the patient establish differential access controls. This limitation is addressed in Ibraimi el al (2010) by extending the identity based encryption scheme (Boneh et al 2001) to a type-and-identity based proxy re-encryption algorithm. In this method the patient can categorize the data into different types corresponding to different levels of sensitivity using one key-pair and delegate the decryption key of each type to a different healthcare professional thorough a proxy. This has the advantage that if the proxy and the delegatee are corrupted only one a subset of the data will be compromised. Also, the patient can control access to his/her data based on the level of sensitivity they associate with different subsets. It also has the advantage of giving the patient more access control over their private data, which should enhance their trust in the system. In this mechanism the proxy maintains the list of re-encryption keys that should not be made public. However, the proxy cannot decrypt any of the data by themselves because they do not have access to the private keys of the delegates.

CLINICAL DECISION SUPPORT

Computational methods have long been studied for developing tools and techniques to support decision making in healthcare. However, recent advancement in information technology has generated tremendous opportunities sharing, designing, and integrating information among patients and healthcare professionals in the forms of record sharing, health information networks, and protocols (Feishi et al 2003). In this section we describe a few studies to illustrate the role of information technology in the practice of medicine.

Identifying, Screening, and Testing At-Risk Groups

Zhao et al (2010) describe a two-step branch and bound algorithm to help clinical managers make decisions to identify at-risk population groups and develop strategies for screening and treatment of Chlmydia Trachomatis (CT) and Neisseria Gonorrhoeae (GC), two of the most common sexually transmitted diseases in the United States. Screening for CT and GC is expensive and budget restrictions limit the extent to which clinics can perform expensive screening procedures. In order to be cost effective the Center for Disease Control (CDC 2010) and the U.S. Preventive Services Task Force (USPSTF 2005) have identified the subpopulation of women who are 25 or under for such screening. Although restricting diagnostic tests to a subpopulation reduces the cost of testing, it does not solve the problem of choosing between expensive but sophisticated testing options versus testing wider groups of the population with less expensive and less effective tests. Bundled tests as opposed to single-pathogen tests have also been offered as potential solutions. Zhao et al. (2010) proposed an optimization method to solve the resource allocation problem under cost constraints for two sexually transmitted diseases. The solution is a two-step branch and bound algorithm, and subsequently a dynamic programming algorithm that provides the globally optimal solution that is also computationally efficient. The cubic binary model proposed by the authors is applicable for solving resource allocation problems to manage budgets under a fixed number of groups, screening assays, and treatment regiments for CT and GC.

Clinical errors are the cause of a significant number of deaths in hospitals in the United States (Ludwig et al 2010). Examples of such errors include adverse drug effects and improper transfusions, falls, burns, pressure ulcers, wrong-site surgery, and mistaken patient identities. Errors in intensive care units, operating rooms and emergency department have the most adverse consequences (IM 1999). Clinical decision support systems (Kaplan 2001, Metaxiotis et al 2000) can be decision aids for medical practitioners in various ways such as matching specific patients using a computerized knowledge base, patient-specific assessments and recommendations, pattern recognition, and data visualization. Frtize et al (2010) identify three main areas as critical for the design of a clinical decision support system: data entry and decision algorithms, human factor and usability for data acquisition and data requests, and presentation of the output. Machine learning has been used in clinical decision support systems in mainly two areas: (1) diseases recognition from input sources such as cardiograms, Computed Axial Tomography, and Magnetic Resonance Imaging; (2) bioinformatics such as DNA analysis and interpretation of gene expression data (Li 2011). Lugwig et al (2010) compare machine learning techniques using data from adult intensive care units to predict two outcome measures in two different data sets: death and hours of ventilation needed by the patient. Eight classification algorithms including Bayesian networks, nearest neighbor classifier, decision tree, naïve Bayes classifier, and support vector machines were compared with two new algorithms automatic genetic programming and neural network with weight-elimination.

Implantation of Coronary Stents

Implantation of coronary stents is a regular non-clinical procedure applied to patients with coronary heart disease. Stents are metallic cylinders that can be classified as slotted tubes, coil, or mesh (Xiao *et al.*, 2007). Computer simulations based on the Finite Element method have been developed to study the structural behavior of stents in terms of stresses and strains developed when the device is implanted. The finite element method is used to generate a description of a real structure in terms of discrete finite elements and develop a mathematical model to describe the behavior of the structure. Computational finite element methods generate an approximate numerical solution and the goal is to minimize the modeling error. The better the selected mathematical model describe the physical properties of the structure being analyzed the less the error. A few additional factors such as constraints and loads, coarseness of the mesh that discretizes the structure, mesh dimensions, the number of degrees of freedom, and the simplification of the geometry can affect the modeling error and also runtime accuracy.

Gigliardi (2010) describes a method for optimizing the mesh dimensions and simplification of the geometry using seven different mesh dimensions and three different geometries of a number of commercial stents. Convergence tests were applied to select the best element dimensions for each geometry in order to minimize analysis time. The Newton-Raphson method was used minimize the residual force and moments calculated from the stiffness matrix in each iteration. This work extends previous related research in several ways: by varying element dimensions (as opposed to Xia et al 2007, Feng et al 2008) and performing convergence tests on a larger range of element sizes (as compared to Narracott et al 2007). This paper used the finite element ANSYS software and the author suggests verifying the results with other software packages for finite element analysis. Furthermore balloon expandable stents and contacts between the stent and atherosclerotic plaque should be included in future studies. However, Gigliardi (2010) provides guidelines for correct mesh choice for computational analysis of bare coronary stents.

Aryya Gangopadhyay
University of Maryland Baltimore County, USA

REFERENCES

Agrawal, D., & Aggarwal, C. On the Design and Quantification of Privacy Preserving Data Mining Algorithms. *In Proceedings of the Twentieth ACM PODS*, Santa Barbara, CA, 2001.

Aggarwal, C. & Yu. P. (2008). *Privacy-Preserving Data Mining: Models and Algorithms.* Springer.

Boneh, D., & Franklin, M. K. (2001). Identity-based encryption from the weil pairing. In J. Kilian (Ed.), Proceedings of Crypto 2001 (Vol. 2139 of LNCS) (pp. 213-229). New York: Springer Verlag.

CDC. (2010). *Recommends screening of all sexually active women 25 and under.* Retrieved September 16, 2010, from http://www.cdc.gov/std/infertility/default.htm

Chaovalit, P. (2010, July-September). An Effective Streams Clustering Method for Biomedical Signals. *International Journal of Computational Models and Algorithms in Medicine, 1*(3), 1–30.

Chen, J., Gangopadhyay, A., Banerjee, M., Chen, Z., Yesha, Y., Patel, J., & Seigel, E. (2011). A Novel Algorithm to De-Identify Pixel Data from CT Scans of the Head and Face to Protect against Patient Identification Using a 3D Surface Reconstruction, in the *97th RSNA Annual Scientific Assembly and Annual Meeting.*

Cowley, M. (2006, January 8). *Electrodes, leads & wires: A practical guide to ecg monitoring and recording.* Retrieved August 15, 2010, from www.mikecowley.co.uk/leads.htm

Feng, J., Zihui, X., & Katsuhiko, S. (2008). On the finite element modelling of balloon-expandable stents. *Journal of the Mechanical Behavior of Biomedical Materials, 1*(1), 86–95. doi:10.1016/j.jmbbm.2007.07.002

Dunham (2003). *Data Mining Introductory and Advanced Topics.* Prentice Hall.

Feishi, M., Dufour, J.-C., Stacini, P., Gouvernet, J., & Bouhaddou, O. (2003). Medical Decision Support Systems: Old Dilemmas and new Paradigms?" Tracks for Successful Integration and Adoption. *Methods of Information in Medicine, 3,* 190–198.

Feng, J., Zihui, X., & Katsuhiko, S. (2008). On the finite element modelling of balloon-expandable stents. *Journal of the Mechanical Behavior of Biomedical Materials, 1*(1), 86–95. doi:10.1016/j.jmbbm.2007.07.002

Frize, M., Solven, F. G., Stevenson, M., Nickerson, B. G., Buskard, T., & Taylor, K. B. (1995, July). Computer-Assisted Decision Support Systems for Patient Management in an Intensive Care Unit. In *Proceedings of Medinfo95,* Vancouver, BC, Canada (pp. 1009-1012).

Gagliardi, M. (2010, October-December). Relevance of Mesh Dimension Optimization, Geometry Simplification and Discretization Accuracy in the Study of Mechanical Behaviour of Bare Metal Stents . *International Journal of Computational Models and Algorithms in Medicine, 1*(4), 31–45.

Gangopadhyay, A. Joshi, A., and Wali, R. (2012). A Spectral Clustering Technique for Studying Post-Transplant Kidney Functions, in *Proceedings of the 2nd* ACM SIGHIT International Health Informatics Symposium (IHI 2012), accepted.

Green, M., & Ateniese, G. (2007). Identity-based proxy re-encryption. In J. Katz & M. Yung (Eds.), Proceedings of Applied Cryptography and Network Security (Vol. 4521 of LNCS) (pp. 288-306). New York: Springer Verlag.

Google. (2007). *Google Health.* Accessed November 27, 2011, http://www.google.com/health.

Han, J., & Kamber, M. (2006). *Data Mining: Concepts and Techniques* (2nd ed.). Morgan Kaufmann.

Han, J. Pei J., & Yon, Y. (2000). Mining Frequent Patterns Without Candidate Generation. In *Proceedings of the ACM-SIGMOD International Conference of Data,* 1-12, Dallas, Texas.

Hand (1998). Data Mining: Statistics and More? *The American Statistician,* 52(2): 112-118.

Ibraimi, L. (2010, April-June). Tang, Q., Hartel, P., and Jonker, W. (2010). Exploring Type-and-Identity-Based Proxy Re-Encryption Scheme to Securely Manage Personal Health Records . *International Journal of Computational Models and Algorithms in Medicine, 1*(2), 1–21.

IM. (1999). *To Err Is Human: Building A Safer Health System*. Washington, DC: Institute of Medicine.

Jolliffe, I. T. (2002). *Principal component analysis*. New York: Springer.

Joshi, A., Gangopadhyay, A., Banerjee, M., Mohanlal, V., and Wali, R. (2010). A clustering method to study the loss of kidney function following kidney transplantation. *International Journal of Biomedical Engineering and technology*, 3((1/2)):64–82, 2010.

Kargupta, H., Datta, S., Wang, Q., & Sivakumar, K. (2003). On the Privacy Preserving Properties of Random Data Perturbation Techniques, in *Proceedings of the IEEE International Conference on Data Mining*.

Kaplan, B. (2001). Evaluating informatics applications clinical decision support systems literature review. *International Journal of Medical Informatics, 64*, 15–37. doi:doi:10.1016/S1386-5056(01)00183-6

Kullback, S. & Leibler, R. (1951). On information and sufficiency. *The Annals of Mathematical Statistics,* (1): 7986, 22.

Lee, M., & Pope, K. (2003). Avoiding the dangers of averaging across subjects when using multidimensional scaling. *Journal of Mathematical Psychology, 47*(1), 32–46.

Li, X. (2011). *Privacy Preserving PCA on Distributed Bioinformatics Data*, Ph.D. dissertation, University of Maryland Baltimore County.

Li, X. (2011). Privacy Preserving Clustering for Distributed Homogenous Gene Expression Data Sets. *International Journal of Computational Models and Algorithms in Medicine* 1(3), 31-54, July-September 2010.

Liu, K., Kargupta, H., & Ryan, J. (2006). Random Projection-Based Multiplicative Data Perturbation for Privacy Preserving Distributed Data Mining. *IEEE Transactions on Knowledge and Data Engineering, 18*(1), 92–106.

Lu, Y.-H., & Huang, Y. (2005, August 18-21). *Mining data streams using clustering*. Paper presented at the 4th International Conference on Machine Learning and Cybernatics, Guangzhou, China.

Ludwig, S. A., Roos, S., Frize, M., & Yu, N. (2010, October-December). Medical Outcome Prediction for Intensive Care Unit Patients. *International Journal of Computational Models and Algorithms in Medicine, 1*(4), 19–30.

Mahalanobis, P. C. On the Generalized Distance in statistics. *In Proceedings of the National Institute of Sciences of India*, 12:4955.

Mextaxiotis, K., & Samouilidis, J.E. (2000). Expert systems in medicine: academic illusion or real power? *Information Management and Security*, 75-79.

Microsoft. (2007). *Microsoft HealthVault*, accessed November 27, 2011, http://www.microsoft.com/en-us/healthvault/.

Mukherjee, S., Banerjee, M., Chen, Z., & Gangopadhyay, A. (2008). A Privacy Preserving Technique for Distance-Based Classification with Worst Case Privacy Guarantees. *Data & Knowledge Engineering, 66*, 264–288.

Narracott, A. J., Lawford, P. V., Gunn, J. P. G., & Hose, D. R. (2007). Balloon folding affects the symmetry of stent deployment: Experimental and computational evidence. In *Proceedings of the 29th Annual Inter- national Conference of IEEE-EMBS, Engineering in Medicine and Biology Society, EMBC'07* (pp. 3069-3073).

Ramesh, R. N. *Dynamic Document Clustering using Singular Value Decomposition.* M. S. Thesis, University of Maryland Baltimore County, May 2011.

Samarati, P., & Sweeney, L. (1998). Protecting privacy when disclosing information: k-anonymity and its enforcement through generalization and suppression. In *Proceedings of the IEEE Symposium on Research in Security and Privacy*, Oakland, CA.

Saul, L. K., Roweis, S. T., & Singer, Y. (2003). Think globally, fit locally: Unsupervised learning of low dimensional manifolds. *Journal of Machine Learning Research, 4,* 119–155.

Tan, P.-N., Steinbach, M., & Kumar, V. (2006). *Introduction to Data Mining.* Pearson Education Inc.

Tenenbaum, J. B., Silva, V., & Langford, J. C. (2000). A Global Geometric Framework for Nonlinear Dimensionality Reduction. *Science, 290*(5500), 2319–2323.

Thompson, J. R., & Tapia, R. A. (1990). *Nonparametric Function Estimation, Modeling, and Simulation.* Philadelphia: Society for Industrial and Applied Mathematics (SIAM).

Udommanetanakit, K., Rakthanmanon, T., & Waiyamai, K. (2007, August 6-8). *E-Stream: evolution-based technique for stream clustering.* Paper presented at the 3rd International Conference on Advanced Data Mining and Applications (ADMA'07), Harbin, China.

USPSTF. (2005). *Screen- ing for Gonorrhea.* Retrieved from http://www.uspreventiveservicestaskforce.org/uspstf/uspsgono.htm

Vaidya, J. Clifton. C. W., & Zhu, Y. M. (2006). *Privacy Preserving Data Mining.* Springer.

Xia, Z., Ju, F., & Sasaki, K. (2007). A general finite element analysis method for balloon expandable stents based on repeated unit cell (RUC) model. *Finite Elements in Analysis and Design, 43,* 649–658. doi:doi:10.1016/j.finel.2007.01.001

Verykios, V. S., Bertino, E., Fovino, I. N., Provenza, L. P., Saygin, Y., & Theodoridis, Y. (2004). State-of-the-Art in Privacy Preserving Data Mining. *SIGMOD Record, 33*(1), 50–57.

Yap, M. H., Edirisinghe, E., & Bez, H. (2010, April-June). Computer Aided Detection and Recognition of Lesions in Ultrasound Breast Images. *International Journal of Computational Models and Algorithms in Medicine, 1*(2), 53–81.

Zhao, K., Chen, G., Gift, T., & Tao, G. (2010, October-December). Optimization Model and Algorithm Help to Screen and Treat Sexually Transmitted Diseases . *International Journal of Computational Models and Algorithms in Medicine, 1*(4), 1–18.

Chapter 1
A Formal Approach to Evaluating Medical Ontology Systems using Naturalness

Yoo Jung An
Fairleigh Dickinson University, USA

Kuo-chuan Huang
New Jersey Institute of Technology, USA

Soon Ae Chun
College of Staten Island, USA

James Geller
New Jersey Institute of Technology, USA

ABSTRACT

Ontologies, terminologies and vocabularies are popular repositories for collecting the terms used in a domain. It may be expected that in the future more such ontologies will be created for domain experts. However, there is increasing interest in making the language of experts understandable to casual users. For example, cancer patients often research their cases on the Web. The authors consider the problem of objectively evaluating the quality of ontologies (QoO). This article formalizes the notion of naturalness as a component of QoO and quantitatively measures naturalness for well-known ontologies (UMLS, WordNet, OpenCyc) based on their concepts, IS-A relationships and semantic relationships. To compute numeric values characterizing the naturalness of an ontology, this article defines appropriate metrics. As absolute numbers in such a pursuit are often meaningless, we concentrate on using relative natural-ness metrics. That allows us to say that a certain ontology is relatively more natural than another one.

INTRODUCTION

An ontology represents a data structure that attempts to model human-like knowledge that can be implemented in computational engineering (Gruber, 1993). Concepts (or classes), attributes (or properties) and relationships among concepts that underlie an ontology support the idea of machine-readable data on the Web. The use of ontologies as part of the Web is desirable, since they could support finding answers for users' queries (Sieg et al., 2007; An et al., 2008). Ontologies may supply

DOI: 10.4018/978-1-4666-0282-3.ch001

generalized terms for a user's Web search terms. An answer for a query could be derived by using specialization and/or generalization relationships between the concepts of an IS-A hierarchy. For example, a search for *Amoxicillin* might not give a satisfactory result, but the user might be satisfied with the search result for the more general term *Penicillin*. Finding broader or narrower concepts of a given concept is an important technique, which is recommended as a Web search strategy. According to Kalfoglou & Hu (2006), application ontologies are converging with the Web. Thus the knowledge provided by ontologies should be filtered dynamically by understanding the needs of Web users.

There are several well-known ontologies, which many researchers have used and referenced, such as UMLS, WordNet and OpenCyc. Some researchers have presented modified or enriched ontological models by adding new types and trimming some detailed relationships from existing ontologies (Stone et al., 2004). On the other hand, research that investigates these ontologies not only from the view point of experts but also from the perspective of casual users is rare. Assessing difficulties in understanding and using ontologies for emerging user communities on the Semantic Web should be conducted as a stage of implementing the Semantic Web (Finin et al., 2007).

In his original work on ontologies, Gruber (1993) stressed that ontologies are about knowledge sharing. We raise the question whether existing ontologies are constructed so that they may succeed at knowledge sharing. Zeng et al. (2005) showed that communication through terminologies can be significantly facilitated if words labeling concepts are comprehensible to users. Finding concepts which are likely to be recognized by users is a trend in ontology engineering, which is different from the traditional approach of building terminologies understandable mainly by experts of a domain.

We are focusing on an ontology's role, that is, knowledge sharing supported by an explicit specification of a conceptualization. The key idea of naturalness is based on the need for making terminologies understandable, as described in previous research (An et al., 2006). Some researchers (Staab and Maedche, 2000) have made efforts in making explicit the meaning of some semantic relationships in the form of axioms. However, this declarative knowledge with universal truths about concepts cannot provide answers for all the forms of knowledge inquiries (Mizoguchi, 2004).

It is widely assumed that ontologies represent information in a form that is at least similar to how human knowledge is represented (Smith, 1982). Note that the distinction between primitive and defined concepts (Baneyx et al., 2005) is not employed in this research. It is easy to give precise definitions in mathematically-oriented domains. However, in real world applications this is often not the case.

To many researchers, an ontology concept is a meaningless label, unless it is given a definition. However, any definition itself will contain logical symbols and other labels. Logical symbols do not cause a problem because they are domain independent. However, how can the defining labels themselves be defined? This leads to an infinite regression or circular definitions. Thus, we assume that, at some level, labels have to be understandable by being known to the recipient (program or human). As there are labels that are better known, what we call "more natural," and labels that are less well known to humans, we prefer to use the more natural labels even for programs. We note that the meaning and the naturalness of concepts are orthogonal factors, as will be explained in more detail below. The author of a document usually has very little choice concerning the meaning he needs to get across. However, he can choose the most natural term for a specific meaning.

In related work about the quality of ontologies, Ram & Park (2004) have focused on semantic interoperability. To enhance the semantics of ontologies, a methodology and analysis have been presented in (Supekar et al., 2004; Brachman, 1992). The ontologies that these researchers presented are domain-specific, so the sizes of the ontologies used are relatively small. In a broader view, some existing ontologies are described in (Noy & Hafner, 1997), however, numeric values and classifications of the ontologies are discussed without being supported by a mathematical model.

On the other hand, the importance of interoperability and compatibility of ontologies can be easily verified, since one of the main reasons why we build ontologies is the sharing of knowledge. Burgun & Bodenreider (2001) conducted an analysis of the compatibilities of different ontologies. This topic of semantic interoperability is not included in our analysis. The topic of our research is to evaluate how *people* perceive or understand concepts and their semantic relationships in different ontologies. This involves user-oriented knowledge base engineering (Brewster *et al.* 2002; Seta et al., 1997). The field of ontology evaluation is in its early stages, but has recently received great interest, including the creation of the US National Center for Ontological Research (Obrst et al., 2006). Much work needs to be done on defining *measurable*, desirable properties of ontologies. Even more work is necessary for building the appropriate "measuring instruments."

In previous papers (Lee & Geller, 2005; An et al., 2006), we have pointed out that unnatural concepts make it difficult to use an ontology and they contradict the desiderata of an ontology, which include explanatory power for the purpose of sharing information. McCray et al. (2001) introduced the idea of naturalness as the acceptance of the ontology by domain experts. In this article, we are extending this idea to regular (non-expert) users. Thus the acceptance of an ontology by Web users is desirable. However, it is impossible to consult many users whether they understand ontology concepts and relationships. We need a mechanical way to measure this naturalness.

The contribution of this study has two aspects. First, we present an evaluation methodology for ontologies focusing on the naturalness perspective.

Secondly, we propose an ontology maintenance model implied by this evaluation methodology. The model is practical and desirable, since it is an interactive process supported by the Web users' inputs. Ideally this processing should be done in real time, by employing the Web as the corpus for the evaluation.

In designing our evaluation model for ontologies, we first start with the naturalness of concepts. Secondly, we focus on the explicit conceptualization expressed in IS-A relationships of ontologies. We elaborate on the testable definition of the natural association of concept pairs by IS-A relationships. Lastly, we extend the naturalness evaluation to semantic relationships.

NATURALNESS FORMALIZATION

This section introduces the notion of naturalness as an objective Quality of Ontologies measure based on ontology concepts, IS-A relationships and semantic relationships.

Naturalness of Concepts

Knowledge engineers use formal or semi-formal languages in order to build ontologies (Colomb, 2002). A language provides us with interchangeable words, so the words, which are comprehensible by users, are an important factor when we evaluate ontologies (Lewis, 1983). Naturalness of the concepts used in an ontology is addressed in (An et al., 2006), based on the question whether the concept labels are comprehensible to users.

In (An et al., 2006), the following measure of the naturalness of an ontology was proposed. If an ontology consists of (a majority of) labels that can be found in a dictionary lookup, then this ontology is more natural than an ontology for which this is not the case. In order to assign a numeric value to naturalness, we need to know how often a term is used, e.g. by searching a large corpus. In recent years, the Internet has become popular as an ersatz corpus, and, luckily, Google provides us with frequency information, which is denoted in this article by *Google#*. The *Google#* has been used in ontology evaluation or matches (An et al., 2006; Gligorov et al., 2007).

Thus, we claim that the higher the $Google\#(c_i)$ of a concept c_i is, the more natural it is. For example, a Google search for *DNA* finds $Google\#(DNA) = 118,000,000$ hits, while a search for *Deoxyribonucleic Acid* finds only $Google\#(Deoxyribonucleic\ Acid) = 1,750,000$ instances. Note that naturalness and meaning are orthogonal. Thus, *DNA* and *Deoxyribonucleic Acid* have exactly the same meaning. Yet, *DNA*, commonly used in the popular press nowadays, is a more natural term to most people than *Deoxyribonucleic Acid* (An et al., 2006).

As noted before, one purpose of this article is to formalize the notion of "naturalness." Researchers are often challenged by the existence of a term that is widely used in everyday life, yet no formal definition exists for it. The term "naturalness" seems to be well understood in everyday language. We performed a small pilot experiment (Chun & Geller, 2008) where human subjects were given pairs of semantically equivalent medical terms and were asked to judge which term from each pair was more natural to them. This was done for 37 pairs. Not one of the subjects asked for additional clarification, beyond the one given, what "natural" is supposed to mean. Subjects were also in good agreement with each other concerning naturalness. On average, 78% of subjects agreed on naturalness judgments. One goal of this article is to provide a criterion for naturalness that is independent of human subjects' judgments.

Zeng et al. (2005) stressed the importance of *consumer-friendly display* of medical terms. In their experiment they used medical terms from MedlinePlus and showed that terms more likely to be entered by "end users" as search terms are more likely to be understood by human subjects than less common synonyms of those search terms. Their paper stresses the importance of (medical) concepts being understandable to non-expert hu-

man users. Zeng et al.'s term "consumer-friendly" appears to be roughly equivalent to our use of the term "natural," except that our term does not assume a reference population ("non-expert users").

Regarding the choice of a proper corpus for finding concept pairs, in (Brewster et al., 2002), the Internet and glossaries are reported to be practical resources. That is because concept pairs randomly selected from a domain specific ontology are rarely found in related journals or texts. Practically, the documents on the Internet have been used as alternative corpus to automatically extract hyponyms in (Agirre et al., 2000) and examples of concepts (Mihalcea & Moldovan, 1999). Accordingly, in our analysis, the Web, indexed by Google, is adapted as the benchmark corpus for measuring naturalness.

We settled on the assumption that most people who make the effort of setting up a Web page have the desire to be understood by other Web users, i.e., they would make their best efforts to use understandable terms. Over 1 trillion unique Web pages indexed by Google support this assumption by the law of large numbers. As we will see, understandable terms occur more often than obscure terms. Zeng et al. (2005) made the assumption that users of a Web site prefer familiar expressions as search terms and thus frequency of used words implies the respective degree of user comprehensibility of the words. In (An et al., 2006) our assumption was that a term that is widely used is more likely to be natural. Based on this assumption, the naturalness of a concept is defined as follows.

Let $L = \{l_1, l_2 \cdots, l_n\}$ be a set of labels which appear in an ontology, where l_i is a label and $|L| = n$ is the size of L or the total number of labels. Then the naturalness of concepts for a certain ontology, O is defined as follows:

$$\text{Concept\_Naturalness}(O) = \frac{\sum_{i=1}^{n} Google\#(l_i)}{|L|}$$

(1)

Naturalness of IS-A Relationships using Frequencies of Concept Pairs

We are using a similar but more complex approach for naturalness of IS-A relationships. An IS-A relationship is a binary relationship of two concepts. We will use $X \Rightarrow Y$ to denote that X IS-A Y. If an ontology contains the relationship X IS-A Y then we would consider this a natural relationship if we find many documents that contain both X and Y, i.e., co-occurrences of X and Y. If we find very few documents that contain both X and Y then we would consider X IS-A Y as an unnatural relationship. See a clarification of the symmetry issue below. Our analysis is based on the number of search results for concept pairs returned by Google. For example, let X and Y be two concepts from an ontology in which X and Y are in an IS-A relationship. We will use $Google\#(X \wedge Y)$, called Concept Pair Google Number (CPGN) in this article, indicating the number of co-occurrences of X and Y on the Web pages. CPGN is the number of Web pages found when we query Google for both X and Y in the search. An estimate of this number is reported by Google at the top of every search result.

Let A be a set of IS-A relationships which appear in an ontology, where $a_i = C_i \Rightarrow P_i$ is an IS-A relationship and $|A|$ is the size of A, or the number of IS-A relationships. P_i and C_i are concepts such that C_i IS-A P_i. Then the naturalness of IS-A relationships for a certain ontology, O is defined as follows:

$$\text{ISA\_Naturalness}(O) = \frac{\sum_{i=1}^{|A|} Google\#(P_i \wedge C_i)}{|A|} \quad (2)$$

Clearly, an IS-A relationship is asymmetric. If $X \Rightarrow Y$ holds, then necessarily $Y \Rightarrow X$ does not. CPGN treats the IS-A relationship as a symmetric relationship, where both $X \Rightarrow Y$ and $Y \Rightarrow X$ result in the same value, thus one cannot tell the direction by CPGN. This concern is imperative and problematic in building ontologies using co-occurrences of concept pairs (Maedche & Staab, 2000), but not for evaluating existing ontologies. We stress that our task is *not* finding IS-A relationships by finding co-occurring concepts C and P in the same Web page. Indeed, when finding co-occurring concepts, we cannot know whether $C \Rightarrow P$ holds, $P \Rightarrow C$ holds, no relationship at all holds, or the relationship between C and P is not an IS-A relationship. Rather, *we already know* that an IS-A relation between C and P holds in a given direction. Otherwise we would have to assume that the designers of the ontology that we are evaluating have made a gross mistake.

Assuming that $C \Rightarrow P$ is correct in that an IS-A relationship between these two concepts really holds in the given direction in the ontology, the question we are asking is only whether this is a *natural IS-A relationship*. If our Web search indicates that there are very few Web pages that contain C and P together, then we may conclude that there is no strong evidence that *any* relationship between C and P holds. Thus we reason as follows. If there does not seem to exist any relationship at all between C and P, then it is highly unlikely that an IS-A relationship exists. However, we know that such a relationship was asserted by an ontology designer (who is assumed not to have been grossly negligent). We conclude therefore that the asserted IS-A relationship is correct but is likely not natural in our sense.

One might also wonder why we are allowing the terms X and Y to occur anywhere within the document, possibly not connected by an IS-A link, or worse, possibly not connected at all. Wouldn't it be better to look for a sentence frame of the form "*X* is a *Y*" instead of query terms of the form "*X*" "*Y*"? While this approach has intuitive appeal, there are two problems with it. (1) IS-A relationships can be expressed in many different ways, not just by an explicit statement. Thus "animals such as dogs and cats" expresses two IS-A relationships. (2) We have done a few experiments querying Google with sentence frames such as "*Xes* are

Ys" and found that they work reasonably well for one-word concepts. However, many medical concepts are expressed by two or more words, e.g. *Amino Acid*. For sentence frames involving multi-word X and Y concepts, Google returned small hit counts, and in many cases no hits at all.

For example, Google returns no document with a search string, "*Amino Acid Sequence is a Molecular Sequence*" or "*An Amino Acid Sequence is a Molecular Sequence.*" Note that the two previous search strings need to be passed to Google *with the double quotes.* Google will respond that "No results found for …" It will then suggest results for the same list of words, but *without double quotes,* which means that the words of the search string may appear separately in any place in the document. In contrast to the previous failure, Google returns 1,070,000 Web documents with a search expression consisting of the two strings "*Amino Acid Sequence*" and "*Molecular Sequence,*" again typed in with double quotes.

An Initial Experiment

We are assuming that if X_i and Y_j are indeed in an IS-A relationship then they are closely related and tend to co-occur. In order to support our assumption, one experiment was conducted in which the concept pairs in IS-A relationships and non-relevant concept pairs were compared with respect to CPGN. For each concept pair (X_i, Y_j), we generated a non-relevant concept pair as (X_i, Z_k) or (Z_k, Y_j) where Z_k is a randomly selected concept. A group of these non-relevant concept pairs is the control group to verify the assumption that the naturalness of an IS-A relationship can be approximated by a Google search. The result of the comparison shows that submitting concept pairs with IS-A relationships to Google results in conspicuously higher numbers of frequency results than for random concept pairs. The lists of concept pairs used for this experiment are omitted for space reasons, but they can be found in (An, 2008). Therefore, low CPGN values indicate that the

existence of an IS-A relationship is unlikely. Thus, if we *know* that the IS-A relationship exists, we apply frequencies of co-occurrences by Google search to the measurement of its naturalness.

Naturalness of Concept Pairs Connected by Semantic Relationships

A similar approach as in the previous section is used for pairs of concepts connected by semantic relationships. An ontology contains not only hierarchical classifications but also other relationships which enrich data semantics. In (Seta et al., 1997), taxonomy and axioms are regarded as the major components of an ontology. The taxonomy consists of IS-A relationships and axioms define rules, constraints and relationships among concepts. There are various ways to represent data semantics. Different domain experts may perceive the same domain in slightly different ways (Necib & Freytag, 2003). If an ontology on the same topic is designed by different domain experts and knowledge engineers, there will be natural variations between the results, as each one is bringing his own perspective to the task.

Generally, the knowledge engineers need to explore related concepts (Brewster et al., 2003; Hearst, 1992). In addition, frequencies of co-occurrences of the concepts may be used to compute a "semantic distance" between the non-taxonomic concepts (Brewster, 2003). Thus, in this article, *naturalness of concept pairs connected by semantic relationships* is measured by *CPGN* described in the above section. We obtain $Google \#(X_i \wedge Y_j)$ where X_i and Y_j are semantically related. We assume that if the sampled concepts, which are defined as semantically related in the ontology, have a high frequency in our benchmark corpus, the Web as indexed by Google, the semantic relationship of X_i and Y_j is natural. That is, the higher the $Google \#(X_i \wedge Y_j)$ is, the more natural is the semantic relationship.

Let S be a set of semantic relationships which appear in an ontology where s_i is a semantic relationship $X \Leftrightarrow Y$ and $|S|$ is the size of S, i.e. the number of semantic relationships. Then the naturalness of semantic relationships for a certain ontology O is defined in Equation (3) which is analog to Equation (2):

$$semantic\_Naturalness(O) = \frac{\sum_{i=1}^{|S|} Google\#(s_i)}{|S|}$$

(3)

Let R be the set of all binary relationships of all ontologies in the domain, excluding IS-A and *inverse* IS-A. Note that R is provided by ontologies in two different ways: While some ontologies provide explicit tables listing all binary relationships, others provide a list of functions. The set S for the UMLS is given in (An, 2008, pp.150) and the sets S for WordNet and OpenCyc are described below.

METHODOLOGY

Data Sources

Three major ontologies, UMLS, WordNet and OpenCyc are investigated in this article. A comparison of ontologies is (statistically) only meaningful if they are large. We also would prefer that they are in the same domain, but this is not an absolute requirement. In medicine, the largest (meta) terminology is the UMLS. As there is no other medical terminology of the same size, we are using two other large ontologies that have at least some medical coverage, namely WordNet and CYC.

UMLS (Unified Medical Language System)

The UMLS is a large-scale knowledge base used in Medical Informatics. The UMLS consists of three parts of which we are interested in the Metathesaurus and the Semantic Network with its semantic relationships. The Metathesaurus had 1.9 million concepts (i.e., the preferred terms of concepts) in the version 2008AB (U.S. National Library of Medicine, 2008) and the Semantic Network has 135 semantic types. The Semantic Network contains 133 IS-A relationships organized in two trees rooted in the "Entity" and "Event" semantic types. There are also non IS-A relationships such as treats, prevents, affects, associated-with, etc. to connect semantic types.

The UMLS Semantic Network is used to provide the consistency for the Metathesaurus concepts. Each Metathesaurus concept is assigned at least one semantic type. The relationships between the semantic types provide the structure of the Semantic Network which in turn provides important implications for interpreting the meaning of the Metathesaurus concepts. When assigning semantic types to Metathesaurus concepts, the most specific semantic type in the structure is used. Figures 1 (a), (b), and (c) show examples of IS-A relationships of the Semantic Network, the Metathesaurus and semantic type assignments of the Metathesaurus, respectively.

In the UMLS Metathesaurus, concepts are closely connected by certain relationships since they have common properties even in their definitions. Most of the relationships come from the same sources called intra-source relationships (U.S. National Library of Medicine, 2008). For example, there are over 25 million relationship instances between two concepts in the major relationships files, "mrrel.rrf" and we ignore relationships such as *inverse_isa*, *has_permuted_term*, *permuted_term_of* and *sib_in_isa* in our analysis. The general labels of relationships can be found in the UMLS file, "mrdoc.rrf."

Figure 1. (a) A part of the Semantic Network; (b) an example of parent-child relationships in the Metathesaurus; (c) an example of assignments of semantic types to concepts in the Metathesaurus of the UMLS.

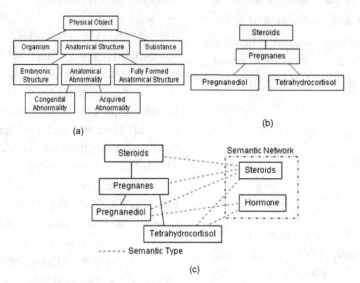

Even though the UMLS is strictly speaking not an ontology, it is close enough for our purposes to treat it in the same way as the other terminologies.

WordNet

WordNet is a large-scale lexical reference system for the purpose of natural language processing. It contains 117,798 nouns in the version 3.0 (Princeton University, 2006). Nouns are hierarchically organized with *hypernym and/or hyponym* relationships. A *hypernym* is a more general concept while a *hyponym* is more specific. We used WordNet 2.0 which is a version for Windows and considered *hypernyms/hyponyms* as IS-A relationships.

In WordNet, there are other relationships, such as *substance_meronym*, *substance_holonym*, *part_meronym*, *part_holonym* and *entailment*, *entailed_by*, *derived* and *cause*. Generally, holonymy is the part-whole relationship such that X is in Y or X is a part of Y. Meronymy is holonymy's inverse. For example, brain cell and brain are in a *part_holonym* relationship while law

of gravitation and gravitational constant are in a *part_meronym* relationship. These relationships and their corresponding concepts are the subjects of our analysis.

OpenCyc

OpenCyc is the open source version of Cyc, which is intended for general knowledge processing. The name CYC is based on the word EnCYClopedia, and CYC was built with the intention of providing encyclopedic knowledge of concepts and reasoning rules. OpenCyc had 47,000 concepts in the initial release, and 300,000 in the release 0.9 (Cycorp, 2005) which was used for our experiment.

Classes provide an abstraction mechanism for grouping resources with similar characteristics. Classes are organized into a superclass-subclass hierarchy, which can usually be shown as a Directed Acyclic Graph structure. Subclasses specialize their superclasses, while superclasses generalize their subclasses. A class maybe associated with a set of individuals, which are the leaves in the hierarchical structure and cannot have any sub-individuals. For example, consider the classes "Canine Animal" and "Dog" and the individual "German Shepherd Dog." Dog is a subclass of Canine Animal; Canine Animal is the superclass of Dog. We can say that, 'All members of the class Dog are members of the class Canine Animal.' German Shepherd Dog is one of the instances of Dog, which cannot have any sub-individuals.

In OpenCyc, *predicate* and *function-denotational* are kinds of *relations* (OpenCyc, 2005) which are constraints and relations between concepts. For example, a predicate, *performedBy* which is preceded by a concept, *PettingAnAnimal* limits a following concept to be a *Person*. So, only if individuals conforming to the above concepts are in a sentence like *PettingAnAnimal performedBy Person* is the sentence semantically well-formed. In our analysis, we will only consider *predicate* relations not *function-denotational* relations since functions are used to generate new concepts.

In summary, we are using five components in this research: (1) UMLS Semantic Network, (2) UMLS Metathesaurus, (3) sets of pairs (p,r) where p is a concept of the UMLS Metathesaurus and r is a semantic type of the UMLS Semantic Network and r is assigned to p in the UMLS, (4) WordNet, and (5) OpenCyc Class.

Phase I: Extracting Data and Computing Naturalness

To retrieve words (concepts) and their relationships from WordNet, we used JWNL (Sourceforge.net, 2008), an *API* (application programming interface) for accessing WordNet-style relational dictionaries and the WordNet database. For Open-Cyc, the database server (Sourceforge.net, 2007) is run on our local host and the OpenCyc API was used to access the database. The UMLS offers an SQL query capability in XML format to directly get records from its database, hosted at umlsks. nlm.nih.gov, by using Java Remote Method Invocation. The table "*mrrel*" in the UMLS database is used to store all IS-A records for the Metath-

esaurus. After all records are stored in our local database, we then build relationships between Metathesaurus concepts and semantic types. We used the UMLS API to retrieve the assignments of semantic types for each Metathesaurus concept. To retrieve relationship between semantic types, the "*srstr*" table in the UMLS database has all the records we need. In a similar way, we extracted all sampled non-IS-A relationships from the UMLS Semantic Network and the UMLS Metathesaurus. Note that the Metathesaurus of the UMLS, which contains IS-A (parent/child) relationships, was used in its entirety. But for efficiency reasons, some semantic relationships mentioned previously were removed in the analysis of semantic relationships. For semantic types, the Semantic Network was also used in its entirety, as it is of moderate size.

Approximating the Naturalness of Concepts for an Ontology

Algorithm 1 for extracting concepts depends on the APIs and the structure of each ontology and can be described as follows.

Note that m is a user-defined sample size. We used $m = 3000$ for each ontology with a very large number of concepts. The details of Algorithm 1 can be found in (An, 2008).

Approximating the Naturalness of IS-A Relationships

Extracting IS-A relationships depends on APIs and the structure of the ontology. Since not all ontologies provide an explicit list of IS-A relationships, we utilize m sample concepts which are produced by Algorithm 1 and find their IS-A relationships.

Note that $|A^1| \leq m$.

We obtain concept pairs, taking an input array which contains the randomly sampled concepts from Algorithm 1. The details of Algorithm 2 can be found in (An, 2008).

Algorithm 1: *Approximating the naturalness of concepts for an ontology*

Input: a certain ontology O, represented as a set of concepts (labels)
$L = \{l_1, l_2 \cdots, l_n\}$

Output: $L' = \{l_1', l_2' \cdots, l_m'\}$ where $l_i' \in L$ where L' is a randomly selected sample set
and $l_i' \in L'$ and $m << n$
of labels from L and

$$\text{Concept\_Naturalness}(O) = \frac{\sum_{i=1}^{m} Google\#(l_i')}{|L'|}$$

Approximating the Naturalness of Semantic Relationships

Semantic relationships are provided by ontologies in different ways; while some ontologies provide an explicit table, *T, listing* all binary relationships, others provide a list of API functions, *F*. When an explicit table of all binary relationships is given, *CP'*, a sample set of concept pairs with semantic relationships, can be easily generated by a random selection excluding the IS-A or *inverse* IS-A relationships. Note that *T*'s schema includes a concept *L*, a concept *R* and a *relationship name*, etc. where *L* and *R* are connected by the relationship. Examples of this kind of ontology are the UMLS Metathesaurus and the UMLS Semantic Network. Alternatively, the API function set, $F = (f_1, f_2, \cdots, f_n, g_1, g_2, \dots g_m)$ may be given, such that each f_i takes a term as an input and returns true if the term is a relationship name (e.g., *binary predicate*). Each g_i takes a *relationship$_i$* as an input and outputs CP_i, a set of all concept pairs consisting of *Ls* and *Rs* connected by this relationship. This kind of ontology is exemplified by OpenCyc. Lastly, when *F* is given without a get_concept_pairs feature, one must try different *Rs* to extract its corresponding *Ls* exhaustively, such that $L = f_i(R)$. An example of this kind of ontology is WordNet.

The details of Algorithm 3 can be found in (An, 2008). The complete lists of the semantic relationships used for the Metathesaurus and for the Semantic Network can be found in (An, 2008, pp.150).

Algorithm 2: *Approximating the naturalness of concept pairs in IS-A relationships*

Input: A certain ontology O, represented as a set of sample concepts
$L' = \{l_1', l_2' \cdots, l_m'\}$ with either an explicit set A of IS-A relationships, or a getParent function.
Output:
$A' = \{(P, C) \mid C \in L' \ \wedge$

1. $((C \Rightarrow P) \in A \ \vee \ P$
   $= getParent(C))\}$

2. CPGN(A'), corresponding CPGNs for each IS-A relationship in A'.

3. $\text{ISA\_Naturalness}(O) = \dfrac{\sum_{i=1}^{|A'|} Google\#(P_i \wedge C_i)}{|A'|}$

Algorithm 3: *Approximating the naturalness of concept pairs in semantic relationships*

Input: A relationship table $T = (L, R, relationship)$ of a certain ontology O or an API function set F of a certain ontology O.

Output:

$$CP = \{(L, R) \mid (L, R, relationship) \in$$

1. $CP' = sampling(CP)$ where $T \; \wedge \; relationship \neq$ 'IS_A' and $\neq$ 'inverse IS_A'}

$$CP = \{(L, R) \mid f_i \in F \; \wedge \; L =$$

or $f_i(R) \; \wedge \; f_i \neq$ 'IS_A' and $\neq$ 'inverse IS_A'}

$$CP = \{(L, R) \mid f_i, g_j \in$$

or $F \; \wedge \; f_i(relationship)$ is true $\wedge$ $(L, R) \in g_j(relationship)\}$

2. $semantic\_Naturalness(O) = \dfrac{\sum\limits_{i=1}^{|CP'|} Google\#(L_i, R_i)}{|CP'|}$

Phase II: Data Analysis

Our definitions for naturalness of concepts, IS-A relationships, and semantic relationships are based on the means of Google#s and CPGNs. These numbers are meaningless for a single ontology and must be compared to other ontologies to become useful. In order to compare two or more means (and mean ranks), we employed the ANOVA test and the Kruskal-Wallis test accordingly. The null hypothesis is that the population mean is the same in all conditions or groups. To test the hypothesis, the *f-statistic* and *chi-square* were computed. In computing the f-statistic and chi-square, we used SAS software.

RESULTS

The Naturalness of Concepts

Descriptive Statistics

Following are the symbols used in this article and their corresponding statistical measurements: "M"

is the mean value of the number of search results for a concept, "SD" is the standard deviation, "R" is the Range (the difference between the minimum and the maximum), and "N" is the sample size.

Following are the symbols used in this article for ontologies: "W" = WordNet, "US" = UMLS Semantic Network, "UM" = UMLS Metathesaurus and "OCC" = OpenCyc. We will also use the abbreviation "UMS" = a set of pairs (X, Y) where X is in UM and Y is in US.

Table 1 shows the descriptive statistics for concept naturalness where "M" is the value of Equation (1). The ontology with the highest mean value, 5,059,901 is the Semantic Network and the ontology with the lowest mean value, 21,499 is the Metathesaurus of the UMLS. This agrees with our intuition, as the Metathesaurus contains many highly specialized medical terms. The result of the *Kolmogorov-Smirnov test*, which is a common normality distribution test shows that the numbers associated with search results returned by Google are not normally distributed. Therefore, to investigate any statistically significant difference among the four groups of ontologies, a non-parametric test for such a non-normal data set, the Kruskal-

Wallis test, was conducted, which is common in medical studies (Kuhnast & Neuhauser, 2008).

Analysis of the Means (Concept Naturalness) for Four Groups of Ontologies

The Kruskal-Wallis test indicated that the mean ranks of numbers associated with search results returned by Google are significantly different in the investigated ontologies (chi-square with 3 degrees of freedom = 2696.89, p=0.0001).

In total, 9,427 labels were sampled from the ontologies. Because of random, independent sampling of the large sample sizes, the result of a parametric test is asymptotically correct. The one-way ANOVA had a result of F-statistic equal to 32.55 at p-value = 0.0001. Therefore, the null hypothesis of equal means for the different ontologies is rejected.

The Naturalness of Concept Pairs in IS-A Relationships

Descriptive Statistics of IS-A Naturalness

Table 2 shows the descriptive statistics. "M" is the naturalness of IS-A relationships and was given in Equation (2). The variable is the number of search results when we send a concept pair to Google, which is denoted as CPGN in Algorithm 2. Note that the CPGNs for IS-A relationships in each investigated component are not normally distributed.

The ontology with the highest mean value, 323,777 is the Semantic Network. On the other hand, the relationship between the Semantic Network and the Metathesaurus of the UMLS has the lowest mean value, 1,410.

Analysis of the Means (Naturalness in IS-A relationship) for the Five Components of Ontologies

The result of the Kruskal-Wallis test indicates that the mean ranks of CPGNs for IS-A relationships are significantly different in the investigated components (chi-square with 4 degrees of freedom = 7030.14 at p=0.0001). Similarly, the one-way ANOVA had a result of F-statistic equal to 38.58 at p=0.0001. Therefore, the null hypothesis that there is no significant difference in the means of IS-A naturalness among the components was rejected.

The Naturalness of Concept Pairs Connected by Semantic Relationships

Descriptive Statistics of Semantic Naturalness

Table 3 shows the descriptive statistics for the naturalness of semantic relationships with M as given in Equation (3). The ontology with the highest mean value, 1,079,738 is the Semantic Network and the ontology with the lowest mean value, 2,759 is the Metathesaurus of the UMLS.

Table 1. The descriptive statistics I: Concept occurrence

	US	UM	W	OCC
N	135	4,858	3,000	1,434
M	5,059,901	21,499	837,584	771,400
SD	16,622,855	313,416	6,841,168	6,983,312
R	116,999,967	16,800,000	195,999,948	182E6

Table 2. Descriptive statistics II: Pair occurrence in IS-a relationship

	US	UM	UMS	W	OCC
N	135	5,000	6,249	3091	7,787
M	323,777	3,752	1,410	86,643	7,867
SD	1,774,338	57,133	62,138	1,094,492	184,993
R	17,699,975	2,500,000	4,500,000	55,099,969	342224E10

Analysis of the Means (Naturalness in Semantic Relationships) in Four Groups of Ontologies

The result of the Kruskal-Wallis test indicates that the mean ranks of CPGNs for semantic relationships are significantly different among the investigated ontologies (chi-square with 3 degrees of freedom = 2003.80 at p=0.0001). Similarly, the one-way ANOVA had a result of F-statistic equal to 18.11 at p=0.0001. Hereby, the null hypothesis that there is no significant difference in the means of naturalness of semantic relationships among the ontologies was rejected.

SUMMARY AND DISCUSSION

Naturalness of Concepts

In summary, the UMLS Semantic Network is the most natural, followed by WordNet, OpenCyc, and the UMLS Metathesaurus.

Naturalness of IS-A Pairs (using Frequencies of Concept Pairs)

The ontologies with the largest naturalness are the UMLS Semantic Network and WordNet, followed by OpenCyc, and the UMLS Metathesaurus. The associations between Semantic Network semantic types and Metathesaurus concepts (UMS) were found to be the least natural pairs. Numbers are based on the means of frequencies.

Naturalness of Pairs with Semantic Relationships

The Semantic Network shows the highest naturalness followed by WordNet, OpenCyc, and the Metathesaurus. Numbers are based on the means of frequencies.

Figure 2 shows how natural each ontology is in three segments: concepts, concept pairs connected by IS-A relationships and concept pairs connected by semantic relationships. Each value in the y-axis, which measures naturalness, is based on the descriptive statistics presented in Tables 1, 2 and 3.

The Table 4 summarizes the results of *Tukey* comparisons. Two ontologies in different groups

Table 3. The descriptive statistics III: Pair occurrence in semantic relationships

	US	UM	W	OCC
N	316	2,171	1,095	414
M	1,079,738	2,759	949,976	157,900
SD	8,323,491	29,666	5,965,384	1,443,433
R	113,999,974	667,000	158,999,952	27,400,000

Figure 2. Descriptive graph to show the naturalness of ontologies

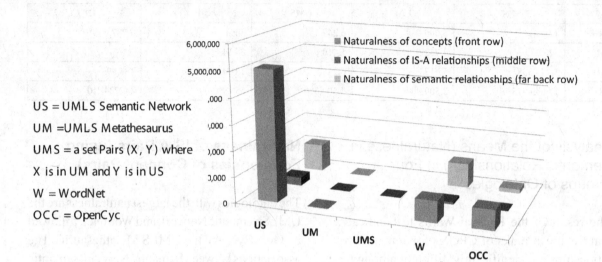

US = UMLS Semantic Network

UM = UMLS Metathesaurus

UMS = a set Pairs (X, Y) where

X is in UM and Y is in US

W = WordNet

OCC = OpenCyc

(Group A, Group B, Group C) are considered significantly different. Two ontologies in the same group are not significantly different. For example, the mean values of Google numbers for concept pairs in semantic relationships among the different ontologies are significantly different. The Semantic Network of the UMLS and WordNet are in group A, while OpenCyc and the Metathesaurus of the UMLS are in group B.

Comparing the results of all three naturalness measures (concepts, IS-A relationships, and semantic relationships) we see that they agree substantially. Thus, no complicated scheme was needed to aggregate results and the overall naturalness is derived based on Table 4 and Figure 2.

Overall Naturalness

The most natural ontology component is the (1) Semantic Network, followed by (2) WordNet and (3) OpenCyc. The least natural ontology (components) are (4) the Metathesaurus and (5) relationships between the Semantic Network and Metathesaurus of the UMLS (i.e., UMS). The Semantic Network is the best, but the number of semantic types in it is comparatively very small,

too small to be useful in practice. We conclude that WordNet, which is the second most natural ontology, can be used to define a likely upper limit of naturalness or at least a reference point.

In addition, improving the naturalness of concepts and relationships in the Metathesaurus of the UMLS and the relationships between the Semantic Network and the Metathesaurus of the

Table 4. Juxtaposing medical language systems in the context of naturalness

	A	B	C
Naturalness of Concepts	- Semantic Network of the UMLS	- WordNet - OpenCyc	- Metathesaurus of the UMLS
Naturalness of Concept Pairs in IS-A relationships	- Semantic Network of the UMLS	- WordNet	- OpenCyc - Metathesaurus of the UMLS - A Set of Concept Pairs (X, Y) where X is in UM and Y is in US
Naturalness of Concept Pairs in semantic relationships	- Semantic Network of the UMLS - WordNet	- OpenCyc - Metathesaurus of the UMLS	

UMLS (i.e., UMS) is desirable to help casual users to utilize medical information systems on the Web. For example, two terms may have identical meanings, however, they may be of vastly different naturalness. Varicella and chicken pox are identical in meaning. However, human subjects (Chun & Geller, 2008) consider chicken pox as much more natural. Thus, we claim that chicken pox should be presented to users, as opposed to varicella.

Practical Implications

The evaluation model experimented with in this article can be useful in personalization of Web search, suggesting more natural terms for a non-expert user, or searching for expert terms when given colloquial search terms. Such transformations are less costly than building separate ontologies for different user groups. The model can also be applied to *ontology maintenance*. If an ontology has lower naturalness compared with another ontology in the same domain, the quality of the first ontology can be improved by replacing unnatural concepts or concept pairs with more natural synonyms, hypernyms or hyponyms from the second ontology. The improvement of the first ontology is easily verifiable by a systematic Google search. This procedure can be further simplified when the necessary synonyms, hypernyms or hyponyms are derived from WordNet or a domain-specific 'gold standard' ontology if such an ontology exists (Castano & Antonellis, 1999).

LIMITATIONS AND FUTURE WORK

One may argue against the reliability of the Internet as corpus by pointing out that there are many noise effects. This is why the research of (Brewster et al., 2003) does not consider the Internet as ideal, but accepts it as the best available source. Search results cannot distinguish terms which have the same spelling but their meaning is different. For example, when 'Jaguar' is sent to Google as a query, Jaguar Cars (http://www.jaguar.com/), Jaguar Animals (http://www.bigcatrescue.org/jaguar.htm), and the Jaguar Sports Team (http://www.jaguars.com/), etc. appear in the about 75,800,000 search results. Considering the limited reliability of our Web sources, we sampled, in total, 9,427 concepts, 22,262 concept pairs in IS-A relationships and 3,996 concept pairs in semantic relationships and used statistical mean comparisons for evaluating ontologies to reduce the effect of this problem.

Five components of three important ontologies have been evaluated in this article. One may argue against the selection of the ontologies by pointing out that our comparative approach would be more proper if two ontologies are in the same domain. Several ontologies in the same domain, "university student" were ranked in (Alani & Brewster, 2005). However, we doubt whether ranking of ontologies with small numbers of concepts is useful and reliable. There are few domains that have several large, well developed ontologies of comparable sizes. Unfortunately, most ontologies available on the Web are not well developed (Ding et al., 2004). Thus we had to use the "best" ontologies with some medical coverage. Our main criteria in selecting ontologies were whether they are actively used by other applications, whether APIs to access their data exist and whether they are of substantial sizes.

As future work, we will investigate whether our methods can be used to actively improve the naturalness of ontologies, e.g. by identifying unnatural parts of an ontology and replacing them by synonyms and alternative structures. Empirical tests with human subjects were conducted by Zeng et al. (2005) to show that human subjects produced significantly higher scores on a set of health literacy questions containing familiar concept labels than for non-familiar concept labels. We intend to conduct thorough human subject tests to validate whether the conclusions of our proposed method are in fact corroborated by human perception. In summary, we expect that natural concepts and concepts pairs, verified by the measurement methods we have developed, will increase knowledge sharing of ontologies between humans and humans as well as between humans and programs.

REFERENCES

Agirre, E., Ansa, O., Hovy, E., & Martinez, D. (2000). Enriching very large ontologies using the WWW. In *Proceedings of ECAI Workshop on Ontology Learning*, Berlin.

Alani, H., & Brewster, C. (2005). Ontology Ranking based on the Analysis of Concept Structure. In *Proceedings of the Third International Conference on Knowledge Capture (K-Cap)* (pp. 51-58), Banff, Alberta, Canada.

An, Y. J. (2008). *Ontology Learning for the Semantic Deep Web*. Doctoral dissertation, New Jersey Institute of technology. Retrieved from NJIT eTD: The New Jersey Institute of Technology's electronic Theses & Dissertations Web site: http://library1.njit.edu/etd/2000s/2008/njit-etd2008-027/njit-etd2008-027.html

An, Y. J., Huang, K.-C., & Geller, J. (2006). Naturalness of Ontology Concepts for Rating Aspects of the Semantic Web. *Communications of the International Information Management Association, 6*(3), 63–76.

Baneyx, B., Charlet, J., & Jaulent, M.-C. (2005). Building Medical Ontologies Based on Terminology Extraction from Texts: An Experimentation in Pneumology. *Studies in Health Technology and Informatics, 116*, 659–664.

Brachman, R. J. (1992). Reducing CLASSIC to practice: Knowledge Representation Theory Meets Reality. In *Proceedings of the Third International Conference on the Principles of Knowledge Representation and Reasoning* (KR-92) (pp. 247-258).

Brewster, C., Ciravegna, F., & Wilks, Y. (2002). User-Centred Onlogy Learning for Knowledge Management. In *Proceedings of the 7th International Workshop on Applications of Natural Language to Information Systems*.

Brewster, C., Ciravegna, F., & Wilks, Y. (2003). Background and Foreground Knowledge in Dynamic Ontology Construction: Viewing Text as Knowledge Maintenance. In *Proceedings of the Semantic Web Workshop (SIGIR)*. Retrieved from AKT EPrint Archiveat Web site: http://eprints.aktors.org/307/

Burgun, A., & Bodenreider, O. (2001). Mapping the UMLS Semantic Network into General Ontologies. In *Proceedings of American Medical Informatics Association (AMIA) Annual Symposium* (pp. 81-85).

Castano, S., & Antonellis, V. D. (1999). A Discovery-Based Approach to Database Ontology Design. *Distributed and Parallel Databases - Special Issue on Ontologies and Databases. 7*(1), 67-98.

Chun, S. A., & Geller, J. (2008). Evaluating Ontologies based on the Naturalness of their Preferred Terms. In *Proceedings of the 41st Annual Hawaii International Conference on System Sciences (HICSS 2008)* (p. 238).

Colomb, R. M. (2002, November). *Quality of Ontologies in Interoperating Information Systems*. Retrieved from the Institute of Cognitive Science and Technology, Laboratory for Applied Ontology Web site: http://www.loa-cnr.it/Papers/ISIB-CNR-TR-18-02.pdf

Cycorp. (2005). *OpenCyc Version 0.9*. Retrieved from http://www.opencyc.org/releases/

Ding, L., Finin, T., Joshi, A., Pan, R., Cost, R., Peng, Y., et al. (2004). Swoogle: a search and metadata engine for the semantic web. In *Proceedings of the 13th ACM Conference on Information and Knowledge Management* (pp. 652-659).

Finin, T., Sachs, J., & Parr, C. S. (2007). Finding Data, Knowledge, and Answers on the Semantic Web. In *Proceedings of the 20th International FLAIRS Conference* (pp. 2-7).

Gligorov, R., Aleksovski, Z., Kate, W., & Harmelen, F. (2007). Using Google Distance to Weight Approximate Ontology Matches. In *16th International World Wide Web Conference* (pp. 767-775).

Gruber, T. R. (1993). Toward principles for the design of ontologies used for knowledge sharing. In *Proceedings of International Workshop on Formal Ontology*, Padova, Italy. Retrieved from Web site: http://www-ksl.stanford.edu/knowledge-sharing/papers/README.html#onto-design

Hearst, M. A. (1992). Automatic Acquisition of Hyponyms form Large Text Corpora. *Proceedings of, COLING-92*, 539–545.

Kalfoglou, Y., & Hu, B. (2006, May). Issues with evaluating and using publicly available ontologies, In *Proceedings of the Fourth International Evaluation of Ontologies for the Web Workshop (EON2006)*, Edinburgh, UK.

Kuhnast, C., & Neuhauser, M. (2008). A note on the use of the non-parametric Wilcoxon-Mann-Whitney test in the analysis of medical studies. *German Medical Science*, 6.

Lee, Y., & Geller, J. (2005). Semantic Enrichment for Medical Ontologies. *Journal of Biomedical Informatics*, *39*(2), 209–226. doi:10.1016/j.jbi.2005.08.001

Lewis, D. (1983). New Work for a Theory of Universals. *Australasian Journal of Philosophy*, *61*, 343–377. doi:10.1080/00048408312341131

Maedche, A., & Staab, S. (2000). Mining Ontologies from Text. *Proceedings of EKAW-2000, Springer Lecture Notes in Artificial Intelligence (LNAI-1937)* (pp. 189-202), Juan-Les-Pins, France.

McCray, A. T., Burgun, A., & Bodenreider, O. (2001). Aggregating UMLS Semantic Types for Reducing Conceptual Complexity. In *Proceedings of Medinfo, 2001*, 171–175.

Mihalcea, R., & Moldovan, D. I. (1999). An Automatic Method for Generating Sense Tagged Corpora. In *Proceedings of American Association for Artificial Intelligence* (pp. 461-466), Orlando, FL.

Mizoguchi, R. (2004). Tutorial on Ontological Engineering: Part 3: Advanced Course of Ontological Engineering. *New Generation Computing, 22*(2).

Necib, C. B., & Freytag, J. (2003). Ontology Based Query Processing in Database Management Systems. In *Proceedings of the 6th International Conference on Ontologies, Databases and Applications of Semantics for Large Scale Information Systems (ODBASE'2003)* (pp. 37-99).

Noy, N. F., & Hafner, C. (1997). The State of the Art in Ontology Design: A Survey and Comparative Review. *AI Magazine, 18*(3), 53–74.

Obrst, L., Hughes, T., & Steve Ray, S. (2006, May). Prospects and Possibilities for Ontology Evaluation: The View from NCOR. In *Proceedings of the Fourth International Evaluation of Ontologies for the Web Workshop* (EON2006), Edinburgh, UK.

OpenCyc. (2005). *Predicates and Denotational Functions of Cyc.* Retrieved from Web site: http://www.cyc.com/doc/tut/DnLoad/TheBasicsOf-PredDenoFun.pdf

Pisanelli, D. M., Gangemi, A., & Steve, G. (1998). An Ontological Analysis of the UMLS Metathesaurus. *Journal of the American Medical Informatics Association, 5,* 810–814.

Princeton University. (2006). *WordNet 2.1 Database Statistics.* Retrieved from Web site: http://wordnet.princeton.edu/man/wnstats.7WN

Seta, K., Ikeda, M., Kakusho, O., & Mizoguchi, R. (1997, June 2-5). Capturing a Conceptual Model for End-User Programming: Task Ontology as a Static User Model. In *Proceedings of the Sixth International Conference on User Modeling* (pp. 203-214). Chia Laguna, Sardinia, Italy.

Sieg, A., Mobasher, B., & Burke, R. D. (2007). Ontological User Profiles for Representing Context in Web Search. In *Proceedings of Web Intelligence/IAT Workshops* (pp. 91-94).

Smith, B. C. (1982). *Reflection and Semantics in a Procedural Language.* PhD thesis. Massachusetts Institute of Technology. MIT-LCS-272:154.

Sourceforge.net. (2007). *OpenCyc.* Retrieved from Web site: http://sourceforge.net/project/showfiles.php?group_id=27274.

Sourceforge.net. (2008). *JWNL – Java WordNet Library.* Retrieved from Web site: http://sourceforge.net/projects/jwordnet.

Staab, S., & Maedche, A. (2000). *Axioms are objects too – Ontology engineering beyond the modeling of concepts and relations.* Research report 399, University of Karlsruhe, Institute AIFB.

Stone, J., Wu, X., & Greenblatt, M. (2004). An Intelligent Digital Library System for Biologists. In *Proceedings of the 2004 IEEE Computational Systems Bioinformatics Conference (CSB 2004)* (pp. 491-492).

Supekar, K., Patel, C., & Lee, Y. (2004). Characterizing Quality of Knowledge on Semantic Web. In *Proceedings of the Seventeenth International Florida Artificial Intelligence Research Symposium Conference* (pp. 220-228).

U. S. National Library of Medicine. (2008). *UMLS Knowledge Sources.* Retrieved from Unified Medical Language System Web site: http://www.nlm.nih.gov/research/umls/umlsdoc.html.

Zeng, Q. T., Tse, T., Crowell, J., Divita, G., Roth, L., & Browne, A. C. (2005) Identifying Consumer-Friendly Display (CFD) Names for Health Concepts. In *Proceedings of the AMIA Annual Symposium* (pp. 859-863).

This work was previously published in International Journal of Computational Models and Algorithms in Medicine, Volume 1, Issue 1, edited by Aryya Gangopadhyay, pp. 1-18, copyright 2010 by IGI Publishing (an imprint of IGI Global).

Chapter 2
A Partial Optimization Approach for Privacy Preserving Frequent Itemset Mining

Shibnath Mukherjee
Yahoo! Research and Development, India

Aryya Gangopadhyay
University of Maryland Baltimore County, USA

Zhiyuan Chen
University of Maryland Baltimore County, USA

ABSTRACT

While data mining has been widely acclaimed as a technology that can bring potential benefits to organizations, such efforts may be negatively impacted by the possibility of discovering sensitive patterns, particularly in patient data. In this article the authors present an approach to identify the optimal set of transactions that, if sanitized, would result in hiding sensitive patterns while reducing the accidental hiding of legitimate patterns and the damage done to the database as much as possible. Their methodology allows the user to adjust their preference on the weights assigned to benefits in terms of the number of restrictive patterns hidden, cost in terms of the number of legitimate patterns hidden, and damage to the database in terms of the difference between marginal frequencies of items for the original and sanitized databases. Most approaches in solving the given problem found in literature are all-heuristic based without formal treatment for optimality. While in a few work, ILP has been used previously as a formal optimization approach, the novelty of this method is the extremely low cost-complexity model in contrast to the others. They implement our methodology in C and C++ and ran several experiments with synthetic data generated with the IBM synthetic data generator. The experiments show excellent results when compared to those in the literature.

DOI: 10.4018/978-1-4666-0282-3.ch002

INTRODUCTION

Knowledge discovery from databases (KDD) and knowledge hiding in databases (KHD) are perhaps oxymoron, yet this is indeed the problem faced by the data mining research community these days. Over the past decade, research in the line was focused primarily in discovery of memory efficient and fast algorithms that could discover patterns in large databases in forms of association rules, classification models and clusters of data values. Today with rigorous improvements in the field of these algorithms (Han & Kamber 2006), the primary area has taken quite a leap forward, but has posed some grave problems as well in terms of security and privacy preservation in the knowledge discovery tasks (Dasseni et al., 2001; Evfimienski et al., 2002; Oliviera et al., 2003a, 2003b; Han et al., 2006). A number of cases have been reported in literature where data mining actually has posed threats to discovery of sensitive knowledge and violating privacy. One typical problem is that of inferencing, which means inferring sensitive information from non-sensitive or unclassified data (Oliviera et al., 2002; Clifton, 2001).

Data mining is part of the larger business intelligence initiatives that are taking place in organizations across government and industry sectors, many of which include medical applications. It is being used for prediction as well knowledge discovery that can lead to cost reduction, business expansion, and detection of fraud or wastage of resources, among other things. With its many benefits, data mining has given rise to increasingly complex and controversial privacy issues. For example, the privacy implications of data mining have lead to high profile controversies involving the use of data mining tools and techniques on data related to drug prescriptions. Two major health care data publishers filed a petition to the Supreme Court on whether commercial use of data mining is protected by the First Amendment[1], an appeal to a controversial ruling by the 1st U.S. Circuit Court of Appeals that upheld a 2006 New Hampshire law that banned the usage of doctor's prescription history to increase drug sales.

Privacy implications are a major roadblock to information sharing across organizations. For example, sharing inventory data might reveal information that can be used to gain strategic advantages by competitors. Unless the actual or perceived implications of data mining methods on privacy issues are properly dealt with, it can lead to sub-optimal decision making in organizations, and reluctance to accept such tools by the public in general. For example there could be benefits in sharing prescription data from different pharmacy stores to mine for information such as the use of generic drugs, socio-demographic and geographic analysis of prescription drugs, which will require moving the data from each store or site to a central location, which increases the risks of litigation. In general several potential problems that have been identified for privacy protection make the case for privacy reserving data mining. These include: legal requirements for protecting data (e.g. HIPAA healthcare regulations in the US) Federal register (2002), liability from inadvertent disclosure of data, risk of misuse of proprietary information (Atallah et al., 2003), and antitrust concerns (Vaidya et al., 2006).

Thus it is of growing importance to devise efficient tradeoffs between knowledge discovery and knowledge hiding from databases so that cost to the involved, in general, gets minimized in the process yet the benefit is maximized. The work that will be presented in this article will focus on formulating a model for sanitization of databases against discovery of restrictive associative patterns, while distorting the databases and legitimate pattern discovery as little as possible. To illustrate the problem, consider a classic example given in (Evfimienski et al., 2002; Oliviera et al., 2002). There is a server and several clients, each having its own set of items. The clients want the server to provide them with recommendations based on statistical information about association among items. However the clients do not want the server to know some restrictive patterns. Now what is sent to the server is the raw database and in its process of searching for frequent patterns the server will discover the restrictive patterns as well. Thus what the client has to send is the raw database, modified in a manner so that the restrictive patterns are not discovered. But this needs distortion to the raw database before sending it to the server and the distortion should be such that it is minimal and hiding of the legitimate patterns is also minimal. Other examples of the problem are given in (Verikyos et al., 2004). The example shows the vulnerability of critical frequent patterns, however it is directly associated with the problems of exposing critical association rules as well since rules are built from patterns. Indeed some of the research work like (Verikyos *et al* 2004) use reduction of support of sensitive frequent patterns as one of the methods to hide association rules that could be generated from them. All these methods are based on modifying the data by reducing the support of the critical frequent patterns while keeping the damage to the legitimate patterns and the database to the minimal extent possible. Unfortunately due to the NP-hard nature of the problem (Dasseni et al., 2001) the literature has a history of using heuristics-only methods. Very few (Menon *et al.,* 2005) used an ILP approach for seeking semi-optimality in transaction selection for sanitization. However the methods are expensive with respect to cost complexity. The novelty of our approach is the use of an extremely cheap integer linear programming (ILP) model as the optimization method so that scalability is not a problem. We use heuristics at the later stage of sanitization (removing items from an identified transaction) once the optimal set of transactions are identified.

The rest of the article is organized as follows: in the next section we discuss some of the relevant previous work, following which we describe the methodology followed by experimental results and conclusions.

PREVIOUS WORK

A rich body of work on privacy preserving mining exists. Depending on the type of data privacy problems being addressed, these studies can be divided into two categories: ones that try to hide the data values when the data is sent to a third party for analyses (Agrawal et al., 2001; Agrawal et al., 2000) and others that try to hide the identity of entities when publishing data (Bayardo & Agrawal, 2005; Samarati, 2001). This article falls in the first category.

To date, existing literature on the first category, focus on random perturbation approaches that add or multiply random noise to the data such that individual data values are distorted while the underlying distribution can be reconstructed with fair degree of accuracy (Agrawal & Srikant, 2000; Rizvi & Haritsa, 2002; Evfimevski et al., 2002).

There has also been work on using secure multi-party computation techniques for a wide range of data mining algorithms to address the privacy issue in distributed environment (Vaidya & Clifton, 2002; Kantarcioglu & Clifton, 2004). They share intermediate mining results to calculate mining functions securely over multiple sources. We refer to (Vaidya et al., 2006) for a detailed discussion on research in PPDM. There has been work for secure association rule mining in distributed environment. These methods build global mining models securely by following secure multi-party computation protocols (Kantarcioglu & Clifton, 2004; Vaidya & Clifton, 2002). However, this article focuses on the case when the data is sent to a third party for analysis and we assume that the data owner either does not have the capability or is not willing to do the mining himself. This assumption is often true in supply chain management environment where there are a large number of small retailers.

Security issues in the general framework of association rule mining have been pursued with much interest in recent years (Atallah et al., 1999; Evfimevski et al., 2002; Kantarcioglu & Clifton,

2004; Lin & Liu, 2007; Menon, 2007; Oliveira & Zaiane, 2002; Rizvi & Haritsa, 2002; Vaidya & Clifton, 2002; Verykios et al., 2004). The bulk of the past work on such issues deals with preventing disclosure of sensitive rules by a potential adversary (Atallah et al., 1999; Menon, 2007; Oliveira & Zaiane, 2002; Verykios et al., 2004). This work complements ours since it addresses concerns about output privacy, whereas our focus is on the privacy of the input data while disclosing the output. Since our proposed approach is more closely related to data hiding, we will limit our discussion on prior work to input data hiding.

Evfimevski et al. (2002), Lin & Liu (2007), Rizvi & Haritsa (2002) propose solutions for mining association rules from transactions where the data is randomized to preserve privacy of individual transactions. However these solutions only work for transactions consisting of categorical items and are not applicable to quantitative data.

Random perturbation has also been used to preserve the privacy of input data in classification rule mining (Agrawal & Aggarwal, 2001; Agrawal & Srikant, 2000). Here the data is predominantly numerical. But, as in the case of categorical data, both privacy and mining results are adversely affected by randomly perturbing quantitative data. Kargupta et al. (2003) show that the privacy in perturbation approaches can be breached by the application of Independent Component Analysis (ICA) which is used extensively to split source signals from output signals. From (Wilson, 2003), it is also clear that both additive and multiplicative perturbation alter the relationships between confidential and non-confidential attributes. Therefore, generating association rules from quantitative data, which is randomly perturbed, is not advisable.

A method that does preserve correlations between attributes is suggested in (Liu, et al., 2006). It multiplies the original data with a lower dimension random matrix, but is also problem-prone, because dimensionality reduction changes the data's original form or domain. Further, this method is suggested for a distributed environment, whereas the focus in the current study is on centralized data.

The research on preserving private information in frequent patter/association rule mining can be categorized into techniques for data randomization, partitioning, and sanitization. This work belongs to the last category—data sanitization, which deals with the problem of limiting the disclosure of sensitive rules with the minimal possible impact on non-sensitive rules and the database itself. The methodology in (Atallah et al., 1999) dealt with modifying a database such that the support of the restrictive rules fall below the minimum support value. The authors proved that optimal sanitization is an NP-hard problem.

In a subsequent work (Verykios et al., 2004), many strategies were developed for hiding sensitive association rules by either hiding the frequent itemsets from which they are derived or by reducing their confidence below a user-specified threshold. The algorithms required multiple scans and modified database values. Another recent article (Menon et al., 2005) devices an ILP formulation to solve the given problem semi-optimally, however the novelty of our method is to modify the formulation such that the cost-complexity can be reduced on a large scale still keeping the formal flavor of optimally solving the problem.

METHODOLOGY

Notation

Before we proceed to describe our optimization algorithm we list down a set of notations that we shall be using throughout the rest of the article in developing the model.

1. D denotes for the original database having N transaction entries or tuples.
2. D' denotes the modified database after sanitization.

3. $T = \{T_1, T_2, ...T_N\}$ denotes the set of transactions in D.

4. $I = \{I_1, I_2, ...I_t\}$ denotes the set of all the items in D.

5. $L = \{L_1, L_2, ...L_l\}$ denotes the set of all legitimate itemsets/patterns mined with a pre-defined minimum support ξ.

6. $R = \{R_1, R_2, ...R_r\}$ denotes the set of all restrictive itemsets/patterns mined with a pre-defined minimum support ξ.

7. $I_R = \{I_{R1}, I_{R2}, ...I_{Rk}\}$ denotes the union of all items contained in all the restrictive patterns of R.

Keeping the above notation in mind we propose our sanitization scheme first in the next section, and the algorithm thereafter sequentially, as the sanitization scheme is intimately related to our definition of costs and benefits for the optimization problem.

The Sanitization Scheme

Let T_i denote a transaction we select for sanitization. The first step of sanitization will be to find the intersection set of items contained in I_R and T_i, that is, to find the common elements between T_i and I_R. The second step will be to remove those common items from T_i. In a worst case scenario a transaction will have all its items from the set I_R. In that case we place a NULL for the transaction. However, the percentage of such transactions is negligible and accounts for approximately 0.05% of the transactions in most of our experiments. We do not add spurious items in its place and frame a false transaction to avoid the possibility of generation of false frequent patterns (Oliviera et al., 2002, Verikyos et al., 2004). The logic behind our proposition of this scheme of sanitization is the fact that we effectively reduce the support of all restrictive itemsets supported by T_i by one, yet at the same time try to make a minimum impact on the support of legitimate itemsets contained

in the transaction by removing only the items contained in I_R. The point of trade off comes since it is possible that some of the legitimate itemsets will also contain some items from I_R. When those items are removed from T_i, both the support for the restrictive itemsets and legitimate itemsets having those items will drop by one. A more effective way would have been to identify the restrictive itemsets associated with each T_i to be sanitized, separately, compute the union of items in each of those sets and remove only those items from T_i. However in such a scheme the computation involved would be too tedious since then, for each transaction to be sanitized, the union item list would have to be constructed. Further, defining costs (as is discussed in the next section) would have been a complicated and tedious issue. Since the number of restrictive itemsets is supposed to be much smaller than that of legitimate itemsets, we may safely assume that in all probability I_R will be a small subset of the entire set of items I in the database. Consequently we adopt the simpler method of finding the union item list, to be removed, considering all the restrictive itemsets together at the very beginning. The additional damage following this method, rather than the more involved one, is expected to be nominal, when weighted against the savings of computational time and resources. Thus we stick to the first method of sanitization for our purposes. However, other sanitizations methods can also be applied in which case the definitions of cost and benefit would change to suit the schemes.

The Optimization Algorithm

Given the sanitization scheme we proposed in the last section, we proceed to define the costs and benefits associated with sanitizing a transaction T_i. Following the scheme, sanitizing a transaction T_i essentially means the following

1. Support of all restrictive patterns associated with it gets reduced by one.

2. Support of those legitimate patterns associated with it, but containing at least one of the items from the set I_R gets reduced by one.
3. Support of all the items of I_R contained in T_i gets reduced by 1.

Considering the three factors stated above the benefit in terms of reducing support of restrictive patterns, cost in terms of reducing support of legitimate patterns, and data damage in terms of reduction of support of the items contained in a transaction terms are defined respectively as follows, where *sup* stands for support:

$$B_{ij} = \frac{1}{\sup(R_j)} \; if \; T_i \supseteq R_j$$
$$= 0 \; otherwise$$

$$C_{ij} = \frac{1}{\sup(L_j)} \; if \; T_i \supseteq L_j \; and \; L_j \cap I_R \neq \varphi$$
$$= 0 \; otherwise$$

$$D_{ij} = \frac{1}{\sup(I_{Rj})} \; if \; I_{Rj} \in T_i$$
$$= 0 \; otherwise.$$

The above parameters are defined based on the concept that if support of a pattern in case of B_{ij} and C_{ij} or an individual item (in case of D_{ij}) is very high, then reducing its support by 1 will have a smaller impact than one with a lower support. The next step in the process is to frame the objective function for the problem.

Let X_i be a binary variable that has a value 1 if transaction i is to be sanitized and 0 otherwise.

Thus our objective will be to maximize the weighted net benefit

$$\sum_{i=1}^{N}\sum_{j=1}^{r} bB_{ij}X_i - \sum_{i=1}^{N}\sum_{j=1}^{l} cC_{ij}X_i - \sum_{i=1}^{N}\sum_{j=1}^{k} dD_{ij}X_i$$

where b c and d are the user defined scalar weights assigned to benefit cost and damage respectively to include the importance of the parameters in the optimization problem. Later while discussing the results we will analyze the variation in results due to the variation of $b{:}c{:}d$ ratio. We will be concerned only with those transactions which support at least one restrictive pattern else there is no reason whatsoever for considering the transaction for sanitization as is quite intuitively obvious.

Thus we have the following constraint

$$i \in \{F : \forall i \; in \; F, \sum_{j} B_{ij} \neq 0\}$$

The above constraint dictates that only those transactions will be considered associated with which there is at least one non zero benefit term that is, it supports at least one restrictive pattern. Let S be the number of such transactions. Further let the set of feasible X_is be $X=\{X_{F1}, X_{F2}, ..., X_{FS}\}$. Finally we have one more constraint which will decide up to what extent the user wants to sanitize the database that is what percentage of S the user want to sanitize. Thus the constraint will look like

$$\sum_{i \in F} X_i = \delta S .$$

Summing up we have the integer programming formulation for the optimization problem as

Maximize
$$Z = \sum_{i=1}^{N}\sum_{j=1}^{r} bB_{ij}X_i - \sum_{i=1}^{N}\sum_{j=1}^{l} cC_{ij}X_i - \sum_{i=1}^{N}\sum_{j=1}^{k} dD_{ij}X_i$$

$$S.T. \quad i \in \{F : \forall i \; in \; F, \sum_{j} B_{ij} \neq 0\} \quad (1)$$

$$\sum_{i \in F} X_i = \delta S \quad 0 \leq \delta \leq 1 \quad (2)$$

$$X_i \in \{0,1\}. \quad (3)$$

A few important features can be intuitively seen from the formulation. First, constraint (1) reduces the search space of the problem drastically. This is due to the fact that given there are very few restrictive patterns, generally, only a small subset of transactions from the entire database will support them. For instance in our experiments it got reduced from 98260 transactions in the entire database to a set of 825 transactions in case of 10 restrictive patters, and 677 in case of 5 restrictive patterns, that we needed to consider for sanitization. This reduced the number of X_i variables in the objective function of the problem by a factor of approximately 100. Further only those $\sum_j C_{ij}$ s need to be calculated whose corresponding $\sum_j B_{ij}$ s are not 0s for the same value of i. Calculation of C_{ij}s, as one can note, is tedious (worst case complexity $O(t^2)$, where t is the total number of items in D) thus constraint (1) in essence reduces that by the same factor as it reduces the number of variables in the objective function. The second constraint (2) gives some sort of flexibility to the user regarding his preferences in how much damage he can tolerate (in number of spoiling tuples) and how many restrictive patterns he may allow to appear even after sanitization. As one goes on increasing δ towards 1 from 0 the number of restrictive patterns exposed post-sanitization decreases while the damage to the database and legitimate patterns increase. Third, the ease of solving this ILP is the novelty of this formulation worth mentioning from the viewpoint of ease of computation as well as memory resources. If one notices the nature of the problem its bogs down to actually searching δS number of feasible X_is (feasibility defined by constraint (1)) having the highest coefficients and setting them to 1. Figure 1 shows the flowchart of the algorithm.

As shown in Figure 1, the algorithm first frames the objective function. This is done by scanning every transaction in the database. For each trans-

action, the algorithm first checks whether any of the restrictive patterns is contained in the transaction (i.e., computing sum of B_j). If the transaction does not contain restrictive patterns (i.e., sum of B_j equals 0), the algorithm simply ignores the transaction. Otherwise, the algorithm finds the legitimate patterns in the transaction as well as the set of items in I_R (i.e., computing sum of C_j and D_j).

Once all transactions are processed, the algorithm computes the coefficient for each transaction containing restrictive patterns. The coefficient of any X_i in the objective function is of form $(bB - cC - dD)$ where B, C and D are the summation of benefit, cost, and damage terms for each X_i over all patterns it contains and b, c and d are the weights assigned to cost, benefit, and marginal frequency damage, respectively. The algorithm then sorts these coefficients in descending order, and picks the first σS of them. These transactions are sanitized by removing any items in I_R.

Let N be the number of transactions, m be the average number of items in each pattern, r be the number of restrictive patterns, l be the number of legitimate patterns, k be total number of items in I_R, and S be the number of transactions containing restrictive patterns. The cost of computing sum B_j is $O(rm)$ for each transaction if hash tree is used to match the transaction against the set of restrictive patterns. Similarly, the cost of computing sum C_j and D_j are $O(lm)$ and $O(km)$, respectively. We only need to compute them for transactions that contain restrictive patterns. Thus the cost of framing the objective function is $O(N r m + S(l+k) m)$. Sorting the coefficients takes time $O(S \log S)$ because there are only S transactions containing restrictive patterns. Finally sanitizing the selected σS transactions takes time $O(\sigma S k)$. The total cost of the algorithm is thus $O(N r m + S(lm+km+\log S + \sigma k))$. The algorithm scales linearly with the number of transactions and the number of restrictive and legitimate patterns.

Figure 1. Flowchart of the optimization algorithm

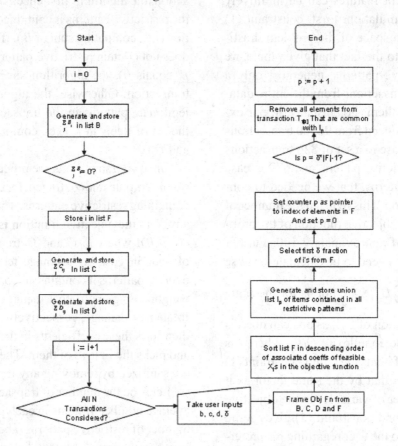

EXPERIMENTAL RESULTS

Details of Experiments

We used IBM synthetic data generator to create about 100K (98,260 to be precise) transactions with 500 different items, with an average of 10 items per transaction. There were 10,440 patterns generated using the *Apriori* algorithm (Goethals) with a minimum support of 0.14%. We conducted two sets of experiments. In the first case 10 patterns having 5 or more items in each were randomly selected as restrictive patterns, which left 10430 legitimate patterns. In the second case 5 patterns having 5 or more items each were randomly selected as restrictive patterns, which left 10435 legitimate patterns. The basis of our selection is

the intuition that typically patterns having large number of item associations and supports just above threshold are likely to be the sensitive ones. A strategy analyst typically would bother about them rather than ones having association of few items and having large supports, since, they are expected to be common knowledge, might be available even from other sources.

The effectiveness of the methodology is measured in three ways: damage done to the database, the number of restrictive patterns disclosed in spite of the sanitization, and the number of legitimate patterns accidentally hidden. In some data sanitization artificial patterns appear in the altered database. Since we are not injecting any new data into the database this is not the case in our methodology.

We evaluated the performance by varying δ from 10% to 90%. The disclosure threshold ψ defined in (Oliviera *et al* 2003a, 2003b) is a decreasing function of δ in our case. The value of δ is specified by the database owner and indicates the extent to which privacy is preserved. For example, $\delta=100\%$ it means that no restrictive association patterns are allowed to be mined. Similarly, $\delta=0\%$ means that there are no restrictions on mining association patterns. In our experiments δ was 90% before all restrictive association patterns got hidden in the worst-case scenario.

The first measure, damage done to the database is expressed as the difference between the original database D and the sanitized database D'. Furthermore, the difference is measured by comparing the sum of frequencies of all items in each of the databases, as shown by Equation (4), taken from (Oliviera *et al* 2002, 2003a, 2003b), where $f_D(I)$ and $f_{D'}(i)$ represent the frequency of the ith item in database D and D' respectively.

$$Dif(D,D') = \frac{1}{\sum_{i=1}^{n} f_D(i)} \times \sum_{i=1}^{n} [f_D(i) - f_{D'}(i)]$$

(4)

Figure 2 shows that the extent of damage caused by our methodology as measured by the difference between D and D' is negligible, ranging from 0.04% in the best case to 0.45% in the worst case. Figure 2 also shows the difference between D and D' for different weights on benefit, cost, and damage. Thus, when $b{:}c{:}d$ was set to *1000:1:1*, which means that there is more weight on benefit than on cost or damage to the database, the difference between D and D' ranged from 0.067% to 0.38%. When $b{:}c{:}d$ was set to *1:1000:1*, which means that there is more weight on cost than on benefit or damage to the database, the difference between D and D' ranged from 0.04% to 0.45%. When $b{:}c{:}d$ was set to *1:1:1000*, which means that there is more weight on damage to database

than on benefit or cost of losing legitimate patterns, the difference between D and D' ranged from 0.04% to 0.45%. Thus, as can be seen from Figure 2, more weight on the cost or damage as compared to benefit resulted in a slightly lower damage curve.

The second measure, number of restrictive patterns disclosed in spite of sanitization, is referred to as *hiding failure* and defined as follows (Oliviera et al., 2002, 2003a, 2003b):

$$HF = \frac{R_{D'}}{R_D},$$

where R_D and $R_{D'}$ stand for the set of restrictive patterns in databases D and D' respectively. Unlike (Oliviera *et al* 2002, 2003a, 2003b), where all supersets of restrictive patterns were also included in the set of restrictive patterns explicitly, we consider only the original set of restrictive patterns to be on the conservative side. The logic behind this is that if a restrictive pattern is hidden, all of its supersets also get hidden automatically. As the support of a restrictive pattern goes below a threshold, the supports of all its supersets go below the threshold as well. As stated above, we varied the $b{:}c{:}d$ ratio in favor of benefit, cost and damage to the database to evaluate the impact of each on hiding failure. As expected, more emphasis on benefit results in a better performance in terms of hiding failure. As shown in Figure 3 the best case sanitizing 70% of S resulted in the value of hiding failure of 0 and in the worst case it took sanitizing 90% of the S to achieve the same result.

We also followed the same definition for the third measure, the number of legitimate patterns accidentally hidden by the sanitization as described in (Oliviera et al., 2002, 2003a, 2003b). It is referred to as *misses cost*, and is defined as follows:

$$MC = \frac{L_D - L_{D'}}{L_D},$$

Figure 2. Damage to the DB based on δ

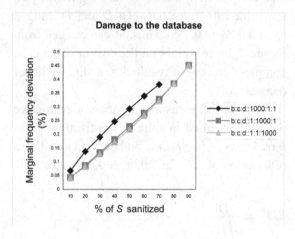

Figure 3. Hiding failure based on δ

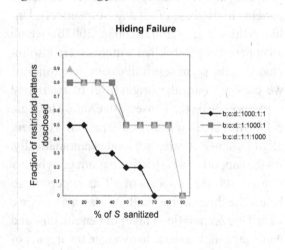

Figure 4. Misses cost based on δ

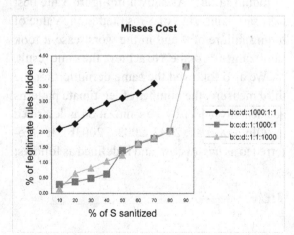

where L_D and $L_{D'}$ stand for the set of restrictive patterns in databases D and D' respectively. In our experimental results shown in Figure 4, we calculated the measure *misses cost* by varying the relative weights benefit, cost, and damage to the database. When maximizing benefit has the highest weight *b:c:d::1000:1:1*, *misses cost* ranged from 2.1% when δ is 90% to 3.6% when δ is 0%. When we put more weight on minimizing cost *b:c:d::1:1000:1*, *misses cost* varied from 0.3% at 90% δ to 4.1% at 0% δ. When the maximum weight is put on minimizing the damage to the database, such that the ratio is equal to *b:c:d::1:1:1000*, the values of *misses cost* ranged from 0.14% at 90% δ to 4% at 0% δ. These results show a significant improvement in our approach in terms of protecting legitimate patterns from being hidden in the process of sanitization.

The experiments were replicated with 5 restrictive patterns with five or more items in each. The results, compared with those with 10 restricted patterns, are shown in Figures 5-7. In all cases the *b:c:d* was set to *1000:1:1*. Figure 5 shows that the damage to the database is smaller when we used 5 restrictive patterns instead of 10. However, the rate of increase with 10 restrictive patterns is slightly higher than that with 5 restrictive patterns initially, but eventually becomes parallel. Figure 6 shows that the two curves are similar with some overlaps. We note that the value for % of *S* for 10 restrictive patterns is slightly higher than that for 5 restrictive patterns, and hence the absolute number of transactions sanitized in the former is slightly higher than in the latter. Figure 7 shows that the *misses cost* for 10 restrictive patterns is roughly parallel to that with 5 restrictive patterns but have a higher *Y*-intercept. These results are intuitive as they suggest that as the number of restrictive patterns increase the performance degrades but the trend remains the same.

Analysis of Experimental Results

During the experimentation, we varied the scalar weight parameters b, c, and d to get our results and curves of performance indicator variables. In this section we will discuss the significance of variation of these parameters on the results. When we are solving the ILP we are essentially finding out δS of the feasible X_is having the highest coefficients in descending order from the lot of S feasible X_i variables (feasibility given by Equation (1)). We consider two typical coefficients of say X_m and X_n. The coefficients will look like $(bB_m - cC_m - dD_m)$ and $(bB_n - cC_n - dD_n)$ respectively where B_i, C_i and D_i stand for the B_{ij}, C_{ij} and D_{ij} coefficient terms added over their respective js. Now if we consider their relative rank-wise positioning as to who comes before the other in the sanitization list then whether $(bB_m - cC_m - dD_m) > (bB_n - cC_n - dD_n)$ or the other way is true is the judgment factor. Given a set of B_m, B_n, C_m, C_n and D_m D_n, the validity of the inequality is governed by relative values of b, c and d that is the $b:c:d$ ratio as can be easily seen. Thus varying the ratio and analyzing the effect on performance indicators to give suggestions to users becomes important.

Conclusions from Experimental Results

To analyze and interpret the above curves a couple of things hinted at earlier in the last section, have to be recalled. First, in maximizing the objective function of the problem, for a given δ, δS number of X_is, having the highest coefficient terms are selected and set equal to 1. Second, the coefficient of any X_i in the objective function is of form $(bB - cC - dD)$ where B, C and D are the summation of benefit, cost and damage terms for each X_i over all patterns it contains and b, c and d are the weights assigned to cost, benefit and marginal frequency damage respectively. *Hiding failure* curves will fall with increase in summation of B terms and *misses cost* will rise with summation of C terms.

Figure 5. Comparison of database damage with number of restrictive patterns

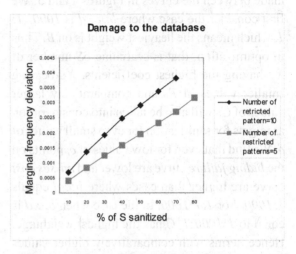

Figure 6. Comparison of hiding failure with number of restrictive patterns

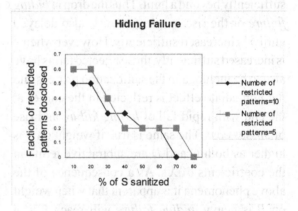

Figure 7. Comparison of misses cost with number of restrictive patterns

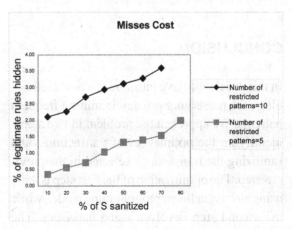

Keeping the above in mind, a comparison is made between the curves in Figures 4 and 5. We first consider the case where *b: c: d* is *1000: 1: 1*, which means the heaviest weight is on *B*. Thus in optimization, that is searching δS number of X_is having the highest coefficients, X_is bearing smaller values of *B*s and comparatively larger values of *C*s will also be taken into consideration as targets for sanitization for even small values of δ. We find that even for low values of δ, points on the *hiding failure* curve are lower and *misses cost* curve are higher than cases where *b:c:d* equals *1:1000:1* or *1:1:1000*. In the case when *b:c:d* is equal to *1:1000:1*, *C* has the highest weightage. Hence, terms with comparatively higher values of *B* and lower values of *C* will also be rejected from the sanitization procedure until δ is increased sufficiently beyond a limit. Thus the drop in *hiding failure* or the rise in *misses cost* is also delayed until δ is increased sufficiently. However when δ is increased sufficiently, those rejected terms have also to be included in the sanitization process and the immediate effect is reflected in the curves at the end with rapid fall of *hiding failure* and rise of *misses cost*. The same is true if weight on *d* is higher as both *C* and *D* are subtractive terms in the coefficients of X_is. As a consequence of the above phenomena it is apparent that when weight on *B* is heavy, *hiding failure* will reach 0 at a lower value of δ than when the weight is heavy on *C* and *D* terms, which is what our experiments suggest as well.

CONCLUSION

In this article we have introduced a new methodology for preserving privacy in mining frequent patterns. We approach the problem in two steps: identifying the optimal set of transactions, and sanitizing the transactions selected in the previous step. The optimization of the first step is done using an integer linear programming model, while the second step is solved using heuristics. The optimization problem is designed to maximize the net benefit of sanitizing a transaction, which is obtained by subtracting the cost and damage from the benefit of sanitization. A user in our methodology can further adjust the relative weights on benefit, cost, and damage. The uniqueness of our approach is in the fact that part of the privacy preservation process has been optimized instead of solving the entire problem with heuristic algorithms, as is the case in previous work in this area.

We ran several experiments by using data generated by the IBM synthetic data generator. There were two sets of restrictive patterns with 10 and 5 items in each. The result showed that the methodology is very effective in hiding restrictive patterns, avoiding inadvertent hiding of legitimate patterns, and causing minimal damage to the database.

There are several possible extensions of this work. These include designing an integrated approach for privacy preserving mining of classification, clustering, and association rules. Another approach could be developing optimization models for quantitative association rules, other types of data such including semi-structured and unstructured data, and application of this technique in domains such as supply chain management, healthcare, and bio-terrorism that may involve mining and hence discovering privacy sensitive information at corporate or individual levels.

REFERENCES

Aggarwal, C. C., & Yu, P. S. (2004). *A Condensation Approach to Privacy Preserving Data Mining.* Paper presented at the 9th International Conference on Extending Database Technology (pp. 183-199).

Agrawal, D., & Aggarwal, C. (2001). *On the design and quantification of privacy preserving data mining algorithms.* Paper presented at the 20th ACM SIGMOD SIGACT-SIGART Symposium on Principles of Database Systems (pp. 247-255).

Agrawal, R., & Srikant, R. (2000). *Privacy preserving data mining.* Paper presented at the 2000 ACM SIGMOD Conference on Management of Data (pp. 439-450).

Atallah, M., Bertino, E., Elmagarmid, A., Ibrahim, M., & Verikyos, V. (1999, November). Disclosure Limitations of Sensitive Rules. In *Proceedings of IEEE Knowledge and Data Engineering Workshop* (pp. 45-52), Chicago, Illinois.

Atallah, M., Elmongui, H. G., Deshpande, V., & Schwartz, L. B. (2003, June 24-27). *Secure Supply-Chain Protocols.* In IEEE International Conference on E-Commerce (pp. 293-302), Newport Beach, California.

Atallah, M. J., Elmagarmid, A. K., Ibrahim, M., & Verykios, V. S. (1999). *Disclosure Limitation of Sesitive Rules.* Paper presented at the IEEE Knowledge and Data Engineering Workshop (pp. 45-52).

Bayardo, R. J., & Agrawal, R. (2005). *Data Privacy through Optimal k-Anonymization.* Paper presented at the ICDE (pp. 217-228).

Chen, Z.-Y., & Liu, G.-H. (2005). *Quantitative Association Rules Mining Methods with Privacy-preserving.* Paper presented at the Sixth International Conference on. Parallel and Distributed Computing, Applications and Technologies, PDCAT.

Clifton, C. (2001). Using Sample Size to Limit Exposure to Data Mining. *Journal of Computer Security, 8*(4), 281–307.

Dasseni, E., Verikyos, V., Elmagarmid, A., & Bertino, E. (2001, April). *Hiding Association Rules by Using Confidence and Support.* In proceedings of the 4th Information Hiding Workshop (pp. 369-383), Pittsburgh, PA.

Evfimevski, A., Gehrke, J., & Srikant, R. (2003). *Limiting privacy breaches in privacy preserving data mining.* Paper presented at the 22nd ACM SIGMOD-SIGACT-SIGART Symposium on Principles of Database Systems, San Diego, CA.

Evfimevski, A., Srikant, R., Agrawal, R., & Gehrke, J. (2002). *Privacy preserving mining of association rules.* Paper presented at the 8th ACM SIGKDD International Conference on Knowledge Discovery and Data Mining (KDD'02) (pp. 217-228).

Federal Register. (2002, August 14). Standard for Privacy of Individually Identifiable Health Information. *Federal Register, 67*(157), 53181–53273.

Goethals. B. (n.d.). http://www.adrem.ua.ac.be/~goethals/software. Last accessed on 05/19/09.

Han, J., & Kamber, M. (2006). Data Mining: Concepts and Techniques (2nd ed.), Morgan Kaufmann.

Kantarcioglu, M., & Clifton, C. (2004). Privacy-preserving distributed mining of association rules on horizontally partitioned data. *IEEE Transactions on Knowledge and Data Engineering, 16*(9), 1026–1037. doi:10.1109/TKDE.2004.45

Kargupta, H., Datta, S., Wang, Q., & Sivakumar, K. (2003). Random data perturbation techniques and privacy preserving data mining. *Knowledge and Information Systems, 7*(4), 387–414. doi:10.1007/s10115-004-0173-6

Li, X. B., & Sarkar, S. A. (2006). Tree-Based Data Perturbation Approach for Privacy-Preserving Data Mining. *IEEE Transactions on Knowledge and Data Engineering, 18*(9), 1278–1283. doi:10.1109/TKDE.2006.136

Lin, J.-L., & Liu, J. Y.-C. (2007). Privacy preserving itemset mining through fake transactions http://doi.acm.org/10.1145/1244002.1244092. In *Proceedings of the ACM symposium on Applied computing* (pp. 375-379), Seoul, Korea: ACM Press.

Liu, K., Kargupta, H., & Ryan, J. (2006). Random projection-based multiplicative data perturbation for privacy preserving distributed data mining. *IEEE Transactions on Knowledge and Data Engineering, 18*(1), 92–106. doi:10.1109/TKDE.2006.14

Mallat, S. G. (1989). A theory for multiresolution signal decomposition: The wavelet representation. *IEEE Transactions on Pattern Analysis and Machine Intelligence, 11*(7), 674–693. doi:10.1109/34.192463

Menon, S., & Sarkar, S. (2007). Minimizing Information Loss and Preserving Privacy. *Management Science, 53*(1), 101–116. doi:10.1287/mnsc.1060.0603

Menon, S., Sarkar, S., & Mukherjee, S. (2005). Maximizing Accuracy of Shared Databases when Concealing Sensitive Patterns. *Information Systems Research, 16*(3), 256–270. doi:10.1287/isre.1050.0056

Oliveira, S., & Zaiane, O. R. (2002). *Privacy Preserving Frequent Itemset Mining.* Paper presented at the IEEE International Conference on Privacy, Security and Data Mining, Maebashi City, Japan.

Oliveira, S., & Zaiane, O. R. (2003a, July). Algorithms for Balancing Privacy and Knowledge Discovery in Association Rule Mining. In *Proceedings of the 7th International Database Engineering and Applications Symposium (IDEAS)* (pp. 54-63), Hong Kong, China.

Oliveira, S., & Zaiane, O. R. (2003b, November). Protecting Sensitive Knowledge by Data Sanitization. In *Proceedings of the 3rd IEEE International Conference on Data Mining* (pp. 613-616), Melbourne, Florida.

Rizvi, S., & Haritsa, J. R. (2002). *Maintaining Data Privacy in Association Rule Mining.* Paper presented at the VLDB.

Samarati, P. (2001). Protecting Respondents' Identities in Microdata Release. *TKDE, 13*(6), 1010–1027.

Vaidya, J., Clifton, C., & Zhu, Y. (2006). *Privacy Preserving Data Mining.* New York: Springer.

Vaidya, J. S., & Clifton, C. (2002). *Privacy preserving association rule mining in vertically partitioned data.* Paper presented at the 8th ACM SIGKDD International Conference on Knowledge Discovery and Data Mining (pp. 639-644).

Verykios, V. S., Elmagarmid, A. K., Elisa, B., Saygin, Y., & Elena, D. (2004). Association Rule Hiding. *IEEE Transactions on Knowledge and Data Engineering, 16*(4), 434–447. doi:10.1109/TKDE.2004.1269668

Wilson, R. L., & Rosen, P. A. (2003). Protecting Data Through 'Perturbation' Techniques: The Impact on Knowledge Discovery in Databases. *Journal of Database Management, 14*(2), 14–26.

Zhang, N., Wang, S., & Zhao, W. (2004). *A New Scheme on Privacy Preserving Association Rule Mining.* Berlin Heidelberg: Springer-Verlag.

ENDNOTE

[1]   http://www.law.com/jsp/article.jsp?id=1202429488883

This work was previously published in International Journal of Computational Models and Algorithms in Medicine, Volume 1, Issue 1, edited by Aryya Gangopadhyay, pp. 19-33, copyright 2010 by IGI Publishing (an imprint of IGI Global).

Chapter 3
Classification Systems for Bacterial Protein–Protein Interaction Document Retrieval

Hongfang Liu
Georgetown University Medical Center, USA

Manabu Torii
Georgetown University Medical Center, USA

Guixian Xu
Minzu University of China, China

Johannes Goll
The J. Craig Venter Institute, USA

ABSTRACT

Protein-protein interaction (PPI) networks are essential to understand the fundamental processes governing cell biology. Recently, studying PPI networks becomes possible due to advances in experimental high-throughput genomics and proteomics technologies. Many interactions from such high-throughput studies and most interactions from small-scale studies are reported only in the scientific literature and thus are not accessible in a readily analyzable format. This has led to the birth of manual curation initiatives such as the International Molecular Exchange Consortium (IMEx). The manual curation of PPI knowledge can be accelerated by text mining systems to retrieve PPI-relevant articles (article retrieval) and extract PPI-relevant knowledge (information extraction). In this article, the authors focus on article retrieval and define the task as binary classification where PPI-relevant articles are positives and the others are negatives. In order to build such classifier, an annotated corpus is needed. It is very expensive to obtain an annotated corpus manually but a noisy and imbalanced annotated corpus can be obtained automatically, where a collection of positive documents can be retrieved from existing PPI knowledge bases and a large number of unlabeled documents (most of them are negatives) can be retrieved from PubMed. They compared the performance of several machine learning algorithms by varying the ratio of the number of positives to the number of unlabeled documents and the number of features used.

DOI: 10.4018/978-1-4666-0282-3.ch003

INTRODUCTION

Protein-protein interaction (PPI) network is essential to understand the fundamental processes governing cell biology. PPI network data for several organisms has already been generated by high-throughput studies and submitted to/or collected by various PPI interaction databases (Morrison et al., 2005). However, the majority of PPIs are reported in the scientific literature. To collect such data in a standardized way and to avoid duplication of efforts, IMEx[1] databases such as IntAct (http://www.ebi.ac.uk/intact), DIP (Database of Interacting Proteins; http://dip.doe-mbi.ucla.edu), MINT (Molecular Interactions Database; http://mint.bio.uniroma2.it/mint) and MPIDB (Microbial Protein Interaction Database; http://www.jcvi.org/mpidb) conduct coordinated manual literature curation. Text mining system to prioritize articles for curators according to their PPI relevance can accelerate such curation processes significantly. For example, MPIDB curators scan a whole issue (20 to 50 articles) of the Journal of Bacteriology or Molecular Microbiology and find approximately 10% of these articles report interaction experiments. Thus, the curators spend roughly 90% of their time reading irrelevant articles. A text mining system to prioritize articles for curators can be developed using supervised classification algorithms that provide certain kinds of confidence scores during classification. In order to build such systems, a class-labeled corpus is needed where PPI-relevant documents are labeled as positive and those irrelevant as negative. In many real-world applications, it is common that positive instances are explicitly included in a designated database, but it is uncommon to also include negatives in the database (Elkan & Noto, 2008). In developing a PPI mining application, PPI-relevant documents can be retrieved from existing PPI knowledge bases and unlabeled documents are available in large literature repositories such as PubMed. Learning with only positively labeled documents has great importance in this application.

We consider learning with only positive labeled documents as learning from a noisy and imbalanced training set where unlabeled documents are considered as negatives with some mislabeled documents. We build a document retrieval system to assist the curation of MPIDB (Goll et al., 2008) and report our investigation of the stability of two document classification algorithms with respect to the ratio of positives and unlabeled documents in the training set and also of the impact of feature selection on the classification performance. We also propose to use different subsets of unlabeled documents and form an ensemble of classifiers.

In the following, we first describe the background of classification algorithms. The experimental methods are introduced next. We then present the results and discussion, and conclude our work.

BACKGROUND

Learning from Positives and Unlabeled

Existing methods for learning from positives and unlabeled (LPU) commonly adopt a two-step strategy where the first step is to obtain a reliable negative data set (RN) based on keywords or available classifiers and the second step is to refine or augment RN using various learning approaches such as clustering or boosting. One popular approach to obtaining RN is to define a classification task which considers unlabelled documents as negatives, build a binary classifier, and treat those predicted negatives as RN. For example, Li and Liu proposed a method where they first build a Rocchio classifier based on positives and regard negatives according to that classifier as RN. Similar technology can be used to augment training data for PPI document classification. For example, Tsai et al. trained a SVM classifier with 3,536 positives (TPs) and 1,959 negatives (TNs) from BioCreAtIvE II workshop.

Then the training set was augmented by applying the SVM classifier to the likely positive data sets and 50,000 unlabeled MEDLINE. Finally, an improved SVM classifier was derived from the original corpus using additional features based on the augmented corpus.

Recently, Elkan and Noto showed that if positive documents were randomly sampled, the conditional probability of a given document being labeled (and thus positive) differ from the conditional probabilities of a given document being positive only by a constant factor (Elkan & Noto, 2008). We have also found that when defining document retrieval as a classification-based ranking task, given a few labeled positives and many unlabeled documents, the performance of a classifier trained from positives and reliable negatives is similar to the performance of a classifier trained by treating unlabeled documents as negatives (Xu et al., 2009). In this study, we define retrieval of documents pertaining to the curation of MPIDB as a classification task where positive documents are those that are referenced in MPIDB and unlabeled documents are abstracts cross-referenced by bacterial protein records in UniProtKB (Wu et al., 2006).

In the general domain, there are some studies focusing on classification with imbalanced training data. For example, it has been shown that skewed training data can negatively impact the performance of identifying instances belonging to the minority class (usually a class of interest). Weiss (Weiss, 2004) and Chawla et al. (Chawla et al., 2004) had investigated the mining framework with rarity. Also, there have been several studies investigating the stability of different classification systems with respect to the size and skewed class distribution of the training set (Yen et al.; Akbani et al., 2004; Estabrooks et al., 2004; Zheng et al., 2004; Visa & Ralescu, 2005; Ng & Dash, 2006; Weng & Poon, 2006; Molinara et al., 2007; Chen & Wasikowski, 2008). Despite the large number of studies on this topic, there is no simple solution as Chawla et al. wrote; "Though all these papers shed

some light on the way various methods compare, there is no single final word on the question. In other words, a number of techniques were shown to be effective if applied in a certain context, where the breadth of the context may vary."

Classification Algorithms

We explored two classification algorithms: Support Vector Machine (SVM) and Logistic Regression (LR). SVM (Vapnik, 2000) is a powerful machine learning paradigm that has been often reported to outperform other machine learning classifiers, e.g., (Joachims, 1999). SVM classifiers can exploit a very large number of features while resisting against over-fitting to training data. Given two sets of instances belonging to two classes, SVM seeks a hyper-plane in the feature space that maximizes the margin between the two sets of instances. When instances are not linearly separable or a large margin is attainable by overlooking (misclassifying) some instances, the soft-margin method can be used to allow misclassification at a defined cost for each misclassified instance. The so-called kernel trick can also be used to derive a non-linear SVM classifier, but the past studies suggest that a linear classifier is usually sufficient for text data, e.g., (Joachims, 1998). The derivation of a hyper-plane is a numerical optimization process that can be computationally expensive, but efficient implementations of SVM have been publicly available, e.g., LibSVM. An output from an SVM classifier reflects the distance of an instance from a derived hyper-plane, but calibration of probabilities for predicted classes has also been studied for SVM (Scholkopf & Smola, 2001; Chang & Lin, 2009). In statistics, LR is used for prediction of binary-event probabilities by fitting a generalized linear model to provided data points. Like many forms of regression analysis, it makes use of several predictor variables that may be either numerical or categorical. LR can be expensive in high-dimension learning but recently with the availability of fast implementations, it has gained popularity for high-dimensional classification such as text processing where linear boundaries are usually adequate to separate the classes (Komarek & Moore, 2005).

LR and SVM have been shown to be competitive for classification tasks. For example, Zhang et al described a modified version of LR algorithm for text classification, which yields an iterative approximation to SVM. Vapnik also compared LR and SVM in terms of their loss functions (Vapnik, 2000).

Feature Selection

Features commonly used for text classifiers are words. Powerful machine learning algorithm such as SVM can accommodate a large number of word features effectively, but they may perform better with a selected subset of available words in terms of computational costs and/or of classification performance (Yang & Pedersen, 1997; Forman, 2003). Information gain (IG) is one of the feature selection methods widely used. Given a class-labeled article set, A, let A_w be a subset of A that contains articles with a feature word, w. Then, IG to measure the utility of the word w for article classification can be calculated as below:

$$IG(A,w) = H(A) - \left[\frac{|A_w|}{|A|} H(A_w) + \frac{|A| - |A_w|}{|A|} H(A - A_w) \right].$$

Here, $|S|$ is the number of instances in an article set S, and H(S) is the entropy of S calculated by $H(S) = -\sum_{class} p_S(class) \log_2 p_S(class)$, where $P_S(class)$ is the ratio of instances (articles) that belong to the specified class in the set S. Entropy is an index of the uncertainty in predicting classes, and IG measures the reduction in entropy after knowing the presence/absence of a word in an article. Therefore, in general, the larger the IG is, the more informative the word is for article classification. There are other methods

to measure the utility of features, such as χ^2 statistics and point-wise mutual information. With these measures, features can be sorted according to their utility, and a selected number of words at the top of the sorted list are used in classifiers.

METHODS

Data Sets

There are two data sets used in our experiments. The first one (DEV_set) consists of 814 positive and 27,140 unlabeled MEDLINE abstracts. The positive data set was compiled based on MPI-LIT (Rajagopala et al., 2008), a literature-curated subset of MPIDB, and the unlabeled data set was compiled based on UniProtKB records for the organisms included in MPIDB (a total of 93 organisms, accessed April 2009). The imbalanced level measured as the ratio of the number of positives to unlabeled is 1/33.6. The second data set (TEST_set) consists of 682 MEDLINE abstracts mostly from two journals Molecular microbiology and Journal of bacteriology. These articles were manually labeled as positive (i.e., bacterial PPI relevant) or negative (i.e., not bacterial PPI relevant) during the period of January 2009 to June 2009. There are 156 positives and 526 negatives with the imbalanced level of 1/3.3.

Classification Algorithm Implementations

LibSVM implementation of soft margin SVM (Chang & Lin, 2009) and LR-TRIRLS implementation of regularized LR (logistic regression) (Komarek & Moore, 2005) were used in our experiments. For LibSVM, the linear (dot product) kernel with the default setting of parameter C=1.0 was employed and also the option ('-b 1') was set to calculate calibrated probabilities, P(positive | document). LR-TRIRLS implements a fast optimization method to fit a logistic model to given data points, and it can accommodate high-dimensional features. To mitigate model over-fitting, it uses ridge regularization. LR-TRIRLS aims to be a parameter-free tool and we did not need to select any model parameter.

Features

Individual words (word unigrams) except for PubMed stopwords[2] and words found in less than three documents in the training corpus were considered for features. Classification models based on selected informative features sometimes perform better than those trained on all available features (Yang & Pedersen, 1997; Forman, 2003). In our study, IG (information gain) measures were calculated for words, and a selected number of words with high IG values were used in a classification model.

With selected word features, each document is converted into a feature vector. Values in a feature vector are commonly binary (representing presence or absence) or weighted word frequencies (e.g., TF-IDF). For SVM, we used three popular types of values: i) normalized TF-IDF, ii) binary, and iii) normalized binary. LR-TRIRLS accepts either dense numeric feature vectors or sparse binary feature vectors, and given high-dimensional features in our problem, the latter was used in our experiments.

We considered two parameters in preparing the training corpus. Given that a set of unlabeled articles substantially larger than that of positive articles, the first parameter was the size of unlabeled articles used in the training corpus. Let N be the number of positive articles available, we randomly select $N \times 2^{(i-1)}$ unlabeled articles for $i=1$, 2, ..., 6 and compile a training corpus consisting of $N + N \times 2^{(i-1)}$ articles. Since the selection of unlabeled articles affects the performance of the resulting classifier, the unlabeled set of $N \times 2^{(i-1)}$ articles was compiled ten times, and mean AUC was calculated for ten resulting classifiers. The second parameter considered in our experiments

was the size of word features selected for IG. We tried $100 \times 4^{(j-1)}$ features for $j=1, 2, ..., 5$. When the size of selected unlabeled articles is small, the number of available feature can be less than $100 \times 2^{(j-1)}$.

Given a document, an output of a trained classifier is a confidence score between 0 and 1 for the both classification algorithm (when using '–b' option in LibSVM). A set of documents can then be ranked based on the assigned confidence scores.

Ensemble

An ensemble classifier can be more accurate than its constituent classifiers when the constituent classifiers are accurate and diverse (Dietterich, 2000). Here, a classifier is called accurate if it is better than random guessing and two classifiers are called diverse if they make different errors. As stated above, for a selected size of unlabeled articles, ten training corpora were generated and ten classification models were trained. While they were used to measure the performance of single models, we also combined them to form as an ensemble model. Specifically, as an ensemble classifier, for each article a mean of confidence scores assigned by differently trained classifiers was calculated.

Evaluation Measure

Performance of the trained classifiers was measured using Area under ROC curve (AUC). Given a ranked list which ranks predicted positives high, AUC is interpreted as the probability that the rank of a positive document d_1 is greater (i.e., more likely to be positive) than that of an unlabeled (or a negative) document d_0, where d_1 and d_0 are documents randomly selected from positive and unlabeled (or negative) document sets, respectively. Generally speaking, the higher the AUC value, the better the classifier. After documents (of size n) are ranked from 1 (least likely to be positive) to n (most likely to be positive), AUC can be calculated as

$$AUC = \frac{S - n_1(n_1 + 1)/2}{n_0 n_1},$$ where S is the sum

of the ranks assigned to positive documents, and n_0 and n_1 are the numbers of unlabeled and positive documents, respectively (see the details in (Hand et al. 2001)).

We conducted 5×2 fold cross-validation tests (Dietterich, 1998) on the obtained positive and unlabeled corpus (DEV_set). As stated above, for a particular choice of the unlabeled article size and the size of features, ten sets of unlabeled articles are randomly sampled, and mean AUC was calculated for ten single classifiers, i.e., a reported AUC is a mean calculated for 5×2×10 classifiers, while one ensemble classifier could be built out of ten single classifiers, i.e., a reported AUC is a mean calculated for 5×2 classifiers. We also obtained AUC measures for classifiers trained using DEV_set and tested using TEST_set.

RESULTS AND DISCUSSION

Table 1 shows the average number of word features available for a particular ratio of the number of positives and unlabeled. Given a ratio 1:1, the average number of features available is 3,954 and all features were selected when the parameter of the size of word features is 6,400 and 25,600.

Figure 1 shows the results of LR classifiers with binary features and SVM classifiers with three types of SVM features (binary, normalized binary, and TF-IDF). Figure 2 shows the results of LR classifiers with binary features and SVM classifiers with normalized binary features on DEV_set and TEST_set. The x-Axis of Figure 2 is logarithm of the ratio of the number of unlabeled documents to the number of positives in the training set plus 1. The value of 3 for x-Axis means the ratio of the number of positives to the number of unlabeled is 1 to 4. Table 2 shows the results of LR and SVM with binary features on DEV_set. Table 3 shows the detailed results of LR and SVM with the best feature value selection (i.e., normalized binary) when trained on DEV_set and tested on TEST_set.

In our experiment, we only changed the imbalance level on the training set while the imbalanced level of the test set stayed unchanged (i.e., 1 positive to 33.6 negatives for DEV_set and 1 positive to 3.3 negatives for TEST_set). In general, the performance of LR classifiers tends to have less variation with respect to the imbalance level. For DEV_set, we observed that SVM classifiers using TF-IDF performed the best when the training set is balanced (i.e., positives to negatives is 1 to 1) while other classifiers performed the best when the ratio of the number of positives to unlabeled is around 1 to 8. When evaluated using an independent test set, TEST_set, both LR and SVM classifiers performed the best when the training set is balanced and the performance decreases when the imbalanced level increases.

In general, the performance of classifiers tends to be stable with respect to the size of word features. Our results indicate that the best performed classifiers are generally not those trained with all features. For example, when using TF-IDF as feature values, the performance of SVM classifiers varied dramatically and the best performed SVM classifiers are those trained with 100 word features.

Table 1. Number of available word features for each setting of the unlabeled data size

Positive: negatives (N:N×2^(i-1))	1:1	1:2	1:4	1:8	1:16	1:32
Max features (avg. in 5×2 fold)	3,954	4,568	6,333	8,797	11,931	17,000

Figure 1. Evaluation results of DEV_set

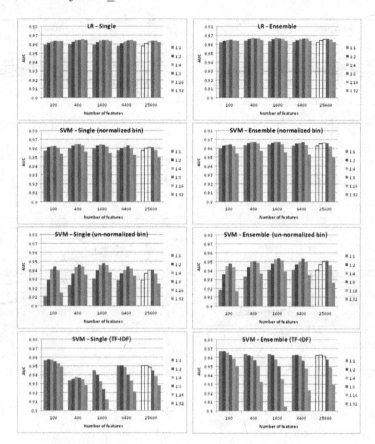

Table 2. Detailed results of LR and SVM using binary features

	FS	100		400		1600		6400		25600	
	ML	LR	SVM	LR	SVM	LR	SVM	LR	SVM	LR	SVM
single	1:1	0.959	0.911	0.960	0.923	0.959	0.931	0.958	0.929	0.958	0.929
	1:2	0.961	0.929	0.963	0.936	0.962	0.940	0.961	0.936	0.961	0.936
	1:4	0.963	0.941	0.964	0.943	0.964	0.946	0.963	0.940	0.963	**0.940**
	1:8	**0.964**	**0.944**	**0.965**	**0.946**	0.964	**0.948**	0.964	**0.944**	**0.964**	**0.940**
	1:16	0.963	0.940	**0.965**	0.944	**0.965**	0.946	**0.965**	0.942	**0.964**	0.936
	1:32	0.963	0.914	0.964	0.935	0.963	0.937	0.963	0.933	0.962	0.925
ensemble	1:1	0.962	0.919	0.964	0.933	0.963	0.941	0.962	0.941	0.962	0.941
	1:2	0.964	0.936	0.966	0.944	0.966	0.948	0.965	0.947	0.965	0.947
	1:4	0.965	0.945	**0.967**	0.950	**0.967**	0.952	0.966	0.951	**0.966**	**0.951**
	1:8	0.965	**0.948**	0.966	**0.951**	0.967	**0.954**	0.967	**0.953**	0.966	**0.951**
	1:16	**0.964**	0.944	**0.967**	0.948	0.966	0.952	0.966	0.950	0.965	0.946
	1:32	**0.964**	0.917	0.965	0.936	0.964	0.939	0.964	0.935	0.962	0.927

Figure 2. Comparison of LR and SVM

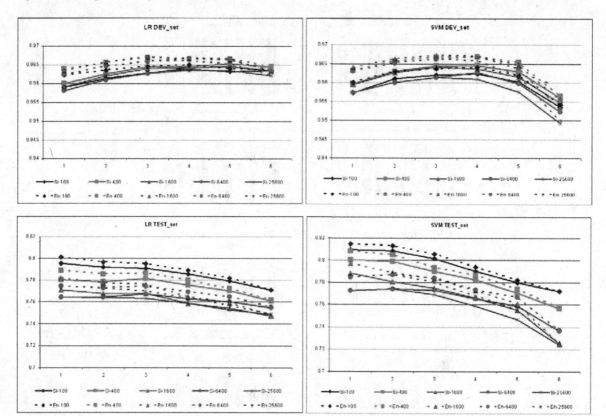

Table 3. Detailed results of LR using binary features and SVM with normalized binary features on TEST_set

	FS	100		400		1600		6400		25600	
	ML	LR	SVM	LR	SVM	LR	SVM	LR	SVM	LR	SVM
single	1:1	**0.796**	**0.810**	**0.780**	**0.800**	**0.771**	**0.788**	0.765	0.773	**0.765**	0.773
	1:2	0.792	0.809	0.779	0.799	0.768	0.781	0.764	**0.775**	0.764	**0.774**
	1:4	0.791	0.802	0.782	0.790	0.768	0.775	**0.768**	0.773	0.763	0.769
	1:8	0.786	0.790	0.776	0.783	0.759	0.766	0.763	0.765	0.759	0.759
	1:16	0.779	0.780	0.770	0.770	0.755	0.755	0.760	0.759	0.753	0.747
	1:32	0.771	0.772	0.761	0.757	0.747	0.725	0.755	0.737	0.749	0.724
ensemble	1:1	**0.801**	**0.815**	**0.789**	**0.808**	**0.782**	**0.798**	**0.775**	0.785	**0.775**	0.785
	1:2	0.797	0.813	0.786	0.805	0.777	0.789	0.773	**0.787**	0.773	**0.787**
	1:4	0.795	0.806	0.786	0.794	0.776	0.783	**0.775**	0.784	0.770	0.780
	1:8	0.789	0.794	0.780	0.787	0.765	0.773	0.769	0.774	0.764	0.768
	1:16	0.782	0.782	0.773	0.775	0.759	0.761	0.765	0.767	0.757	0.756
	1:32	0.771	0.772	0.762	0.757	0.748	0.726	0.756	0.737	0.749	0.725

The appropriate selection of features values is critical for SVM classifiers. For example, the AUC of an LR classifier is 0.02-0.05 higher than that of an SVM classifier when both of them use binary features. While using normalized binary features, SVM classifiers generally achieved comparable performance to LR classifiers.

From Figure 3, we can see that an ensemble classifier consisting of ten classifiers obtained by using different subsets of unlabeled documents tends to perform better than individual classifiers. The proposed approach of forming ensemble classifiers is similar to the traditional bootstrap aggregating (i.e. bagging) way of obtaining ensembles but different from it in the way that only unlabeled (or negative) documents are sampled.

CONCLUSION

In this article, we investigated document retrieval for the curation of bacterial PPI information. We compared classifiers trained using regularized LR (logistic regression) and SVM (support vector machine) by varying the ratio of the number of positives to that of unlabeled documents, feature representation, and the number of features used. We have shown that classifiers trained with LR tend to yield stable performance, while the selection of feature values is critical for SVM classifiers. The imbalance level of the training data impacts the performance of both classifiers. Our results indicate that ensemble classifiers trained using differently sampled unlabeled documents can be superior to single classifiers. When the classifiers were evaluated on the reserved test set, the best performance was observed for the ensemble derived from classifiers trained on the equal size of positive and unlabeled documents. In our future study, we plan to investigate the practical usability of the classification system for the curation of MPIDB in a systematic manner.

REFERENCES

Akbani, R., Kwek, S., & Japkowicz, N. (2004). Applying support vector machines to imbalanced datasets. *Lecture Notes in Computer Science, 3201*, 39–50.

Chang, C.-C., & Lin, C.-J. (2009). *LIBSVM: A library for support vector machines.* Software available at http://www.csie.ntu.edu.tw/~cjlin/libsvm/.

Chawla, N. V., Japkowicz, N., & Kotcz, A. (2004). Editorial: special issue on learning from imbalanced data sets. *ACM SIGKDD Explorations Newsletter, 6*(1), 1–6. doi:10.1145/1007730.1007733

Chen, X., & Wasikowski, M. (2008). *FAST: a roc-based feature selection metric for small samples and imbalanced data classification problems.*

Dietterich, T. G. (1998). Approximate statistical tests for comparing supervised classification learning algorithms. *Neural Computation, 10*(7), 1895–1923. doi:10.1162/089976698300017197

Dietterich, T. G. (2000). Ensemble methods in machine learning. *Lecture Notes in Computer Science, 1857*, 1–15. doi:10.1007/3-540-45014-9_1

Elkan, C., & Noto, K. (2008). *Learning classifiers from only positive and unlabeled data.*

Estabrooks, A., Jo, T., & Japkowicz, N. (2004). A multiple resampling method for learning from imbalanced data sets. *Computational Intelligence, 20*(1), 18–36. doi:10.1111/j.0824-7935.2004.t01-1-00228.x

Forman, G. (2003). An extensive empirical study of feature selection metrics for text classification. *Journal of Machine Learning Research, 3*, 1289–1305. doi:10.1162/153244303322753670

Goll, J., Rajagopala, S. V., Shiau, S. C., Wu, H., Lamb, B. T., & Uetz, P. (2008). MPIDB: the microbial protein interaction database. *Bioinformatics (Oxford, England)*, *24*(15), 1743–1744. doi:10.1093/bioinformatics/btn285

Hand, D. J., Mannila, H., & Smyth, P. (2001). *Principles of Data Mining*. MIT Press.

Joachims, T. *(1998)*. Text categorization with Support Vector Machines: Learning with many relevant features. *In* Proc of Tenth European Conference on Machine Learning (ECML-98).

Joachims, T. (1999). *Making large-Scale SVM Learning Practical*. Advances in Kernel Methods - Support Vector Learning. MIT-Press.

Komarek, P., & Moore, A. (2005). *Making logistic regression a core data mining tool: A practical investigation of accuracy, speed, and simplicity* (pp. 685-688). Institute, Carnegie Mellon University.

Molinara, M., Ricamato, M. T., & Tortorella, F. (2007). *Facing Imbalanced Classes through Aggregation of Classifiers*. IEEE Computer Society Washington, DC, USA.

Morrison, J. L., Breitling, R., Higham, D. J., & Gilbert, D. R. (2005). GeneRank: using search engine technology for the analysis of microarray experiments. *BMC Bioinformatics*, *6*, 233. doi:10.1186/1471-2105-6-233

Ng, W., & Dash, M. (2006). *An Evaluation of Progressive Sampling for Imbalanced Data Sets*. IEEE Computer Society Washington, DC, USA.

Rajagopala, S. V., Goll, J., Gowda, N. D., Sunil, K. C., Titz, B., & Mukherjee, A. (2008). MPI-LIT: a literature-curated dataset of microbial binary protein--protein interactions. *Bioinformatics (Oxford, England)*, *24*(22), 2622–2627. doi:10.1093/bioinformatics/btn481

Scholkopf, B., & Smola, A. J. (2001). *Learning with Kernels: Support Vector Machines, Regularization, Optimization, and Beyond*. MA, USA: MIT Press Cambridge.

Vapnik, V. N. (2000). *The Nature of Statistical Learning Theory*. Springer.

Visa, S., & Ralescu, A. (2005). *Issues in mining imbalanced data sets-a review paper*.

Weiss, G. M. (2004). Mining with rarity: a unifying framework. *ACM SIGKDD Explorations Newsletter*, *6*(1), 7–19. doi:10.1145/1007730.1007734

Weng, C. G., & Poon, J. (2006). A Data Complexity Analysis on Imbalanced Datasets and an Alternative Imbalance Recovering Strategy. IEEE Computer Society Washington, DC, USA.

Wu, C. H., Apweiler, R., Bairoch, A., Natale, D. A., Barker, W. C., & Boeckmann, B. (2006). The Universal Protein Resource (UniProt): an expanding universe of protein information. *Nucleic Acids Research*, *34*(Database issue), D187–D191. doi:10.1093/nar/gkj161

Xu, G., Niu, Z., Uetz, P., Gao, X., Qin, X., & Liu, H. (2009). Semi-Supervised Learning of Text Classification on Bacterial Protein-Protein Interaction Documents. *International Joint Conference on Bioinformatics, Systems Biology and Intelligent Computing (IJCBS'09)*.

Yang, Y., & Pedersen, J. O. (1997). A comparative study on feature selection in text categorization. *Fourteenth International Conference on Machine Learning.*

Yen, S. J., Lee, Y. S., Lin, C. H., & Ying, J. C. (n.d.). *Investigating the Effect of Sampling Methods for Imbalanced Data Distributions.*

Zheng, Z., Wu, X., & Srihari, R. (2004). Feature selection for text categorization on imbalanced data. *ACM SIGKDD Explorations Newsletter, 6*(1), 80–89. doi:10.1145/1007730.1007741

ENDNOTES

[1] The International Molecular-Interaction Exchange consortium (http://imex.sourceforge.net/).

[2] http://www.ncbi.nlm.nih.gov/bookshelf/br.fcgi?book=helppubmed&part=pubmed help&rendertype=table&id=pubmedhelp.T43

This work was previously published in International Journal of Computational Models and Algorithms in Medicine, Volume 1, Issue 1, edited by Aryya Gangopadhyay, pp. 34-44, copyright 2010 by IGI Publishing (an imprint of IGI Global).

Chapter 4
Modeling a Classification Scheme of Epileptic Seizures Using Ontology Web Language

Bhaswati Ghosh
Cleveland State University, USA

Partha S. Ghosh
Cleveland Clinic Foundation, USA

Iftikhar U. Sikder
Cleveland State University, USA

ABSTRACT

Ontology-based disease classification offers a way to rigorously assign disease types and to reuse diagnostic knowledge. However, ontology itself is not sufficient for fully representing the complex knowledge needed in classification schemes which are continuously evolving. This article describes the application of SWRL/OWL-DL to the representation of knowledge intended for proper classification of a complex neurological condition, namely epilepsy. The authors present a rigorous and expandable approach to the ontological classification of epileptic seizures based on the 1981 ILAE classification. It provides a classification knowledge base that can be extended with rules that describe constraints in SWRL. Moreover, by transforming an OWL classification scheme into JESS (rule engine in Java platform) facts and by transforming SWRL constraints into JESS, logical inferences and reasoning provide a mechanism to discover new knowledge and facts. The logic representation of epileptic classification amounts to greater community understanding among practitioners, knowledge reuse and interoperability.

INTRODUCTION

In recent years there is a growing trend towards developing semantic interface for clinical diagnostic decision support systems (Asuman, 2006; Miller & Geissbuhler, 2007; Stephens, Morales, & Quinlan, 2006). As health practitioners are relying more and more on software systems for automating tasks such as electronic medical records maintenance and the implementation of treatment guidelines, there is increasing demand for knowledge integration in such systems. How-

DOI: 10.4018/978-1-4666-0282-3.ch004

ever, there are many issues involved including the complexity of knowledge representation and information encoding which includes (i) definition, (ii) composition, (iii) scale, and (iv) context (Lussier & Bodenreider, 2007). Due to multiple definitions of clinical phenotypes, diagnostic specifications often lack precision. Researchers have reported at least five different definitions of phenotypes in the literature (Mahner & Kary, 1997). To enforce semantic specification, ontology has been widely used in many clinical diagnostic decision support systems (Yu, 2006). In particular, neurology, as a subspecialty, has many native built in semantics. Additionally, neurological conditions are unique and may not be very familiar to other medical specialists. The medications prescribed by neurologists and the investigations (e.g. Electroencephalogram (EEG), Magnetic Resonance Imaging (MRI), Nerve Conduction Study/ Electromyography (NCS/ EMG) etc) are often different from other medical subspecialties. Hence, having a specialty specific ontology is essential to integrate neurology with other medical software systems. It is particularly important when developing a specific ontology system for epilepsy, a subspeciality within neurology. Epilepsy is a condition which is frequently encountered by general practitioners before these patients get referred to a neurologist. Epilepsy is a chronic neurological condition with significant morbidity and increased risk of mortality compared to the general population. Proper diagnosis and management is of essential importance not only in the short term but also for long term prognosis.

In this article we present a rigorous and expandable approach to ontological classification of the epileptic seizures based on the 1981 ILAE classification. Section 2 identifies the role of ontology for developing knowledge specification of domain concept, particularly in the context of clinical decision support systems, by a literature review. Section 3 outlines the complexities involved in classification of epilepsy type and syndrome.

Section 4 describes the development of epilepsy ontology for knowledge modeling and reasoning. Finally, we evaluate the ontology in the context of clinical decision making.

ONTOLOGY FOR CRAFTING SPECIFICATIONS OF DOMAIN CONCEPTS

Historically, expert systems have been used to assist in medical decision making involving diagnosis, prediction, evaluation, monitoring (Heathfield, 1999; Hernandez, Sancho, Belmonte, Sierra, & Sanz, 1994; Keles & Keles, 2008; Liebowitz, 1997; Tsumoto, 2003). By encapsulating domain knowledge into a set of rules, expert systems simulate the performance of one or more human experts with expert knowledge and experience in a specific problem domain. With the advent of Semantic Web movement, a growing interest in ontologies is being noticed as means of representing human knowledge and as critical components in knowledge management over the Web. Various research communities commonly assume that ontologies are the appropriate modeling structure for representing knowledge. While expert systems emphasize technology, ontologies emphasize knowledge. Ontologies make a domain specific knowledge base reusable, sharable and interoperable. Domain-specific questions can then be answered by reasoning over such highly specialized knowledge. Ontologies have evolved in computer science as computational artifacts to provide computer systems with a conceptual yet computational model of a particular domain of interest. While expert systems provide excellent tools for reasoning with domain rules, they often lack the means to resolve semantic ambiguities inherent in the predicates and related facts. Hence, a key requirement is to reason in a semantically consistent way is to exploit both the ontology and the rule-based knowledge to draw inferences.

ONTOLOGY AS SEMANTIC LAYER FOR CLINICAL DECISION SUPPORT: RELATED WORKS

Lussier & Bodenreider (2007) provides an extensive list of clinical ontology which includes Medical Subject Headings (MeSH), International Classification of Primary Care, Second Edition (ICPC-2), Diagnostic and Statistical Manual of Mental Disorders (DSM-IV), Logical Observation Identifiers Names and Codes (LOINC), Unified Medical Language System® (UMLS®), National Cancer Institute (NCI) Metathesaurus. These ontologies differ in term of functionality, concept orientation and contexts. Cimino (1998; 2006) proposed the following list of properties of ontology:

- **Concept-Oriented:** the preferable unit of symbolic processing is the concept.
- Formal semantic definition: the semantic definition of concepts in ontology.
- **Concept permanence:** the meaning of a concept should not change over time and obsolete concepts are retired, not deleted.
- **Non-redundancy:** the definition of a concept should be unique.
- **Non-ambiguity:** distinct concepts should not share the same terminology or code.
- **Relationships:** between concepts differentiate expressiveness of ontologies.

Dieng-Kuntz et al.(2006) translated medical databases to RDF to reconstitute a medical ontology. They presented the construction of a tool called "Virtual Staff", enabling a cooperative diagnosis by some of the health care network actors, by relying on this medical ontology and on the creation of SOAP and QOC graphs. ONTODerm (Eapen, 2008) is grounded on DOLCE Lite foundational ontology and its purpose is to address the unique needs of dermatology as a medical specialty. It is represented in Web Ontology Language (OWL) using the Protégé OWL Plugin. ONTODerm is a system with which other software systems can interact. Potential uses of ONTODerm include teaching, decision support for clinical practice, and semantic assistance for data processing tools. Existing context-sensitive image search and medical resource search systems can be made more efficient with ONTODerm. ONTODerm has an important application in decision support systems for clinical practice and clinical guideline systems. Rajapakse et al. (2008) has deployed a generic infrastructure to facilitate data integration and knowledge sharing in the domain of dengue. It illustrates a simplified search and discovery on dengue information derived from distributed resources and aggregated according to dengue ontology. Also, it apply data mining to the instantiated ontology to elucidate trends in the mentions of dengue serotypes in scientific abstracts since 1974. The system illustrates the ability to aggregate distributed content and semantically index it according to a domain-specific query model. Coupled with an A-box visual query/reasoning tool, the platform facilitates easy access to information that may otherwise be available only in legacy or non-digital data formats. Using this query paradigm it has illustrated that complex queries can be easily constructed using the semantics of the ontology.

CLASSIFICATION SCHEMES OF EPILEPTIC SEIZURES

A classification system is aimed at providing a logical, organized approach and serves as a universal language shared among health professionals all over the world (Commission on Classification and Terminology of the International League Against Epilepsy, 1981, 1989). Epilepsy is a disorder characterized by the occurrence of at least two unprovoked seizures 24 hours apart. Seizures are the manifestation of abnormal hypersynchronous discharges of cortical neurons. The clinical signs or symptoms of seizures depend on the location of the epileptic discharges in the cortex and the extent and pattern of the propagation of the epileptic discharge in the brain. The epilepsies are a diverse group of disorders, with some shared features and some that are distinctly different. The classification criteria of epileptic seizures and syndrome is a complex process (Seino, 2006). The classification scheme evolved through many revisions involving multiple organizations and standards (Fisher et al., 2005; Gastaut, 1970). In 1981, the International League Against Epilepsy (ILAE) developed an international classification of epileptic seizures. This classification divides seizures into three types, with subtypes of each:

- Partial (seizures involving only part of the brain)
- Generalized (seizures involving both sides of the brain)
- Unclassifiable

The usefulness of this classification stems from the fact that seizures can be classified relatively easily and the choice of medication is dependent on seizure type. However, the problem associated with this simplistic classification system is that the same patient may have more than one type of seizure, either together or in sequence. Many patients' seizures also change over the natural course of their illness. These questions are addressed in another system of classification: the ILAE Classification of Epilepsies and Epileptic Syndromes(Epilepsy, 1989). This system is meant to supplement the previous classification, not to replace it. An epileptic syndrome is defined as a disorder characterized by a cluster of signs and symptoms occurring together. According to this system, epilepsies are divided into four broad groups:

1. Localization-related (involves one or more distinct parts of the brain)
2. Generalized (involves both sides of the brain at the same time)
3. Undetermined whether localized or generalized
4. Special syndromes.

Within the localized and generalized groups, there are further subdivisions into idiopathic (unknown cause), symptomatic (identifiable cause), or cryptogenic (hidden cause). This classification system is complex and many syndromes are not adequately defined. It has to be borne in mind that when seizures first begin, physicians may be able to identify the syndrome. Not all patients fit into a specific syndrome and some need to be classified into nonspecific categories, so this classification also is not perfect. Luders et al. (1998) proposed another classification of epilepsy known as semiological seizure classification which aims at addressing the previously unanswered questions.

Partial-onset seizures begin in a focal area of the cerebral cortex, whereas generalized-onset seizures have an onset recorded simultaneously in both cerebral hemispheres. Partial-onset seizures are further classified as simple partial seizures, complex partial seizures, or secondarily generalized tonic-clonic seizures. The simple partial seizure is a seizure with preserved consciousness. Many patients with complex partial seizures have an aura prior to their seizure. An aura is basically a simple partial seizure. The types of simple partial seizures include sensory, motor, autonomic, and psychic. The diagnosis is based on the recurrent, stereotypic occurrence of the sequence of events in association with focal EEG changes. Consciousness is impaired during a complex partial seizure. In practice, assessing the patient's history to determine whether consciousness was impaired is sometimes very difficult. The most common way to assess preserved consciousness is asking patients if they remembered the event. Patients might be able to remember their aura but are unaware that they were briefly unable to respond to the environment because of the amnesia of the event. Secondarily, generalized seizures often begin with an aura that evolves into a complex partial seizure and then into a generalized tonic-clonic seizure. However, a complex partial seizure may evolve into a generalized tonic-clonic seizure, or an aura may evolve into a generalized tonic-clonic seizure without an obvious complex partial seizure. Clinically, classifying a generalized tonic-clonic seizure as being secondarily generalized (partial onset) or primarily generalized is difficult on the basis of the history alone as the patient cannot give the proper history. The history from the bystanders who have observed the event together with the EEG findings often clinches the correct diagnosis.

Generalized-onset seizures are classified into 6 major categories: (1) absence seizures, (2) tonic seizures, (3) clonic seizures, (4) myoclonic seizures, (5) primary generalized tonic-clonic seizures, and (6) atonic seizures. Absence seizures are brief episodes of impaired consciousness with no preceding aura or postictal confusion. They typically last less than 20 seconds and are accompanied by few or no automatisms. Sudden decline in scholastic performance may be a subtle manifestation of frequent absence seizures. Myoclonic seizures consist of brief, arrhythmic, jerking, motor movements that last less than a second. Usually there is no loss of consciousness. Myoclonic seizures often cluster within a few minutes. If they evolve into rhythmic, jerking movements, they are classified as evolving into a clonic seizure. The classic ictal correlate of myoclonic seizures in the EEG consists of fast polyspike-and–slow wave complexes. Clonic seizures consist of rhythmic, motor, jerking movements with or without impairment of consciousness. Clonic seizures can have a focal origin with or without impaired consciousness. The typical generalized clonic seizures simultaneously involve the upper and lower extremities. The ictal EEG correlate (a measure of brain activity during a seizure) consists of bilateral rhythmic epileptic form discharges. Tonic seizures consist of sudden-onset tonic extension or flexion of the head, trunk, and/or extremities for several seconds. These seizures typically occur in relation to drowsiness, shortly after the person falls asleep, or just after

he or she awakens. They are often associated with other co-morbid neurologic abnormalities. Tonic-clonic seizures are commonly referred to as grand mal seizures. They consist of several motor behaviors, including generalized tonic extension of the extremities lasting for few seconds followed by clonic rhythmic movements and prolonged postictal confusion. The ictal correlate of generalized tonic-clonic seizures consists of generalized (bilateral) complexes of spikes or polyspike and slow waves. Generalized tonic-clonic seizures can be primarily generalized (no preceding aura) or secondarily generalized from a focal area of the brain (may have a preceding aura) and then spread to bilateral cerebral hemispheres. Atonic seizures occur in people with clinically significant neurologic abnormalities. These seizures consist of brief loss of postural tone, often resulting in falls and injuries. The ictal EEG correlate is similar to abnormalities observed in tonic seizures.

BUILDING EPILEPSY ONTOLOGY FOR KNOWLEDGE MODELING AND REASONING

In this section we present a description of the ontology construction, semantic translation and system configuration for reasoning and inference. It outlines the rationale behind adopting Web Ontology Language (OWL) supported by enhancement of class semantics through Description Language (DL), incorporation of domain constraints in SWRL (Semantic Web Rule Language) and finally the creation of an interface for inference engines through Java APIs.

Knowledge Engineering Constructs of Ontology

Much work has been done on the advantage of developing ontologies expressed in the Web Ontology Language (OWL) (Stevens et al., 2007), which is due to the OWL's capacity for expressing meaning and semantics better than other ontology languages like XML, RDF, and RDF-S. The Web Ontology Language provides richer schema for expressing meaning and semantics than other ontology languages like XML, RDF, and RDF-S. RDF is a data model for objects and relations between them; it provides a simple semantics for this data model that can be represented in XML syntax. OWL adds more vocabulary for describing properties and classes: among others, relations between classes, cardinality, equality, richer typing of properties, characteristics of properties, and enumerated classes. RDF Schema is a vocabulary for describing properties and classes of RDF resources, with a semantics for generalization-hierarchies of such properties and classes. Thus, OWL goes beyond these languages in its ability to represent machine interpretable content, especially on the Web.

The Web Ontology Language has 3 sublanguages: in order of decreasing expressiveness, they are OWL Full, OWL DL, and OWL Lite. OWL Lite primarily supports classification hierarchy with simple constraints providing a quick migration path for thesauri and other taxonomies. OWL Full guarantees maximum expressiveness and the syntactic freedom from RDF at the cost of computational completeness and undecidability. In OWL Full, a class can be considered as an individual in its own right and at the same time as a collection of individuals. The reasoning support is less predictable as it is not possible to implement reasoning software that supports reasoning for every feature of OWL Full. In contrast, OWL-DL is underpinned by a Description Logic (DL) (Baader, Calvanese, McGuinness, Nardi, & Patel-Schneider, 2003), supporting well-defined semantics and automated reasoning by virtue of being a subset of first order logic. OWL DL supports the maximum expressiveness while retaining computational completeness (i.e., all conclusions are guaranteed to be computable) and decidability (i.e., all computations will finish in finite time). OWL DL includes all OWL language constructs,

but they can be used only under certain restrictions (for example, while a class may be a subclass of many classes, a class cannot be an instance of another class).

Given the ontological requirement posed by classification scheme of epilepsy, we have chosen OWL DL to explore how well OWL DL's model corresponds to those of domain requirements. To overcome the OWL DL's limitation of expressing deductive knowledge in the form of rule types, SWRL (Semantic Web Rule Language) (I. Horrocks et al., 2004), a rule language based on OWL, is used to express various clinical knowledge in the form of rules. SWRL is a Semantic Web Rule Language based on a combination of the OWL DL and OWL Lite sublanguages of the OWL Web Ontology Language with the Unary/Binary Datalog RuleML sublanguages of the Rule Markup Language. It thus enables Horn clause-like (a disjunction of literals with at most one positive) rules to be combined with an OWL knowledge base that can be expressed in terms of OWL concepts and can reason about OWL individuals. Another attractive feature is that SWRL provides deductive reasoning capabilities that can infer new knowledge from an existing OWL ontology. For example, a SWRL rule expressing that a person with a male sibling has a brother would require capturing the concepts of 'person', 'male', 'sibling' and 'brother' in OWL. Intuitively, the concept of person and male can be captured using an OWL class called Person with a subclass Man; the sibling and uncle relationships can be expressed using OWL properties hasSibling and hasUncle, which are attached to Person. The rule in SWRL would be as follows:

hasParent(?x, ?y) ^ hasSibling(?y,?z) -> hasUncle(?x,?z)

Executing this rule would have the effect of setting the hasUncle property of x to z. Similarly, a rule that asserts that all persons who own a car should be classified as drivers can be written as follows:

Person(?p) ^ hasCar(?p, true) -> Driver(?p)

This rule would require that the property hasCar and the class Driver exist in OWL ontology. Executing this rule would have the effect of classifying all car-owner individuals of type Person to also be members of the class Driver. One of SWRL's most powerful features is its ability to support user-defined methods or *built-ins* (O'Connor & Das, 2006). SWRL allows new libraries of built-ins to be defined and used in rules. Users can define built-in libraries to perform a wide range of tasks, which could include currency conversion libraries, and libraries including statistical, temporal or spatial operations. A number of core built-ins for common mathematical and string operations are defined in the SWRL proposal. For example, the built-in greaterThan can be used to determine if one number is greater than another. A sample SWRL rule using this built-in to help classify persons aged greater than 17 as adults can then be written as follows:

Person(?p)^ hasAge(?p,?age) ^
swrlb:greaterThan(?age,17) -> Adult(?p)

When executed, this rule would classify individuals of class Person with a hasAge property value greater than 17 as members of the class Adult. For some application, it may be necessary to transfer characteristics across participating properties which only OWL DL can't facilitate (Ian Horrocks, Patel-Schneider, Bechhofer, & Tsarkov, 2005).

We used SWRL Editor available as an extension to Protégé-OWL(Knublauch, Fergerson, Noy, & Musen, 2009) that permits the interactive editing of SWRL rules. The advantage of user-defined methods is that they can be used in rules, which can be then used to interoperate with third-party inference engines through a Java APIs. The SWRL-based constraint knowledge is then transformed into JESS (Java Expert System Shell) (Friedman-Hill, 2003) facts and JESS rules, respectively. For reasoning and inference with SWRL rules, the Jess rule engine is integrated with Protégé-OWL. The classes defined in OWL are then mapped onto the JESS templates. Figure 1 shows the system configurations of the epileptic classification modeling system.

STRUCTURAL MODELING OF EPILEPSY ONTOLOGY

The structural modeling of the epilepsy ontology is founded upon the notion of computational completeness and decidability of reasoning systems. The combination of the OWL framework with highly expressive description logics (DLs) provides appropriate modeling artifact. We have also included SWRL, a Semantic Web Rule Language combining OWL and RuleML. The basic building blocks of OWL are classes, properties, individuals and the relationships between them. Classes are interpreted as sets containing individuals and they may be organized as a taxonomic hierarchy. Subclasses specialize their superclasses. For example, Epilepsy is a top level class in our ontology and then different types have been included as subclasses in the taxonomy to specialize Epilepsy. Properties can be categorized as object properties, which relate individuals to other individuals and datatype properties, which relate individuals to datatype values, such as integers, floats, and strings. A property can have a domain and range associated with it. There are various special types of properties such as functional, inverse functional, symmetric and transitive. A functional property can take only one value while two different individuals cannot have the same value in an inverse functional property. If a symmetric property links A to B, then one can infer that it links B to A. If a property links A to B and B to C, then if one can infer that it links A

Figure 1. *System configuration of ontology-based epileptic modeling and inference engine*

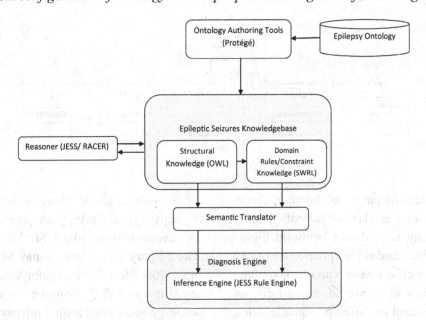

to C, that property is transitive. Individuals are instances of classes; properties can relate one individual to another. Various restrictions can be applied to classes and properties. Cardinality restrictions specify the number of relationships in which a class of individuals can participate. Existential restriction specifies the existence of at least one relationship along a given property to an individual that is a member of a specific class. To restrict the relationship for a given property to individuals that are members of a specific class, a universal restriction must be used.

Figure 2 shows the class structure of Epilepsy ontology. The Epilepsy class contains the hierarchy of epileptic seizures types, Patient is used to hold patient instances; Symptoms is the root for epileptic seizures related symptoms classification; History is used to denote patient history; Reasons are probable reasons behind the disease; EEGPatient is used to hold result of our inference; and EEGReport holds the result of an EEG related to a patient. Figure 4 shows the expanded view of the Epilepsy class showing different types:

We followed the ontology building guideline developed by Noy and McGuinness (2001). The process involves initially determining the domain and scope of the ontology since our objective is to make ontology relevant to many different category uses (e.g., providing clinical diagnose of epileptic syndrome). Some examples of competency questions that we found are as follows:

1. Can jerky movements be a symptom of Epilepsy?
2. Can taking alcohol lead to Epilepsy?
3. Can childcare immunization prevent epilepsy?

We have used nouns describing generic types of Epilepsy like Generalised, Focal/Partial, Primary, Secondary etc. Characteristics of Epilepsy terms like Abnormal movement, Abnormal Sensation, Source of Discharge, etc. Our approach is top-down development process that starts with the definition of the most general concepts in the domain and subsequent specialization of the concepts. The Epilepsy classification super class Epilepsy and associated subclasses is shown in Figure 3a. The characteristics of Epilepsy are shown in that we have super class Symptoms

Figure 2. Epilepsy ontology classes

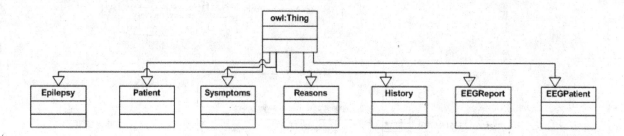

with an associated hierarchy as shown in Figure 3b. History is a super class of patients' history and its hierarchy is as shown below in Figure 3c. The probable reasons for epilepsy are drawn under the super class Reasons and its taxonomy are shown below in Figure 3d. Since Epilepsy types are dependent on different characteristics, patients who have epilepsy have some history, and History must have some reason that we created a few properties to link between the required classes. hasSymptom is a property that relates the class patient to the class Epilepsy. Figure 3e displays the hierarchy of Epilepsy class sub properties hasSymptoms. Moreover, the "CausedBy" and "Causes" properties are inverse type.

Properties can have different facets describing the value type, allowed values, the number of the values (cardinality), and other features of the values the property can take. We have implemented a few value type restrictions that actually help differentiate among several types of Epilepsy. For example, Focal_Partial type of Epilepsy has the restriction "hasHemisphereIncluded some Partial" meaning that for this type of epilepsy, any of the brain hemispheres may be responsible, and for Generalised type of Epilepsy, we have restriction "hasHemisphereIncluded some Bilateral" meaning both hemispheres at the same time are responsible. We have several restrictions for subclasses of History and subclasses of Reasons too, restricting a particular history caused by a particular type of reason. Figure 5 shows the expanded view of Symptom

class with different characteristics related to Epilepsy types. Epilepsy may be caused by any of several reasons like a Stroke, Brain Tumor, Head Injury which in turn may be caused by an unhealthy lifestyle or a Motor Vehicle Accident, etc. Figures 6 & 7 show the causal disorder or etiology associated with Epilepsy class patient history.

Figure 8 shows classification types of epileptic seizures. For example, the hasSymptom property relates individuals from an Epilepsy class with that of a Symptoms class signifying that Epilepsy has different characteristics. More specifically, a Generalised type of epileptic seizures has discharges from both the hemispheres (mentioned as Bilateral), while the Focal_Partial type is associated with discharges from either one of the hemispheres. Primary and Secondary are types of "Generalised" and when the discharge simultaneously starts in both the hemispheres, it's the primary type; for secondary type, it starts at any hemisphere and then spreads to both of them. Simple and Complex being types of Focal_Partial epileptic seizures are differentiated by nonimpaired and impaired consciousness respectively. The Absence and Atonic are types of Primary Generalised seizures. Absence seizures are marked by face loss of consciousness along with eyelid flattering. An atonic seizure are marked by the loss of consciousness along with sudden loss of tone leading to the patient's falling down.

Figure 3. Classes & object properties of epilepsy ontology

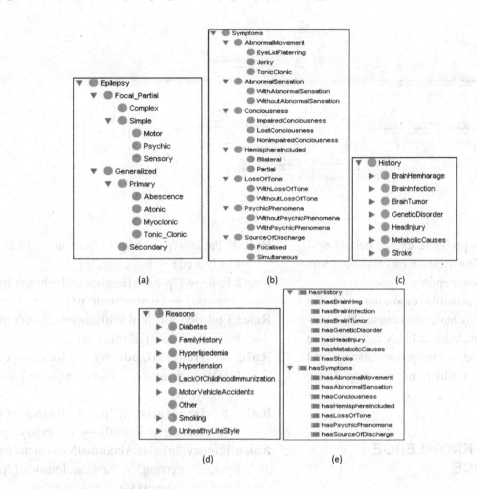

Figure 4. Expanded view of the epilepsy class with multiple types

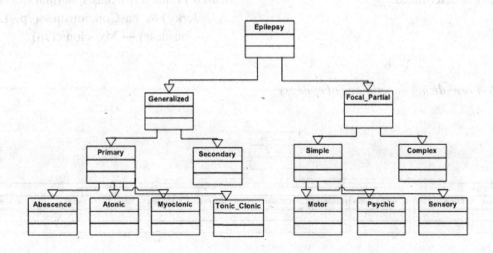

Figure 5. Mapping symptoms of Epilepsy through Symptoms class

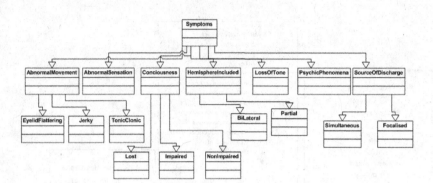

Figure 9 shows probable causes behind epilepsy and how a classification can assist doctors in diagnosing a proper epilepsy type.

For example, a possible reason may be brain hemorrhage that may have been caused by a motor vehicle accident. Another likely cause may be the lack of childhood immunization that may lead to a brain infection which in turn may cause Epilepsy.

CONSTRAINT KNOWLEDGE AND INFERENCE

The system configuration constraints are expressed in SWRL. The following rule shows how given an individual patient's EEG result, the type of epilepsy is determined.

Rule 1: Patient(?p) ∧ hasEEGResult(?p, EEG_Confirmed) → Epilepsy(?p)

Rule 2: Epilepsy(?p)∧hasHemisphereIncluded(?p, Bilateral) → Generalized(?p)

Rule 3: Epilepsy(?p)∧hasHemisphereIncluded(?p, Partial) → Focal_Partial(?p)

Rule 4: Generalized(?p) ∧ hasSourceOfDischarge(?p, Simultaneous) → Primary(?p)

Rule 5: Generalized(?p) ∧ hasSourceOfDischarge(?p, Partial) → Secondary(?p)

Rule 6: Primary(?p)∧hasAbnormalMovement(?p, EyeLidFlaterring) ∧ hasConciousness(?p, LostConciousness)→ abescence(?p)

Rule 7: Primary(?p) ∧ hasLossOfTone(?p, WithLossOfTone) ∧ hasConciousness(?p, LostConciousness) → Atonic(?p)

Rule 8: Primary(?p)∧hasAbnormalMovement(?p, Jerky) ∧ hasConciousness(?p, LostConciousness) → Myoclonic(?p)

Figure 6. Formalizing the etiology of epilepsy

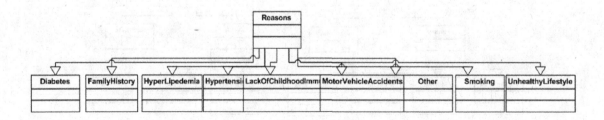

Rule 9: Primary(?p) ∧ hasAbnormalMovement(?p, TonicClonic) ∧ hasConciousness(?p, LostConciousness) → Tonic_Clonic(?p)

Rule 10: Focal_Partial(?p) ∧ hasConciousness(?p, NonImpairedConciousness) → Simple(?p)

Rule 11: Focal_Partial(?p) ∧ hasConciousness(?p, ImpairedConciousness) → Complex(?p)

Rule 12: Simple(?p) ∧ hasAbnormalMovement(?p, Jerky) → Motor(?p)

Rule 13: Simple(?p) ∧ hasAbnormalSensation(?p, WithAbnormalSensation) → Sensory(?p)

Rule 14: Simple(?p) ∧ hasPsychicPhenomena(?p, WithPsychicPhenomena) → Psychic(?p)

It should noted that classification of the seizures into appropriate categories needs not only a thorough history and physical examination of the patient but also requires relevant history from the people who have observed the event to get a clear picture of the semiology of the seizures. Classifying the seizures into proper subtype needs additional investigations that include EEG and sometimes neuro-imaging studies e.g., MRI. The correct diagnosis is of prime importance because further management will be guided by the specific subtype of the seizures. An antiepileptic drug which is suitable for a particular seizure type may be contraindicated in other types.

Regardless of types of Epilepsy, one can diagnose it by analyzing the symptoms of a patient and with help of EEG test results. However, a closer inspection of ontology reveals that certain symptoms are enough to determine an Epilepsy type. For example, if a person goes through episodes of sudden loss of tone that leads to falling down and also occasional loss of consciousness, looking at the ontology we can say this person has Atonic type of Epilepsy. But there are few types that cannot be differentiated from each other like Myoclonic type and Motor type of Epilepsy unless a MRI is performed. Both have jerky movement episodes as symptom and for Motor type consciousness is non-impaired where as for Myoclonic type consciousness may be impaired or non-impaired. Therefore, only EEG test, in this case, can find that which brain hemisphere is source of discharge, and if it is any one of them it has to Motor type and Myoclonic type if both lobes are included. An inference can be run that only EEG test can determine between Myclonic and Motor type of Eplilepsy. The inference rule looks like:

Patient(?p) ∧ hasAbnormalMovement(?p, Jerky) ∧ hasConciousness(?p, NonImpairedConciousness) → EEGPatient(?p)

By using inference it is evident that EEG testing becomes mandatory for specific cases and those patients become members of EEGPatient. EEGReport contains the result of EEG test for any patient who may or may not be a member of EEGPatient.

Figure 7. Mapping patient's history through the History class

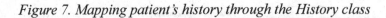
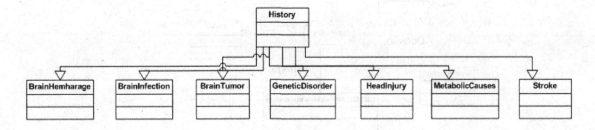

Figure 8. Classification types of epileptic seizures

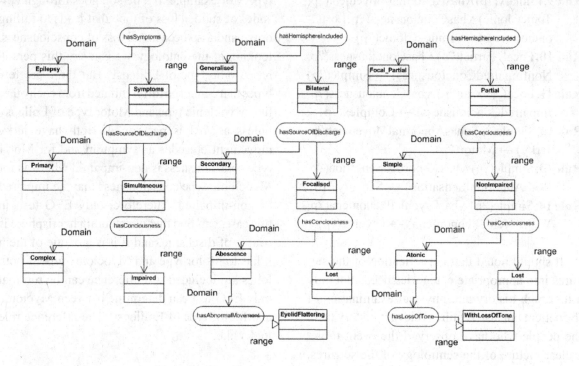

DISCUSSION

Medical information systems need to be able to communicate complex medical terminology unambiguously. Physicians developed their own specialized languages and lexicons to help them store and communicate general medical knowledge and patient-related information efficiently. Medical information systems need to be able to communicate complex and detailed medical infor-

Figure 9. Mapping probable causal structure (with 'causedBy' class) and associated patient history

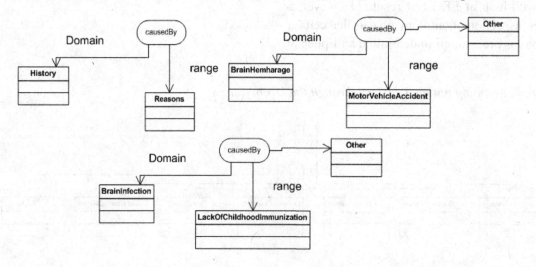

mation unambiguously. This is a difficult task and requires a profound analysis of the structure and the concepts of medical terminologies. Ontology-based disease classification offers a way to reuse diagnostic knowledge by constructing medical domain ontologies for representing medical terminology systems thereby making it easier to model subsequent clinical decisions and management of diseases. The experience in implementing the ontology for a complex neurological disease like epilepsy in the form of an OWL shows the rich expressivity of the semantic language. The well-defined semantics and schematic richness are based on OWL-DL that supports the maximum expressiveness while retaining computational completeness and decidability. Additionally, integration of SWRL provides the additional advantage of expressing deductive knowledge in the form of rule types supporting interfaces for logical reasoning and inference. The ontology structure is expandable and can accommodate revision and expansion with changing knowledge bases of classification types of epilepsy. OWL-DL's logic representation amounts to greater community understanding among practitioners, knowledge reuse and interoperability. It provides the means to convert such computationally amenable aspects of classification to discover new knowledge through inference and reasoning..

CONCLUSION

In this article, an approach to modeling a classification scheme of epilepsy is presented through the application of Semantic Web technique and a standard ontology language. The article outlines the evolving knowledge base of different classification schemes of epilepsy. We present a well-formed and rigorous approach to ontological classification of seizures based on the 1981 ILAE classification. The ontology system facilitates the proper classification of seizure types and associated clinical management. Since the classifica-

tion scheme of epilepsy will continue to evolve, we have developed an expandable and modular ontological structure that can accommodate revision and expansion. The classification knowledge bases could be extended with rules that describe constraints in SWRL. Additionally, transforming OWL classification schemes into JESS facts and SWRL constraints into JESS (a rule engine for the Java platform) rules, logical inference and reasoning allow researchers to discover new knowledge and facts. From the practitioner's point of view, such systems can assist in unambiguous diagnosis and assignment of appropriate classification type of epilepsy and thus provide further insight into clinical management and intervention.

REFERENCES

Asuman, D. (2006). Artemis: Deploying semantically enriched Web services in the healthcare domain. *Information Systems*, *31*(4), 321–339. doi:10.1016/j.is.2005.02.006

Baader, F., Calvanese, D., McGuinness, D., Nardi, D., & Patel-Schneider, P. F. (Eds.). (2003). *The Description Logic Handbook: Theory, Implementation, and Applications*. Cambridge: Cambridge University Press.

Cimino, J. J. (1998). Desiderata for controlled medical vocabularies in the twenty-first century. *Methods of Information in Medicine*, *37*(4-5), 394–403.

Cimino, J. J. (2006). In defense of the Desiderata. *Journal of Biomedical Informatics*, *39*(3), 299–306. doi:10.1016/j.jbi.2005.11.008

Commission on Classification and Terminology of the International League Against Epilepsy. (1981). Proposal for revised clinical and electroencephalographic classification of epileptic seizures. *Epilepsia*, *22*, 489–501. doi:10.1111/j.1528-1157.1981.tb06159.x

Commission on Classification and Terminology of the International League Against Epilepsy (1989). Proposal for revised classification of epilepsies and epileptic syndromes. *Epilepsia, 30*(4, August), 389-399.

Dieng-Kuntz, R., Minier, D., Růžička, M., Corby, F., Corby, O., & Alamarguy, L. (2006). Building and using a medical ontology for knowledge management and cooperative work in a health care network. *Computers in Biology and Medicine, 36*(7-8), 871–892. doi:10.1016/j. compbiomed.2005.04.015

Eapen, B. R. (2008). ONTODerm - A domain ontology for dermatology. *Dermatology Online Journal, 14* (6:16).

Fisher, R. S., van Emde Boas, W., Blume, W., Elger, C., Genton, P., & Lee, P. (2005). Epileptic seizures and epilepsy: definitions proposed by the International League Against Epilepsy (ILAE) and the International Bureau for Epilepsy (IBE). *Epilepsia, 46*, 470–472. doi:10.1111/j.0013-9580.2005.66104.x

Friedman-Hill, E. (2003). *Jess in Action: Rule-Based Systems in Java*: Manning Publications.

Gastaut, H. (1970). Clinical and electro-encephalographical classification of epileptic seizures. *Epilepsia, 11*, 102–113. doi:10.1111/j.1528-1157.1970.tb03871.x

Heathfield, H. (1999). The rise and 'fall' of expert systems in medicine. *Expert Systems: International Journal of Knowledge Engineering and Neural Networks, 16*(3), 183–188. doi:10.1111/1468-0394.00107

Hernandez, C., Sancho, J. J., Belmonte, M. A., Sierra, C., & Sanz, F. (1994). Validation of the medical expert system RENOIR. *Computers and Biomedical Research, an International Journal, 27*(6), 456–471. doi:10.1006/cbmr.1994.1034

Horrocks, I., Patel-Schneider, P. F., Bechhofer, S., & Tsarkov, D. (2005). OWL rules: A proposal and prototype implementation *Web Semantics: Science. Services and Agents on the World Wide Web, 3*(1), 23–40. doi:10.1016/j.websem.2005.05.003

Horrocks, I., Patel-Schneider, P. F., Boley, H., Tabet, S., Grosof, B., & Dean, M. (2004). SWRL: A Semantic Web Rule Language Combining OWL and RuleML. Retrieved May, 2008, from http://www.w3.org/Submission/2004/SUBM-SWRL-20040521/

Keles, A., & Keles, A. (2008). ESTDD: Expert system for thyroid diseases diagnosis. *Expert Systems with Applications, 34*(1), 242–246. doi:10.1016/j.eswa.2006.09.028

Knublauch, H., Fergerson, R. W., Noy, N. F., & Musen, M. A. (2009). *The Prot'eg'e OWL Plugin: An Open Development Environment for Semantic Web Applications* [Electronic Version]. Retrieved May 2009 from http://protege.stanford.edu/plugins/owl/publications/ISWC2004-protege-owl.pdf.

Liebowitz, J. (1997). *The Handbook of Applied Expert Systems*. Boca Raton, FL: CRC Press.

Lüders, H., Acharya, J., Baumgartner, C., Benbadis, S., Bleasel, A., & Burgess, R. (1998). Semiological seizure classification. *Epilepsia, 39*, 1006–1013. doi:10.1111/j.1528-1157.1998.tb01452.x

Lussier, Y., & Bodenreider, O. (2007). Clinical Ontologies for Discovery Applications. In C. J. O. Baker & K.-H. Cheung (Eds.), *SEMANTIC WEB Revolutionizing Knowledge Discovery in the Life Sciences* (pp. 101-121). NY, USA: Springer.

Mahner, M., & Kary, M. (1997). What exactly are genomes, genotypes and phenotypes? And what about phenomes? *Journal of Theoretical Biology, 186*(1), 55–63. doi:10.1006/jtbi.1996.0335

Miller, R. A., & Geissbuhler, A. (2007). Diagnostic Decision Support Systems. In E. S. Berner (Ed.), *Clinical Decision Support Systems Theory and Practice* (pp. 99-125). NY: Springer.

Noy, N. F., & McGuinness, D. L. (2001). *Ontology Development 101: A Guide to Creating Your First Ontology*. Stanford Knowledge Systems Laboratory & Stanford Medical Informatics Technical Report

O'Connor, M. J., & Das, A. (2006). *A Mechanism to Define and Execute SWRL Built-ins in Protégé-OWL* [Electronic Version]. Retrieved May, 2009 from http://protege.stanford.edu/conference/2006/submissions/abstracts/7.3_Martin_oConnor_BuiltInBridge.pdf.

Rajapakse, M., Kanagasabai, R., Ang, W. T. T., Veeramani, A., Schreiber, M. J. J., & Baker, C. J. O. J. (2008). Ontology-centric integration and navigation of the dengue literature *Journal of Biomedical Informatics, 41*(5, October), 806-815.

Seino, M. (2006). Classification criteria of epileptic seizures and syndromes. *Epilepsy Research, 70*(2-3 – Supplement), S27-S33.

Stephens, S., Morales, A., & Quinlan, M. (2006). Applying semantic Web technologies to drug safety determination. *Intelligent Systems IEEE, 21*(1), 82–88. doi:10.1109/MIS.2006.2

Stevens, R., Aranguren, M. E., Wolstencroft, K., Sattler, U., Drummond, N., & Horridge, M. (2007). Using OWL to model biological knowledge. *International Journal of Human-Computer Studies, 65*(65), 583–594. doi:10.1016/j.ijhcs.2007.03.006

Tsumoto, S. (2003). Automated extraction of hierarchical decision rules from clinical databases using rough set model. *Expert Systems with Applications, 24*(2), 189–197. doi:10.1016/S0957-4174(02)00142-2

Yu, A. (2006). Methods in biomedical ontology. *Journal of Biomedical Informatics, 39*(3), 252–266. doi:10.1016/j.jbi.2005.11.006

This work was previously published in International Journal of Computational Models and Algorithms in Medicine, Volume 1, Issue 1, edited by Aryya Gangopadhyay, pp. 45-60, copyright 2010 by IGI Publishing (an imprint of IGI Global).

Chapter 5
Prevalence of Metabolic Syndrome in Subjects with Osteoarthritis Stratified by Age and Sex:
A Cross Sectional Analysis in NHANES III

Ashish Joshi
Department of Information Systems, UMBC, USA

ABSTRACT

The aim of the study was to determine association between osteoarthritis and metabolic syndrome stratified by age and gender categories. A final sample of 16,149 US residents aged 17 years or older was analyzed using the database National Health and Nutrition Examination Survey (NAHNES III). Variables assessed include age, gender, race, education, poverty income ratio, body mass index, smoking history, metabolic syndrome and its risk components. Continuous and categorical variables were compared in the 2 groups using T and chi-square statistics as appropriate. Multivariate analysis was performed after adjusting for the potential confounders. Five percent subjects self-reported of having osteoarthritis. The prevalence of metabolic syndrome in subjects with osteoarthritis was 40% compared to 21% with no osteoarthritis. Subjects with osteoarthritis were significantly older; were females, non-Hispanic whites, less educated and had high prevalence of diabetes, hypertension and high cholesterol. Age, being female, higher education, being non-Hispanic White, absence of osteoporosis, and body mass index were significant predictors of osteoarthritis. Metabolic syndrome was a risk factor for osteoarthritis in males.

INTRODUCTION

Osteoarthritis (OA) is the most common type of arthritis affecting older people. OA affects different people differently. There are several risk factors associated with the development of OA. These include ethnicity, age, gender, genetic factors, bone density, nutritional factors, obesity, prior joint injuries and occupational factors. Obesity, hypertension, dyslipidemia, diabetes and insulin resistance tend to cluster into the so-called metabolic syndrome (MS). There are not

DOI: 10.4018/978-1-4666-0282-3.ch005

many studies that have explored the relationship between MS and OA. The motivation for the study was to determine if there was an increased risk of cardiovascular diseases in subjects with OA.

Epidemiology of OA

Osteoarthritis (OA) is the most prevalent form of arthritis and a major cause of disability in people aged 65 and older (Lawrence, 1998). Osteoarthritis is a clinical syndrome of joint pain and dysfunction caused by joint degeneration. Current estimates are that 27 million people in the United States have OA (Helmick, 2008) and this number is expected to reach 60 million by the year 2020 (CDC, 1996). Approximately 10-30% of those affected with OA in the United States have significant pain and disability (Garstang, 2006). It has been estimated that by the year 2020, 12 million Americans are estimated to have limitation in some aspect of function because of OA (CDC, 1996). OA symptoms typically begin after age 40 and progress slowly (Arthritis Foundation, 2008). OA typically affects only certain joints, such as the hips, hands, knees, low back and neck. After age 50, women are more affected by OA than men (Lawrence, 1998). Loss of joint function as a result of OA overall is a major cause of work disability and reduced quality of life (Arthritis Foundation, 2008) The CDC estimates that OA and related arthritic conditions cost the U.S. economy nearly $128 billion per year in direct medical care and indirect expenses, includding lost wages and productivity (MMWR, 2007). The total annual cost of a person living with OA is approximately $5700 (Maetzel, 2004).

Pathogenesis of OA

The pathogenesis of OA is not fully understood, although multiple contributing factors are recognized including genetic, environmental, metabolic, and biomechanical factors (Kraus, 1997). Osteoarthritis can affect any synovial joint (Mandelbaum

and Waddell, 2005). The normal joint is protected by biomechanical factors such as alignment and muscle strength, the lubrication provided by the synovial fluid, and the shock-absorbing function of bone and cartilage (Mandelbaum and Waddell, 2005). These functions get altered at both the macroscopic and cellular levels resulting in further joint destruction. It involves both destructive and reparative metabolic processes, with a variety of biochemical triggers in addition to mechanical injury of the joint (Mandelbaum and Waddell, 2005). The increased prevalence, chronic nature, lack of preventive services or cure of OA makes it a substantial economic burden for patients and healthcare systems (Brooks PM, 2006).

Risk Factors of OA

The risk factors can be divided into two major types including systemic factors (associated with the development of OA and local factors, (tend to result in abnormal biomechanical loading of affected joints) (Felson, 2004). The systemic factors include ethnicity, age, gender and hormonal status, genetic factors, bone density, nutritional factors, and other factors. Local biomechanical factors include obesity, altered joint biomechanics, prior joint injuries, occupational factors, the effects of sports and physical activities and the result of developmental abnormalities. However, the most important risk factor in all populations is age (Felson, 2004).

Metabolic Syndrome (MS) and Osteoarthritis

Several studies have shown that individuals with obesity or overweight have increased risk of OA in the knee (Oliveria SA, Felson DT, Cirillo PA, Reed JI & Walker AM, 1999 & Gelber AC, Hochberg MC, Mead LA, Wang NY, Wigley FM, Klag MJ, 1999) and hip (Flugsrud GB, Nordsletten L, Espehaug B, Havelin LI, Engeland A & Meyer HE, 2006); however the role of obesity for the development of OA in the hip is unclear. Obesity, hypertension, dyslipidemia, diabetes and insulin resistance tend to cluster into the so-called metabolic syndrome (MS) (Grundy SM, Cleeman JI, Daniels SR, Donato KA, Eckel RH, Franklin BA, Gordon JD, Krauss MR, Savage JP, Smith C S, Spertus AJ & Fernando Costa, 2005). These risk factors are more prevalent in patients with OA (Singh G, Miller JD, Lee FH, Pettitt D & Russell MW, 2002). Obesity and the MS could also be associated with OA through atherogeneic effects of the metabolic factors, resulting in microvascular changes in the subchondral bone (Findlay DM, 2007)

The purpose of the study was to determine associations between metabolic syndrome and osteoarthritis stratified by age and gender categories in the third National Health and Nutrition Examination Survey (NHANES III) sample.

MATERIALS AND METHODS

We estimated the prevalence of Metabolic syndrome using NCEP ATP III criteria (National Cholesterol Education Program (NCEP) Expert Panel on Detection, Evaluation, and Treatment of High Blood Cholesterol in Adults, 2002) among US adults who self-reported having osteoarthritis stratified by age (65 and less and 65+ years) and gender (males and females) using survey data from National Health and Nutritional Examination Survey (NHANES) III. NHANES is one of the major programs in the series of health-related studies conducted by the National Center for Health Statistics, part of the US Centers for Disease Control and Prevention (NHANES III, 2005). NHANES is designed to assess the health and nutritional status of adults and children in the United States through interviews and direct physical examinations. The survey is unique in that it combines a home interview with physical examinations and a variety of diagnostic and laboratory tests conducted in a mobile examina-

tion center. NHANES III, a complex, stratified, multistage probability cluster sampling design conducted from 1988 to1994. Variables assessed included socio-demographic characteristics such as age, gender, race/ethnicity, poverty income ratio, years of education, body mass index, smoking history, waist circumference, systolic/diastolic blood pressure, fasting blood glucose levels, serum high density lipoprotein cholesterol and total triglyceride levels that can classify subjects with/without metabolic syndrome, osteoarthritis (yes/no), diabetes (yes/no), hypertension (yes/no), and high cholesterol (yes/no). Each of these variables is described below in detail. Missing data for any of these variables was excluded from the analyses. A final analyzable sample of 16,149 US residents aged 18 years or older were analyzed after excluding the missing data from any of these variables.

Variable Assessment

Arthritis status was derived from the arthritis section of the health assessment questionnaire (HAQ) in NHANES III where subjects self report if they have been diagnosed with physician confirmed osteoarthritis.

Socio-Demographics

The continuous variables include age (years), education (years), poverty income ratio, body mass index, weight (kg) and waist circumference. Categorical variables include gender (male/female), race/ethnicity (Non-Hispanic white/Non-Hispanic Black and Mexican American). Smoking history was assessed by the question "Do you smoke now (Yes/No)?

Other Risk Variables Assessment

Other risk factors examined in this study include systolic blood pressure (SBP) and diastolic blood pressure (DBP), total and high-density lipoprotein (HDL) cholesterol, physician diagnosed diabetes mellitus, hypertension and high cholesterol, and current cigarette smoking. Information was gathered if subjects had diabetes, hypertension or high cholesterol by gathering self-report responses to the questions

Metabolic Syndrome Assessment

We used NCEP ATP III criteria to classify subjects with/without MS by the presence of 3 or more of the following abnormal physiological parameters: waist circumference of 40 inches or greater for males or 35 inches or greater for females; systolic blood pressure of 135 mm Hg or greater or diastolic blood pressure of 85 mm Hg or greater; fasting blood glucose level of 100 mg/dL or greater (6.1 mmol/L); serum high-density lipoprotein cholesterol level of 40 mg/dL or less (1.03 mmol/L) in males or 50 mg/dL or less (1.29 mmol/L) in females; and total triglyceride level of 150 mg/dL or greater (1.69 mmol/L).

STATISTICAL ANALYSIS

Descriptive analysis was performed using univariate statistics with means, standard deviations and medians reported for the continuous variables and frequency distributions for the categorical variables. Each patient was characterized as having metabolic syndrome by using the threshold criteria as described in the variables assessment in the methods section. We used t-statistics and chi-square test to compare individual demographics, cardiovascular risk assessment, and prevalence of metabolic syndrome in patients with or without osteoarthritis. The results of these comparisons have been reported as frequency distributions, means and standard deviations and significant differences between the variables in these groups have been reported as p-values. Variables with missing information were excluded from the analysis and only those subjects having complete information were included in the final analysis.

Several multivariate adjusted analysis models were performed using logistic regressions to determine association between osteoarthritis and metabolic syndrome (yes/no) after adjusting for potential confounders including age, gender, race/ethnicity, poverty income ratio, years of education, diabetes, hypertension and high cholesterol. A base model was created and several variables were added individually and those variables that resulted in a 10% change in the odds ratio of the metabolic syndrome were kept in the final model. The relationship between these parameters was determined by using logistic regression. A sub-analysis was performed to determine association between subjects with/without osteoarthritis and metabolic syndrome stratified by age (65 and less and 65+ years) and gender (male and female) categories. All analysis performed was 2-tailed and results have been reported as p-values and 95% CI. Statistical analysis was performed in SAS, version 9.1 (SAS Institute Inc, Cary, NC)

RESULTS

The distribution of the analyzable sample and the prevalence of MS are shown in subjects with osteoarthritis stratified by age and gender categories in Figure 1. There were overall 33,199 subjects in NHANES III. Of these subjects, 13,581 were excluded from the analysis as they were in the age category of less than or equal to 17 years leaving 19,618 subjects for the analysis. Further, 3,469 subjects were excluded from the sample because of the missing values leaving 16,149 as the final analyzable sample.

Descriptive Analysis Overall Population

Descriptive analysis was performed for 16,149 subjects using univariate statistics to describe characteristics in NHANES III. Figure 1 describes the analyzable sample in NHANES III with age

Figure 1. Flow of the analyzable sample in NHANES III (1988-1994)

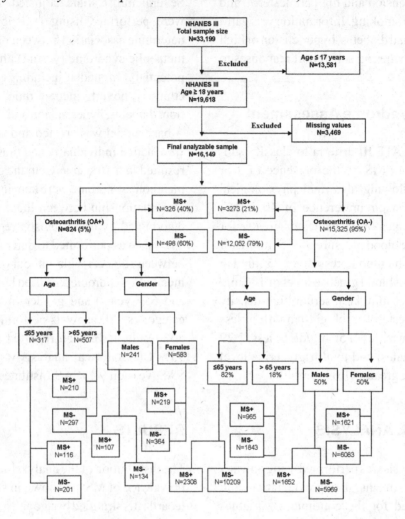

greater than 17 years. The average age of the analyzed subjects was 45 years (SD=20), 51% (n=8287) were females, 41% (n=6611) were non-Hispanic whites. The average poverty income ratio was 2.45 (SD=1.79) and average education was 11 (SD=3.80) years and 53% (n=4196) of them were current smokers. The prevalence of diabetes, hypertension and high cholesterol in the overall subjects was 6% (n=1049), 23% (n=3728) and 30% (n=2294). The prevalence of metabolic syndrome in these subjects was 22% (n=3599).

Subjects With/Without Osteoarthritis

The prevalence of self-report osteoarthritis in this analyzable sample was 5% (n=824). The subjects were older with an average age of 66 (SD=15) years, 71% (n=583) were females, 77% (n=630) were non-Hispanic whites and 66% (n=542) had education less than or equal to 12 years. There were 23% (n=185) who had osteoporosis as compare to 1% (n=104) who did not have osteoarthritis.

Prevalence of Risk Variables in Subjects with/without Osteoarthritis

Subjects with osteoarthritis had a significant increase in the prevalence of diabetes (12% vs. 6%; p<0.0001), hypertension (46% vs. 22%; p<0.0001) and high cholesterol (37% vs. 30%) as compared to those who did not have osteoarthritis. (Table 1). There was a significant increase in the average systolic and diastolic blood pressure measurements, HDL, fasting blood glucose and triglycerides assessments in subjects with osteoarthritis compared to those who did not have osteoarthritis (Figure 2).

Prevalence of Metabolic Syndrome and its Risk Components

The prevalence of metabolic syndrome was 40% (n=326) in subjects with osteoarthritis as compared to 21% (n=3273) in those without osteoarthritis. There was a significant increase in the prevalence of MS risk components in subjects with osteoarthritis including categories of high blood pressure (64% vs. 34%), increase fasting blood glucose levels (40% vs. 27%), increase triglycerides levels (43% vs. 30%) and waist circumference (62% vs. 36%0. No significant difference was seen in the

HDL levels in subjects with or without osteoarthritis (Table 2).

RISK FACTORS OF OSTEOARTHRITIS AFTER ADJUSTING FOR THE POTENTIAL CONFOUNDERS

Logistic regression analysis was performed after adjusting for potential confounders including age, gender, race/ethnicity, poverty income ratio, education, smoking history, CRP levels, diabetes, hypertension, high cholesterol, osteoporosis, fasting blood glucose levels, HDL, triglycerides, waist circumference, body mass index. Several models were performed to determine if metabolic syndrome was a significant predictor of osteoarthritis after adjusting for the potential confounders. Results found that metabolic syndrome was a predictor of osteoarthritis but was insignificant when body mass index was added into the model. The odds of having osteoarthritis increased 1.05 times (95% CI 1.06; 1.10) with each unit increase in age. Similarly the odds of likely to have osteoarthritis increased 1.11 times (95%CI 1.06; 1.17) with each unit increase in year of education. The likelihood of having osteoarthritis increased 2.50

Figure 2. Average cardiovascular Risk Variable assessments in subjects with and without Osteoarthritis SBP; Systolic blood pressure, DBP: Diastolic blood pressure; HDL: High density lipoprotein; FBS: Fasting blood glucose

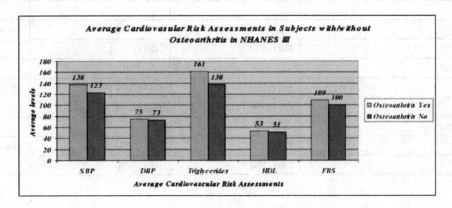

Table 1. Comparing Socio-demographic characteristics, CVD risk variables in subjects with/without Osteoarthritis. * Poverty Income Ratio, ^ Body Mass Index and ' C Reactive protein

Variables	Osteoarthritis		p-value
	Yes N=824 (5%)	No N=15,325 (95%)	
A. Socio-demographics			
Age, years; Mean (SD)	66; (15)	44; (19)	<0.0001
Less than or equal to 65 years	317 (38%)	12517 (82%)	
Greater than 65 years	507 (62%)	2808 (18%)	
Gender			
Male	241 (29%)	7621 (50%)	<0.0001
Female	583 (71%)	7704 (50%)	
Race			
Non-Hispanic White	630 (77%)	5981 (41%)	<0.0001
Non-Hispanic Black	119 (15%)	4293 (29%)	
Mexican American	63 (8%)	4408 (30%)	
Urbanization classification			
Metro Areas	382 (46%)	7907 (52%)	0.003
All other areas	442 (54%)	7418 (48%)	
Education, years; Mean (SD)	11.71; (3.3)	11.06; (3.81)	<0.0001
Less than or equal to 12 years	542 (66%)	10862 (71%)	<0.0001
Greater than 12 years	282 (34%)	4463 (29%)	
PIR*; Mean (SD)	3.00; (2.01)	2.42; (1.77)	<0.0001
BMI^; Mean (SD)	28.5; (6.65)	26.61; (5.66)	<0.0001
CRP'; Mean (SD)	0.59; (0.84)	0.45; (0.76)	<0.0001
Osteoporosis			
Yes	185 (23%)	104 (1%)	<0.0001
No	633 (77%)	14397 (99%)	
B. CVD Risk Assessment			
Diabetes			
Yes	100 (12%)	949 (6%)	<0.0001
No	724 (88%)	14358 (94%)	
Hypertension			
Yes	383 (46%)	3345 (22%)	<0.0001
No	440 (54%)	11803 (78%)	
High Cholesterol			
Yes	246 (37%)	2048 (30%)	0.0001
No	425 (63%)	4867 (70%)	
Current smoking			
Yes	120 (29%)	4076 (54%)	<0.0001
No	296 (71%)	3404 (46%)	

times (95%CI 1.82; 3.43) in females, 5.34 times (95% CI 1.20; 23.75) in non-Hispanic Whites, 1.48 times (95%CI 1.08; 2.04) in current smokers and 1.06 times (95%CI 1.01; 1.12) with each unit increase in body mass index. However, osteoporosis had a protective effect in getting osteoarthritis (OR=0.06; 95%CI 0.04; 0.11) (Table 3)

Sub-Analysis

We performed multivariate logistic regression analysis to determine association between osteoarthritis and prevalence of metabolic syndrome stratified by age (≤65 years and 65+) and gender (male and female) categories (Table 4)

Stratification by Age

In subjects with age ≤65 years, the likelihood of having osteoarthritis increased 1.08 times (95%CI 1.06; 1.10) with each unit increase in age, 1.16 times (95%CI 1.07; 1.25) with each unit increase in education. Similarly we found that females (OR=3.28), current smokers (OR=1.77) were significant predictors of osteoarthritis. However osteoporosis (OR=0.03) had a protective effect on osteoarthritis (Table 4). Similarly in subjects with age 65+ years, gender (OR=1.62), education (OR=1.08), poverty income ratio (OR=1.13) and osteoporosis (OR=0.09) were significant predictors of osteoarthritis (Table 4).

Table 2. Prevalence of metabolic syndrome, high blood pressure, fasting blood glucose levels, total trigylcerides, high density lipoprotein, and waist circumference in subjects with and without osteoarthritis

Metabolic Syndrome and components	Osteoarthritis		p-value
	Yes N=824 (5%)	No N=15,325 (95%)	
Metabolic Syndrome, (%)			
Yes	326 (40%)	3273 (21%)	<0.0001
No	498 (60%)	12052 (79%)	
High Blood Pressure (135/85 mm Hg), (%)			
Yes	510 (64%)	5143 (34%)	<0.0001
No	290 (36%)	9922 (66%)	
Fasting Blood glucose levels (>100mg/dl), (%)			
Yes	267 (40%)	3369 (27%)	<0.0001
No	398 (60%)	9016 (73%)	
Total Triglyceride levels (>150 mg/dl), (%)			
Yes	300 (43%)	3878 (30%)	<0.0001
No	398 (57%)	9203 (70%)	
High density lipoprotein (HDL) 40 mg/dl or less, (%)			
Yes	267 (38%)	4624 (36%)	0.13
No	430 (62%)	8395 (64%)	
Waist Circumference, (%) (M 40 inch or > ; F 35 inch or >)			
Yes	398 (62%)	4753 (36%)	<0.0001
No	245 (38%)	8327 (64%)	

Table 3. Adjusted analysis using logistic regression was performed in the overall analyzable sample to determine risk factors of osteoarthritis after adjusting for the potential confounders

Variables	Parameter estimate	Standard Error	Odds Ratio	95% CI	p-value
Age	0.05	0.005	1.05	1.05; 1.07	<0.0001
Education	0.11	0.02	1.11	1.06; 1.17	<0.0001
Gender	0.92	0.16	2.50	1.82; 3.43	<0.0001
Race/ethnicity; Non-Hispanic White	1.67	0.76	5.34	1.20; 23.75	0.03
Smoking History; Current smokers	0.39	0.16	1.48	1.08; 2.04	0.02
Osteoporosis; yes	-2.79	0.28	0.06	0.04; 0.11	<0.0001
BMI	0.06	0.03	1.06	1.01; 1.12	0.03

Stratification by Gender

In males, the likelihood of having osteoarthritis increased age (OR=1.07), education (OR=1.13) and osteoporosis (OR=0.03) were significant predictors of osteoarthritis. The odds of osteoarthritis increased 1.66 times (95%CI 1.07; 2.59) in subjects who had metabolic syndrome compared to those who did not have metabolic syndrome.

In females, age (OR=1.05), education (OR=1.09), current smokers (OR=1.69), osteoporosis (OR=0.07) and body mass index (OR=1.06) were significant predictors of osteoarthritis. Metabolic syndrome was not a significant predictor of osteoarthritis (p>0.05) (Table 4)

Discussion

The purpose of this study was to determine association between metabolic syndrome and osteoarthritis stratified by age and gender categories in the third National Health and Nutrition Examination Survey (NHANES III) sample. Results show that the subjects with osteoarthritis were old, predominantly females, non-Hispanic Whites, and had high body mass index as compared to subjects in the general population.

Results show an increase prevalence of MS in subjects with OA as compared to the general population. Similarly, results also show an increase prevalence of diabetes, hypertension and high cholesterol in subjects with osteoarthritis. These results are similar to an earlier study that have shown increase prevalence of MS in subjects with OA (Korochina, 2007). 1350 individuals were evaluated who were diagnosed with OA and the frequency of metabolic syndrome among these individuals was found to be 62.56% (Korochina, 2007). In another prior study, patients suffering from OA with MS had stage IV of erosive knee joint cartilage lesion significantly more frequently. In addition, results have shown that the presence of MS in patients with OA is accompanied by more severe cartilage lesions, which are associated with the development of oxidative stress against the background of dyslipidemia (Kratnov AE, Kuryleva KV & Kratnov AA, 2007).

Our results showed MS as a significant risk factor of OA; however its effect became insignificant once BMI was kept in the model. These results were similar to another study by (Engstrom G, Gerhardsson de Verdier M, Rollof J, Nilsson PM & Lohmander LS, 2009) where results showed that after adjustment for age, sex, smoking, physical activity and CRP, presence of MS was associated with significantly increased risk of knee OA (relative risk [RR]: 2.1, 95%confidence interval [CI]: 1.3-3.3). However, this relationship was attenuated and non-significant after adjustment for body mass index (BMI) (RR: 1.1, 95% CI: 0.7-1.8).

Table 4. Adjusted analysis using logistic regression was performed to determine risk factors of osteoarthritis after adjusting for the potential confounders stratified by age ($\leq$ 65 years and > 65 years) and gender (males and females) categories

Variables	Parameter estimate	Standard Error	Odds Ratio	95% CI	p-value
Age $\leq$ 65 years	0.08	0.01	1.08	1.06; 1.10	<0.0001
Education	0.15	0.04	1.16	1.07; 1.25	0.0002
Gender	1.19	0.24	3.28	2.07; 5.21	<0.0001
Smoking History	0.57	0.21	1.77	1.16; 2.69	0.007
Osteoporosis	-3.56	0.49	0.03	0.01; 0.08	<0.0001
Age > 65 years					
Gender	0.48	0.23	1.62	1.02; 2.56	0.04
Education	0.07	0.03	1.08	1.01; 1.15	0.02
Poverty Income ratio	0.12	0.05	1.13	1.02; 1.25	0.02
Osteoporosis	-2.37	0.34	0.09	0.05; 0.18	<0.0001
Males					
Age	0.06	0.008	1.07	1.05; 1.08	<0.0001
Education	0.12	0.03	1.13	1.06; 1.21	0.0004
Metabolic Syndrome	0.51	0.23	1.66	1.07; 2.59	0.03
Osteoporosis	-3.57	0.63	0.03	0.008; 0.09	<0.0001
Females					
Age	0.05	0.006	1.05	1.04; 1.07	<0.0001
Education	0.09	0.03	1.09	1.02; 1.17	0.01
Smoking History	0.52	0.21	1.69	1.13; 2.53	0.01
Osteoporosis	-2.64	0.31	0.07	0.04; 0.13	<0.0001
BMI	0.06	0.03	1.06	1.00; 1.13	0.05

Obesity could be associated with OA through atherogeneic effects of the metabolic factors, resulting in microvascular changes in the subchondral bone (Findlay DM, 2007). Relationships between obesity and OA in the knee or hip have been earlier reported (Pottie P, Presle N, Terlain B, Netter P, Mainard D & Berenbaum F, 2006). It has been proposed that metabolic risk factors and systemic low-grade inflammation, which often is increased in obesity, could contribute to this relationship (Findlay DM, 2007 & Pottie P, Presle N, Terlain B, Netter P, Mainard D & Berenbaum F, 2006).

We performed age stratified analysis ($\leq$65 years and >65 years) and did not find MS as a risk factor for OA. However, gender, education and osteoporosis were significant predictors of OA in subjects in the age groups $\leq$65 years and >65. The only difference in these two groups was that in subjects in the age group of $\leq$65 years, the odds to have OA increased 1.77 times (95% CI 1.16; 2.69) if the subjects were current smokers. Compared to the subjects in the age group of >65 years, the odds of having OA increased 1.13 times (95% CI 1.02; 1.25; p=0.02) with each unit change in poverty income ratio. This could be explained due to the fact that large number of subjects in the age group of >65 years could have smoked in the past and were not current smokers.

Similarly gender stratified analysis was performed to determine risk factors of OA in males and females. Our results found that the odds of having OA increased 1.66 times (95% CI 1.07; 2.59; p=0.03) if subjects had MS in males as compared to females where MS was not significant. BMI was not a significant predictor of OA in males while it was a significant predictor in females (OR=1.06; 95% CI 1.00; 1.13; p=0.05). This is similar to the findings in the previous study where in the univariate analysis, women who developed severe knee OA had higher prevalence of the MS, hypertension, hyperglycemia and high CRP (>3 mg/L) than women without OA during follow-up. However, these relationships were attenuated and non-significant when BMI was taken into account in the multivariate analysis (Engstrom G, Gerhardsson de Verdier M, Rollof J, Nilsson PM & Lohmander LS, 2009). Results also show that 79% of the variance of MS was unique for that variable and only 21% could be explained by all other independent variables (Engstrom G, Gerhardsson de Verdier M, Rollof J, Nilsson PM & Lohmander LS, 2009). The components of the MS are well-known atherosclerotic risk factors. Prevalence of atherosclerotic risk factors is high in individuals with OA, and it has been proposed that vascular pathology of subchondral small vessels could play an etiological role in the development of OA(Engstrom G, Gerhardsson de Verdier M, Rollof J, Nilsson PM & Lohmander LS, 2009).

There are several limitations of the current study. Firstly, the NHANES III is a cross sectional data and so it is difficult to establish cause-effect relationships. Secondly, there may be inaccuracies in methods of data collection since the information about their health status was gathered through self-report measures. Thirdly, we did not characterize the types of osteoarthritis in these subjects such as hip, knee, hand, or spine that could potentially confound the results. Fourthly, we did not control for the severity of the OA and the medications that these subjects were taking which could possibly bias our results. Lastly, there may not be adequate power to demonstrate this association after adjusting for the potential confounders in this analyzable sample.

However several important themes emerge from this analysis. Firstly there are not many studies that have explored the relationship between MS and OA. Our results show increase prevalence of MS in overall OA subjects and also those stratified by gender and age categories. Findings suggest that these may be at an increased risk of cardiovascular diseases compared to those subjects who do not have OA. Our findings also suggest that the prevalence of diabetes and hypertension is significantly greater among OA subjects compared to those without arthritis. These results coincide with previous studies (Gabriel SE, Crowson CS & O'Fallon WM, 1999 & Singh G, Miller JD, Lee FH, Pettitt D, Russell MW, 2002). Similarly our results showed high prevalence of increased cholesterol levels in subjects with arthritis as compared to those with no arthritis. (Singh G, Miller JD, Lee FH, Pettitt D, Russell MW, 2002). The prevalence of diabetes, hypertension, high cholesterol, low HDL, and increased prevalence of MS demonstrate the need for enhanced public health surveillance systems to monitor, track and detect longitudinally the cause effect relationship between OA and the cardiovascular diseases and its effect on health outcomes so that interventions can be done in a timely manner and OA subjects at high risk of MS can be aggressively managed.

REFERENCES

Brooks, P. M. (2006, November). The burden of musculoskeletal disease--a global perspective. *Clinical Rheumatology*, *25*(6), 778–781. doi:10.1007/s10067-006-0240-3

Centers for Disease Control and Prevention (CDC). (1996). Prevalence and impact of arthritis by race and ethnicity-United States. *MMWR Morb Mortal Wkly*, *45*, 373–378.

Engström, G., Gerhardsson, de Verdier., M., Rollof., J., Nilsson, P.M., & Lohmander, L.S. (2009). C-reactive protein, metabolic syndrome and incidence of severe hip and knee osteoarthritis. A population-based cohort study. *Osteoarthritis and Cartilage*, *17*(2), 168–173. doi:10.1016/j.joca.2008.07.003

Felson, T. D. (2004, October). Risk factors for osteoarthritis: understanding joint vulnerability. *Clinical Orthopaedics and Related Research*, (427), S16–S21. doi:10.1097/01.blo.0000144971.12731.a2

Findlay, D. M. (2007). Vascular pathology and osteoarthritis. *Rheumatology, 46,* 1763e8. Oxford

Flugsrud, G.B., Nordsletten, L., Espehaug, B., Havelin, L.I., Engeland, A., & Meyer, H.E. (2006). The impact of body mass index on later total hip arthroplasty for primary osteoarthritis: a cohort study in 1.2 million persons. *Arthritis Rheum, 54,* 802e7.

Gabriel, S. E., Crowson, C. S., & O'Fallon, W. M. (1999). Co morbidity in arthritis. *The Journal of Rheumatology*, *26*, 2475–2479.

Garstang, S. V., & Stitik, T. P. (2006). Osteoarthritis: epidemiology, risk factors and pathophysiology. *American Journal of Physical Medicine & Rehabilitation, 85*(11 Suppl), S2–S11. doi:10.1097/01.phm.0000245568.69434.1a

Gelber, A.C., Hochberg, M.C., Mead, L.A., Wang, N.Y., Wigley, F.M., & Klag, M.J. (1999). Body mass index in young men and the risk of subsequent knee and hip osteoarthritis. *Am J Med, 107,* 542e8

Grundy, S.M., Cleeman, J.I., Daniels, S.R., Donato, K.A., Eckel, R.H., Franklin, B.A., Gordon, J.D., Krauss, M.R., Savage, J.P., Smith, C. S., Spertus, A.J., & Fernando, C. (2005). Diagnosis and management of the metabolic syndrome. An American Heart Association/National Heart, Lung and Blood Institute Scientific Statement. Executive Summary. *Circulation, 112,* 2735e52.

Helmick, C., Felson, D., Lawrence, R., Gabriel, S., Hirsch, R., & Kwoh, C. K. (2008). National Arthritis Data Workgroup. Estimates of the Prevalence of Arthritis and Other Rheumatic conditions in the United States. *Arthritis and Rheumatism*, *58*(1), 15–25. doi:10.1002/art.23177

Korochina, I. E., & Bagirova, G. G. (2007). Metabolic syndrome and a course of osteoarthritis. *Terapevticheskii Arkhiv, 79,* 13–20.

Kratnov, A. E., Kuryleva, K. V., & Kratnov, A. A. (2007). Association between primary osteoarthrosis and metabolic syndrome according to data from arthroscopic and cytochemical studies. *Klinicheskaia Meditsina, 84*(6), 42–46.

Kraus, V. B. (1997). Pathogenesis and treatment of osteoarthritis. *Adv Rheumatol, 81,* 85–112.

Lawrence, R. C., Helmick, C. G., Arnett, F. C., Deyo, R. A., Felson, D. T., & Giannini, E. H. (1998). Estimates of the prevalence of arthritis and selected musculoskeletal disorders in the United States. *Arthritis and Rheumatism*, *43*, 778–779. doi:10.1002/1529-0131(199805)41:5<778::AID-ART4>3.0.CO;2-V

Maetzel, A., Li, L. C., Pencharz, J., Tomlinson, F., & Bombardier, C. (2004). The economic burden associated with osteoarthritis, rheumatoid arthritis, and hypertension: A comparative study. *Annals of the Rheumatic Diseases, 63*(4), 395–401. doi:10.1136/ard.2003.006031

Mandelbaum, B., & Waddell, D. (2005, February). Etiology and pathophysiology of osteoarthritis. *Orthopedics, 28*(2Suppl), s207–s214.

MMWR. (2007). *Data Source: 2003 Medical Expenditure Panel Survey, 56*(01), 4-7. Available at: http://www. cdc.gov/nchs/nhanes.htm.

National Cholesterol Education Program (NCEP). (2002). Expert Panel on Detection, Evaluation, and Treatment of High Blood Cholesterol in Adults (Adult Treatment Panel III). Third Report of the National Cholesterol Education Program (NCEP) Expert Panel on Detection, Evaluation, and Treatment of High Blood Cholesterol in Adults (Adult Treatment Panel III) final report. *Circulation, 106*, 3143–3421.

Oliveria, S.A., Felson, D.T., Cirillo, P.A., Reed, J.I., & Walker, A.M. (1999). Body weight, body mass index, and incident symptomatic osteoarthritis of the hand, hip, and knee. *Epidemiology; 10*, 161e6.

Osteoarthritis Fact sheet (2008). *News from the Arthritis Foundation.*

Pottie, P., Presle, N., Terlain, B., Netter, P., Mainard, D., & Berenbaum, F. (2006). Obesity and osteoarthritis: more complex than predicted. *Ann Rheum Dis, 65*, 1403e5.

Singh, G., Miller, J.D., Lee, F.H., Pettitt, D., & Russell, M.W. (2002). Prevalence of cardiovascular disease risk factors among US adults with self-reported osteoarthritis: data from the Third National Health and Nutrition Examination Survey. *Am J Manag Care, 8*(Suppl 15), S383e91.

This work was previously published in International Journal of Computational Models and Algorithms in Medicine, Volume 1, Issue 1, edited by Aryya Gangopadhyay, pp. 61-73, copyright 2010 by IGI Publishing (an imprint of IGI Global).

Chapter 6
Exploring Type–and–Identity–Based Proxy Re–Encryption Scheme to Securely Manage Personal Health Records

Luan Ibraimi
University of Twente, The Netherlands

Qiang Tang
University of Twente, The Netherlands

Pieter Hartel
University of Twente, The Netherlands

Willem Jonker
University of Twente, The Netherlands

ABSTRACT

Commercial Web-based Personal-Health Record (PHR) systems can help patients to share their personal health records (PHRs) anytime from anywhere. PHRs are very sensitive data and an inappropriate disclosure may cause serious problems to an individual. Therefore commercial Web-based PHR systems have to ensure that the patient health data is secured using state-of-the-art mechanisms. In current commercial PHR systems, even though patients have the power to define the access control policy on who can access their data, patients have to trust entirely the access-control manager of the commercial PHR system to properly enforce these policies. Therefore patients hesitate to upload their health data to these systems as the data is processed unencrypted on untrusted platforms. Recent proposals on enforcing access control policies exploit the use of encryption techniques to enforce access control policies. In such systems, information is stored in an encrypted form by the third party and there is no need for an access control manager. This implies that data remains confidential even if the database maintained by the third party is compromised. In this paper we propose a new encryption technique called a type-and-identity-based proxy re-encryption scheme which is suitable to be used in the healthcare setting. The proposed scheme allows users (patients) to securely store their PHRs on commercial Web-based PHRs, and securely share their PHRs with other users (doctors).

DOI: 10.4018/978-1-4666-0282-3.ch006

INTRODUCTION

Recently, healthcare providers have started to use electronic health record systems which have significant benefits such as reducing healthcare costs, increasing the patient safety, improving the quality of care and empowering patients to more actively manage their health. There are a number of initiatives for adoption of electronic health records (EHRs) from different governments around the world, such as the directive on privacy and electronic communications in the U.S. known as the Health Insurance Portability and Accountability Act (HIPAA) (The US Department of Health and Human Services, 2003), which specify rules and standards to achieve security and privacy of health data. While EHR systems capture health data entered by health care professionals and access to health data is tightly controlled by existing legislations, personal health record (PHR) systems capture health data entered by individuals and stay outside the scope of this legislation. Before going into details on how to address the confidentiality issues, let us introduce the definition of PHR system (The personal health working group final report, 2004):

An electronic application through which individuals can access, manage and share their health information, and that of others for whom they are authorized, in a private, secure, and confidential environment.

PHR systems are unique in their design since they try to solve the problem that comes from scattering of medical information among many healthcare providers which leads to unnecessary paper work and medical mistakes (The personal health working group final report, 2004). The PHR contains all kinds of health-related information about an individual (say, Alice) (Tang, Ash, Bates, Overhage & Sands, 2006). Firstly, the PHR may contain medical data that Alice has from various medical service providers, for example about

surgery, illness, family history, vaccinations, laboratory test results, allergies, drug reactions, etc. Secondly, the PHR may also contain information collected by Alice herself, for example weight change, food statistics, and any other information connected with her health. Controlling access to PHRs is one of the central themes in deploying a secure PHR system. Inappropriate disclosure of the PHRs may cause an individual serious problems. For example, if Alice has some disease and a prospective employer obtains this, then she might be discriminated in finding a job.

Commercial efforts to build Web-based PHR systems, such as Microsoft HealthVault (Microsoft, 2007) and Google Health (Google, 2007), allow patients to store and share their PHRs with different healthcare providers. In these systems the patient has full control over her PHRs and plays the role of the security administrator - a patient decides who has the right to access which data. However, the access control model of these applications does not give a patient the flexibility to specify a fine-grained access-control policy. For example, today's Google Health access control is *all-or-nothing* - so if a patient authorizes her doctor to see only one PHR, the doctor will be able to see all other PHRs. Another problem is that the data has to be stored on a central server locked by the access control mechanism provided by Microsoft HealthVault or Google Health, and the patient loses control once the data is sent to the server. PHRs may contain sensitive information such as details of a patients disease, drug usage, sexual preferences, therefore, many patients are worried whether their PHRs will be treated as confidential by companies running data centers. Inappropriate disclosure of a PHR can change patients life, and there may be no way to repair such harm financially or technically. Therefore, it is crucial to protect PHRs when they are uploaded and stored in commercial Web-based systems.

PROBLEM STATEMENT

The problem addressed in this paper is the confidentiality of patient PHRs stored in commercial Web-based PHR systems. A solution to the problem is a system which would have the following security requirements:

- Protect patient PHRs from third parties (from the commercial Web-based PHR systems)
- Provide end-to-end security
- Allow only authorized users to have access to the patient PHRs
- Allow the patient to change the access policy dynamically

Contributions

To solve the identified problem we propose a new public key encryption scheme called type-and-identity-based proxy re-encryption which helps patients to store their PHRs on commercial Web-based PHR systems, and to share their PHRs securely with doctors, family and friends. In public key encryption, each user has a key pair (private/public key) and everyone can encrypt a message using a public key, also referred to as the encryption key, but only users who have the associated private key, also referred to as the decryption key, can decrypt the encrypted message. Proxy re-encryption is a cryptographic method developed

to delegate the decryption right from one party, the delegator, to another, the delegatee. In a proxy re-encryption scheme, the delegator assigns a key to a proxy to re-encrypt all messages encrypted with the public key of the delegator such that the re-encrypted ciphertexts can be decrypted with the private key of the delegatee. The Proxy is a semi-trusted entity i.e. it is trusted to perform only the ciphertext re-encryption, without knowing the private keys of the delegator and the delegatee, and without having access to the plain text. In the context of public key encryption, proxy re-encryption is used to forward encrypted messages without revealing the plaintext. For example, in Figure 1, Alice (delegator) is president of a company who wants to allow her secretary, Bob (delegatee), to read encrypted emails from Charlie when Alice is on vacation (Alice cannot give to Bob her private key). Using proxy re-encryption Alice can compute a re-encryption key which would allow the Proxy to transform a ciphertext for Alice generated by Charlie into a ciphertext for Bob, thus, Bob can decrypt the re-encrypted data using his private key. In practice the role of the Proxy can be played by a commercial enterprise which has enough computation power to perform re-encryption services for a large number of users. Our proposed scheme is suitable for the healthcare setting and has the following benefits:

- Allow the patient to store her PHRs in a protected form on semitrusted commercial

Figure 1. Proxy re-encryption

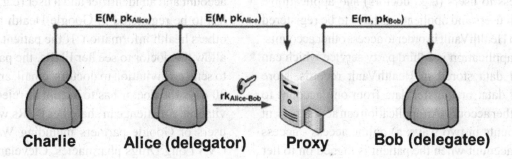

Web-based PHR system. The commercial Web-based PHR system cannot access the data since the data is stored in an encrypted form.

- Allow the patient to define a fine-grained access control policy. The patient only has to compute the re-encryption key and forward it the Proxy which will re-encrypt the data without decrypting them such that the intended user (e.g., doctor) can decrypt the re-encrypted data using his private key. In addition to that, the scheme allows the patient to change dynamically the access policy without necessarily decrypting the data.
- Allows the patient to categorize her messages into different types, and delegate the decryption right of each type to the doctor through a Proxy. Data categorization is needed since different data may have different levels of privacy requirements.

WEB-BASED PHRS

In this section we discuss current Web-based PHRs systems such as Microsoft HealthVault and Google Health and their access control mechanisms. Moreover, we discuss existing techniques to enforce access policies using cryptography and discuss their limitations.

In Microsoft HealthVault each patient has an account and an identifier. Each account has a special role called a *custodian* who has the right to view and modify all records, and grant or revoke access to users (e.g., doctors) and applications. Both users and applications have to be registered with HealthVault in order to access other accounts. An application is a third party service which can read data stored in HealthVault records, store new data, or transfer data from one account to another account. An application can access patient accounts in two ways: a) online access - access the account when the patient is logged on to her

account, and b) offline access – access the account at any time. If the patient uses an application for the first time, and the application requires access to a health record, the application sends an access request to the patient. After the patient approves the request, the application can access the health information. HealthVault uses discretionary access control (DAC) (Graham and Denning, 1971) where access to a patient PHR is based on user identity (e.g. email). For example, if the patient wants to allow the doctor to see her record, the patient has to send a sharing invitation to the doctors' email and within 3 days the doctor has to accept or reject the invitation. The doctor may have one of the following permissions: a) view patient information, b) view and modify patient information or, c) act as a custodian. Microsoft HealthVault defines 74 types of information and allows granular access control for non-custodians. For example, the patient can allow the doctor to have access only to records of type *Allergy*, and block access to records of type *Family History*. However, the patient does not have the flexibility to grant access to the doctor to an individual record. When the patient grants access to the doctor to her health information, the patient can also specify an expiration date. After the expiration date, the doctor would not be able to access the patient information. However, the patient has the option to remove sharing access at any time (even before the expiration date).

Similar to Microsoft HealthVault, Google Health allows a patient to import her PHRs, add test results and add information about allergies, among others. In Google Health each patient has an account and an identifier and a user (e.g., doctor) has to be registered to Google Health to access others health information. If the patient wants to allow the doctor to see her PHRs, the patient has to send an invitation to doctors' email, and within 30 days the doctor has to accept or reject the invitation. A patient can share her PHRs with other users or Google partners including Walgreens, CVS Long Drugs pharmacies, Cleveland Clinic and etc. However, data sharing in Google Health is *all-or-nothing*. The patients does not have the flexibility to chose a fine-grained access policy to share her data. For example, once the patient allows the doctor to see her blood result test, the doctor can access all health information of the patient.

In the access-control mechanisms of Microsoft HealthVault and Google Health the receiving end of the information must provide a set of credentials to the access control manager (ACM) who is responsible for enforcing the access control policies. The ACM checks whether user credentials satisfy the access control policy. If so, the user can read the resource, otherwise not. However, the main limitation of this is that the patient still needs to trust the Microsoft HealthVault and Google Health to enforce access control policies when disclosing data, and specially the access control decisions and privacy enforcement has to be enforced when the data is moving from one enterprise to another. Another limitation is that despite the privacy policy the leakage of confidential information can happen due to compromise of the database maintained by the enterprise. Therefore, to solve the aforementioned problem, recent proposals on enforcing access control policies exploit the use of encryption techniques. In such systems, information is stored in an encrypted form by an enterprise and there is no need for an access control manager to check user credentials. Thus, each user can get the encrypted data, but only users who have the right credentials (the right key) can decrypt the encrypted data. This implies that data confidentiality is preserved even if the database maintained by the enterprise is compromised.

Current Solutions (And Their Drawbacks) Which Enforce Access Control Policies Using Encryption

To prevent commercial Web-based PHR systems to access the content of patients PHRs, the patient can encrypt her data using traditional public key encryption algorithms and store the encrypted data (ciphertext) in a database, and then decrypt the ciphertext on demand. In this case, the patient only needs to assume that Microsoft HealthVault and Google Health will properly store her encrypted data, and even if Microsoft HealthVault and Google Health get corrupted, patients PHR will not be disclosed since the data is stored in an encrypted form. The problem with this solution is that the patient needs to be involved in every request (e.g., from her doctor, hospital) and perform the decryption. This is because only the patient knows the decryption key.

One possible solution is to use more advanced public key encryption schemes such as Ciphertext-Policy Attribute-Based Encryption (CP-ABE) scheme (Bethencourt, Sahai, & Waters, 2007), (Cheung & Newport, 2007), (Ibraimi, Tang, Hartel, & Jonker, 2009). The CP-ABE scheme is a type of attribute-based encryption scheme in which the data owner encrypts the data according to an access control policy τ defined over a set of attributes, and where the receiving end can decrypt the encrypted data only if his private key associated with a set of attributes satisfies the access control policy τ. For example, suppose Alice encrypts her data according to an access policy $\tau = (a_1$ AND $a_2)$ OR a_3. Bob can decrypt the encrypted data only if his private key is associated with a set of attributes that satisfy the access policy. To satisfy the access control policy τ, Bob must have a private key associated with at least one from the following attribute sets: $(a_1, a_2), (a_3)$ or (a_1, a_2, a_3). In CP-ABE the mapping user-attribute is many-to-many, which means that one user may possess many attributes and one attribute may be possessed by many users. The main drawbacks of using CP-ABE to securely manage PHRs are: a) the patient has to know the list of users associated with an attribute, and b) an attribute is possessed by many users. Therefore, using CP-ABE, the patient cannot encrypt a PHR such that only one healthcare provider, with whom the patient has contract, can access it at a time.

This is because one attribute can be possessed by many healthcare providers. This is one of the main reasons why both Microsoft HealthVault and Google Health use DAC where access to patients records is based on doctors identity, instead of using Attribute-Based Access Control (ABAC) where access to patients records is based on doctors attributes.

Another solution is to use existing identity-based proxy re-encryption schemes (Green and Ateniese, 2007), in which the patient assigns a re-encryption key to the Proxy which re-encrypts the encrypted PHR under patients' public key into encrypted PHR under doctors' public key. However this approach has the following drawbacks:

- The Proxy is able to re-encrypt all cipher-texts of the patient such that the doctor can decrypt all ciphertexts using his private key. Thus, the patient does not have the flexibility to define fine-grained access control.

- If the Proxy and the delegatee get corrupted, then all PHRs may be disclosed to an illegitimate entity based on the fact that the re-encryption key can re-encrypt all ciphertexts.

THE CONCEPT OF TYPE-AND-IDENTITY-BASED PROXY RE-ENCRYPTION

In order to solve the aforementioned problems a new encryption scheme which would crypto-graphically enforce access policies is needed. We propose a type-and-identity-based proxy re-encryption scheme which consists of six algorithms: Setup, Extract, Encrypt, Pextract, Preenc and Decrypt.

The basic building block of the type-and-identity-based proxy re-encryption scheme is the

Identity-Based Encryption (IBE) scheme (Figure 2). The concept of IBE was proposed by Shamir (Shamir, 1985), however IBE has become practical only after Boneh and Franklin (Boneh and Franklin, 2001) propose the first IBE scheme based on bilinear pairings on elliptic curve (In appendix A we review in more detail the concept of bilinear pairing). The IBE scheme consist of four algorithms: Setup, Extract, Encrypt and Decrypt. Unlike a traditional public key encryption scheme, an IBE does not require a digital certificate to certify the encryption key (public key) because the public key of any user can be an arbitrary string such as an email address, IP address, etc. Key escrow is an inherent property in IBE systems, i.e., the trusted authority (TA), also referred to as Key Generation Center (KGC), can generate each users' private key, because the TA owns the master key mk used to generate users' private keys. IBE is a very suitable technique to be used in healthcare to exchange emails more securely. For example, in Figure 2, when Alice (the patient) wants to send an encrypted email to Bob (the doctor), Alice can encrypt an email using the encryption key derived from the doctors identity and send the email via an insecure channel. The doctor can authenticate himself to the TA to get the decryption key (private key). After the private key is generated the doctor can decrypt the encrypted email. Unlike in traditional public-key encryption schemes where the private key and the public key has to be created simultaneously, in IBE the private key can be generated long time after the corresponding public key is generated.

A type-and-identity-based proxy re-encryption scheme extends the IBE scheme by adding the Proxy entity to the existing two entities: the TA and users. Another type of extension has been made to the number of algorithms. In addition to the four algorithms of IBE scheme, the type- and-identity-based proxy re-encryption scheme uses Pextract algorithm to generate a re-encryption

Figure 2. Identity-based encryption

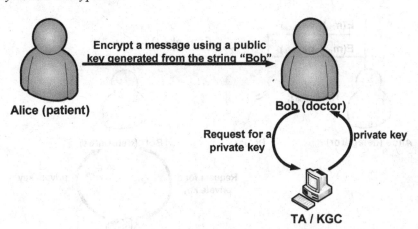

key, and Preenc algorithm to re-encrypt the ciphertext. These algorithms are needed to enable the patient (delegator) to specify a fine-grained access control policy for her PHRs.

In the type-and-identity-based proxy re-encryption scheme (Figure 3), Alice (delegator) using one key-pair can categorize messages (data) into different types and delegate the decryption right of each type to Bob (delegatee) through a Proxy. Grouping the data into different categories is needed since different PHRs may have different levels of privacy requirements. For example, Alice may not be seriously concerned about disclosing her food statistics to other persons, but she might wish to keep her illness history as a top secret and only disclose it to the appropriate person. In addition to categorizing her PHRs according to the sensitivity level, Alice may categorize her PHRs according to the type of information or according to the device which generated the PHR. There are a number of measurement devices in the market which can be used by the patient and can be connected via home hubs to remote back-end servers. Such examples are disease management services (such as Philips Motiva and PTS) or emergency response services (Philips Lifeline) in which the healthcare provider can remotely access the measurement data and help the patients. As illustrated in Figure 3, Alice uses only one public key to encryp all messages, and delegates her decryption right (computes a re-encryption key) only for one type (type 1), and Bob can use his private key to access only messages which belong to type 1. If the Proxy and Bob get corrupted, then only health records belonging to type 1 may be disclosed to an illegitimate entity, while the other types of information remains secure. A full construction of the type-and-identity based re-encryption scheme is given in Appendix B.

The six algorithms are defined as follows:

- Setup(k): run by the TA, the algorithm takes as input a security parameter k and outputs the master public key pk and the master private key mk. pk is used in the encryption phase by each user, and mk is used by the TA to generate users private keys.
- Extract(mk, id): run by the TA when a user request a private key. The algorithm takes as input the master key mk and an user identity id, the algorithm outputs the user private key sk_{id}.
- Encrypt(m, t, pk_{id}): run by the encryptor, the algorithm takes as input a message to be encrypted m, a type t, and an the public key pk_{id} associated with the identity id, and outputs the ciphertext c.

Figure 3. A type-and-identity-based proxy re-encryption

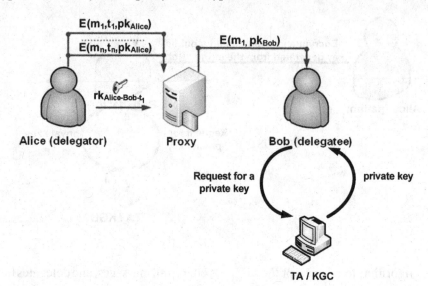

- Pextract(id_i, id_j, t, sk_{id_i}) run by the delegator, this algorithm takes the delegator's identifier id_i, the delegatee's identifier id_j, the type t, and the delegator's private key sk_{id_i} as input and outputs the re-encryption key $rk_{id_i \to id_j}$.

- Preenc($c_i, rk_{id_i \to id_j}$) run by the Proxy, this algorithm, takes as input the ciphertext c_i and the re-encryption key $rk_{id_i \to id_j}$, and outputs a new ciphertext c_j

- Decrypt(c_j, sk_{id_j}) run by the decryptor, the algorithm takes as input the ciphertext c_j and the private key sk_{id_j}, and output a message m.

A formal security model and a formal security proof is given in appendix B.1. and B.2.

Applying the Scheme in Practice

Figure 4 illustrates a general architecture of a PHR system that uses our type-and-identity-based proxy re-encryption scheme. The architecture consists of Trusted Authorities (TAs), a patient, an application hosting device, a Web PHR, a Proxy and a doctor. The TAs are used to generate key pairs for the patient, respectively the doctor. We assume that the patient and the doctor are from different security domains. The application hosting device can be implemented on a home PC of the data source (a patient) or as a trusted service. Its role is to encrypt PHRs and forward them to the Web PHR. The Web PHR stores encrypted PHRs, and Proxy is used to re-encrypt encrypted data and forward them to the doctor. There are five basic processes in the management of PHRs:

- **Setup:** In this phase, TAs run the Setup and Extract algorithm and distribute the public parameters needed to run the algorithms of the type-and-identity-based proxy re-encryption scheme, and distributes the private keys, which are needed to decrypt encrypted messages, to the patient and doctor (1). We assume that there is a secure channel between the TA and the user, respectively the doctor. Note that the doctor can get his key pair during the decryption phase, while the Proxy can per-

Figure 4. Secure management of PHR

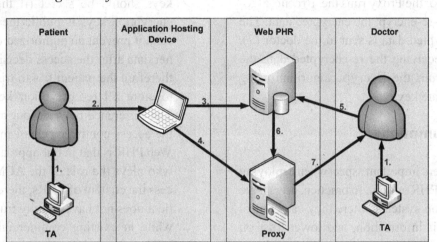

form re-encryption of encrypted data under doctors public key, even if the doctor does not have a private key. This is possible since the doctors public key can be computed by everyone who knows doctors' identity. The TA does not have to be online as long as each user gets his/her key pair.

- **Data creation:** The patient uses a number of healthcare devices and creates measurement data and forwards them to the application hosting device (2). In addition to that, the patient can forward to the application hosting device all kinds of information that the patient has from various medical service providers.

- **Data protection:** The patient categorizes her PHR according to her privacy concerns. For instance, she can set her illness history as type t_1, her food statistics as type t_2, and the necessary PHR data in case of emergency as type t_3. Then the patient generates the encryption key (public key) derived from her identity (identity can be any type of public string) and run the Encrypt algorithm using the generated public key. After the encryption is performed, the patients uploads the encrypted data to Web PHR (3). As in the previous

step, all this (data categorization, data encryption and data uploading) can be done by a hosting device on behalf of the patient.

- **Data Sharing (allow the doctor to see patient data):** In this phase, the patient runs the Pextract algorithm and generates the re-encryption key which will be used by the Proxy to re-encrypt encrypted data under patients public key to encrypted data under doctors public key, such that the doctor can decrypt the encrypted data using his private key. The generated key is forwarded to the Proxy (4). As in the above steps, all this can be done by a hosting device on behalf of the patient who specifies the access control policy.

- **Data consumption (doctors' request-response):** When a doctor wants to use patient data, he contacts the Web PHR and specifies the ciphertext that he wants to decrypt (5). We assume that each ciphertext is associated with appropriate metadata - descriptive information about the patient. The encrypted data is forwarded to the Proxy (6). The Proxy checks if the doctor is allowed to see patient data (checks if it has a re-encryption key $rk_{Patient \rightarrow Doctor}$), and, if so, the Proxy runs the Preenc algorithm to re-encrypt the encrypted data. The re-encrypted data is sent to the doctor (7). After receiving the re-encrypted data the doctor runs the Decrypt algorithm using his private key.

Trust Assumptions

User trust is very important aspect when deploying a Web-based PHR system. In practice, users have greater trust on systems where they can control access to their information, and lower trust on systems where they have to trust someone else to control access to their information (e.g., the user has to trust the access control manager of the Web PHR). Therefore in this paper we provide a solution which compared to existing solutions reduces the trust that patients need to have on commercial Web-based PHR systems. As mentioned above, in our proposal the role of the Web PHR is twofold: a) to provide storage for PHRs, and b) to maintain the Proxy. Next to that, the patient has to put the following trust on Web PHR:

- The Web-based PHR system is trusted to store PHRs in publicly accessible storage only in an encrypted form, therefore the patient does not have to trust the Web-based PHR system to provide data confidentiality service. The data confidentiality service is provided by the patient at the moment when the data is encrypted. Encryption prevents sniffing software to access the data when the data travels from the user to the storage, and the storage cannot decrypt the data without having the private key.

- The Proxy is trusted to maintain a list of re-encryption keys, and to enforce the access policy by properly re-encrypting the encrypted data when the identity of the doctor (requester) is part of the re-encryption key. Note that, the list of re-encryption

keys should be secret (if the list of re-encryption keys is public then the patient cannot prevent an authorized doctor to see her data after the access decision is made), therefore the patient has to trust the Proxy to store all re-encryption keys securely. The difference between our approach and the access control mechanisms in existing Web PHR is that in our approach the Proxy who plays the role of the ACM cannot access the content of PHRs, therefore, the patient does not have to fully trust the Proxy, while in existing commercial Web-based PHR systems the patient has to fully trust the ACM because the ACM can access the content of PHRs.

- The user should trust the Proxy to securely delete re-encryption keys when the user wants to prevent an authorized doctor to access users data further. For example, a patient might change her healthcare provider, and after some time she wants to prevent the doctor from an old healthcare provider to access her data.

Policy Updating

To allow someone to access her data, the patient has to compute a new re-encryption key. For example, if Alice wants to allow Bob and Charlie to see her PHRs belonging to category t_{Alergy}, Alice has to create two re-encryption keys: $rk_{Alice \to Bob}$ and $rk_{Alice \to Charlie}$. Transmission of the re-encryption keys to the Proxy should be secured using cryptographical protocols such as Transport Layer Security (TLS) which allows two entities to securely communicate over the internet.

In practice the patient might want to update her access policy. Using our approach the patient might do this task without entirely decrypting the ciphertext. To update an access policy means to create new, and delete old, re-encryption keys. For example, if Alice wants to update her access policy from $\tau = Bob\ OR\ Charlie$ (this access policy implies that Bob and Charlie can access the data) to a different access policy $\tau' = Bob\ OR\ Dave$ (this access policy implies that Bob and Dave can access the data), she has to follow the following two procedures:

- Notify the Proxy to delete (revoke) the re-encryption key $rk_{Alice \rightarrow Charlie}$. This would prevent the Proxy to re-encrypt encrypted data under Alice's public key to encrypted data under Charlie's public key.
- Create a new re-encryption key $rk_{Alice \rightarrow Dave}$ and send it to the Proxy. This would allow the Proxy to re-encrypt encrypted data under Alice's public key to encrypted data under Dave's public key.

RELATED WORK ON PROXY RE-ENCRYPTION

Since (Mambo and Okamoto, 1997) first proposed the concept, a number of proxy re-encryption schemes have been proposed. (Blaze, Bleumer, and Strauss, 1998) introduce the concept of atomic Proxy cryptography which is the current concept of proxy re-encryption. In a proxy re-encryption scheme, the Proxy can transform ciphertexts encrypted with the delegator's public key into ciphertexts that can be decrypted with the delegatee's private key. (Blaze, Bleumer, & Strauss, 1998) propose a proxy re-encryption scheme based on the (ElGamal, 1985) encryption scheme. One property of this scheme is that, with the same re-encryption key, the Proxy can transform the ciphertexts not only form the delegator to the delegatee but also from the delegatee to the delegator. This is called the "bi-directional" property in the literature. Bi-directionality might be a problem in some applications, but it might also be a desirable property in some other applications. (Jakobsson, 1999) addresses this "problem" using a quorum controlled asymmetric proxy re-encryption where the Proxy is implemented with multiple servers and each of them performs partial re-encryption.

(Ivan & Dodis, 2003) propose a generic construction method for proxy re-encryption schemes and also provide a number of example schemes. Their constructions are based on the concept of secret splitting, which means that the delegator splits his private key into two parts and sends them to the Proxy and the delegatee separately. During the re-encryption process the Proxy performs partial decryption of the encrypted message using the first part of the delegator's private key, and the delegatee can recover the message by performing partial decryption using the second part of the delegator's private key. One disadvantage of this method is that it is not collusion-safe, i.e. the Proxy and the delegatee together can recover the delegator's private key. Another disadvantage of this scheme is that the delegatee's public/private key pair can only be used for dealing with the delegator's messages. If this key pair is used by the delegatee for other encryption services, then the delegator can always decrypt the ciphertexts.

(Ateniese, Fu, Green, & Hohenberger, 2006) propose several proxy re-encryption schemes based on the (ElGamal, 1985) scheme. In their schemes, the delegator does not have to interact and share his private key with the delegatee. The delegator stores two private keys, a master private key and a "weak" private key. The ciphertext can be fully decrypted using either of the two distinct keys. Their scheme is collusion safe, since only the "weak" private key is exposed if the delegatee and the Proxy collude but the master key remains safe. In addition, (Ateniese, Fu, Green, & Hohenberger, 2006) also discuss a number of properties for proxy re-encryption schemes.

Recently, two IBE proxy re-encryption schemes were proposed by (Matsuo, 2007) and (Green & Ateniese, 2007), respectively. The Matsuo scheme assumes that the delegator and the delegatee belong to the same KGC and use the (Boneh & Boyen, 2004) encryption scheme.

The (Green & Ateniese, 2007) scheme assumes that the delegator and the delegatee can belong to different KGCs but the delegatee possess the public parameter of the delegator's KGC.

(Sahai and Waters, 2005) introduce the concept of Attribute-Based Encryption (ABE) which is a generalized form of IBE. In ABE the ciphertext and user private keys are associated with a set of attributes. A user can decrypt the ciphertext if the user private key has the list of attributes specified in the ciphertext. In Ciphertext-Policy Attribute-Based Encryption (CP-ABE) the user private key is associated with a set of attributes and a ciphertext is associated with an access control over some attribute. The decryptor can decrypt the ciphertext if the list of attributes associated with the private key satisfies the access policy. In Key-Policy Attribute-Based Encryption (KP-ABE) (Goyal, Pandey, Sahai, & Waters, 2006) the idea is reversed and the private key is associated with an access control over some attributes and the ciphertext is associated with a list of attributes. The decryptor can decrypt the ciphertext if the list of attributes associated with the ciphertext satisfy the access policy associated with the private key. (Liang, Cao, Lin, & Shao, 2009) proposed an attribute-based proxy re-encryption scheme. The scheme is based on the (Cheung & Newport, 2007) CP-ABE scheme and inherits the same limitations that (Cheung & Newport, 2007) has: it supports only access policies with AND boolean operator, and the size of the ciphertext increases linearly with the number of attributes in the system.

Proxy re-encryption has many promising applications including access control in file storage (Ateniese, Fu, Green, & Hohenberger, 2006), email forwarding (Wang, Cao, T. Okamoto, Miao & E. Okamoto, 2006), and law enforcement (Mambo & Okamoto, 1997). With the increasing privacy concerns over personal data, proxy re-encryption, in particular IBE proxy re-encryption schemes, will find more and more applications. As we show in this paper, proxy re-encryption is a powerful tool for patients to enforce their PHR disclosure policies.

CONCLUSION

This paper presents a new approach for secure management of PHRs which are stored and shared from a semitrusted web server (the server is trusted to perform only the ciphertext re-encryption, without having access to the plain text). We gave an overview of access control mechanisms employed in current commercial Web-based PHR systems and show that traditional access control mechanisms as well as traditional encryption techniques which enforce access control policies are not suitable to be used in scenarios where the data is outsourced to a third party data center. In this paper we propose a type-and-identity-based proxy re-encryption scheme which allow patients to reduce the trust on commercial Web-base PHR systems and enable patients to provide different re-encryption capabilities to the Proxy while using the same key pair. This property has been shown to be useful in our PHR disclosure system, where an individual can easily implement fine-grained access control policies to her PHRs.

REFERENCES

Ateniese, G., Fu, K., Green, M., & Hohenberger, S. (2006). Improved proxy re-encryption schemes with applications to secure distributed storage. *ACM Transactions on Information and System Security*, 9(1), 1–30. doi:10.1145/1127345.1127346

Bethencourt, J., Sahai, A., & Waters, B. (2007). Ciphertext-policy attribute-based encryption. In D. Shands (Ed.), *Proceedings of the 28th IEEE Symposium on Security and Privacy* (pp. 321-334). Oakland, CA: Citeseer.

Blaze, M., Bleumer, G., & Strauss, M. (1998). Divertible protocols and atomic proxy cryptography. In K. Nyberg (Ed.), *Proceeding of Eurocrypt 1998* (Vol. 1403 of LNCS) (pp. 127-144). New York: Springer Verlag.

Boneh, D., & Boyen, X. (2004). Efficient selective-id secure identity-based encryption without random oracles. In C. Cachin & J. Camenisch (Eds.), *Proceedings of Eurocrypt 2004* (Vol. 3027 of LNCS) (pp. 223-238). New York: Springer Verlag.

Boneh, D., & Franklin, M. K. (2001). Identity-based encryption from the weil pairing. In J. Kilian (Ed.), *Proceedings of Crypto 2001* (Vol. 2139 of LNCS) (pp. 213-229). New York: Springer Verlag.

Chen, L. (2007). An interpretation of identity-based cryptography. In A. Aldini & R. Gorrieri (Eds.), *Foundations of Security Analysis and Design, IV FOSAD 2006/2007 Tutorial Lectures* (Vol. 4677 of LNCS) (pp. 183-208). New York: Springer Verlag.

Cheung, L., & Newport, C. (2007). Provably secure ciphertext policy ABE. In P. Ning (Ed.), *Proceedings of the 14th ACM Conference on Computer and Communications Security* (pp. 456–465). New York: ACM.

ElGamal, T. (1985). A public key cryptosystem and a signature scheme based on discrete logarithms. In G. R. Blakley & D. Chaum (Eds.), *Proceedings of Crypto 1984* (Vol. 196 of LNCS) (pp. 10-18). New York: Springer Verlag.

Google. (2008). *Google Health*. Retrieved September 15, 2009 from http://www.google.com/health

Goyal, V., Pandey, O., Sahai, A., & Waters, B. (2006). Attribute-based encryption for fine-grained access control of encrypted data. In A. Juels (Ed.), *Proceedings of the 14th ACM Conference on Computer and Communications Security* (pp. 89-98). New York: ACM.

Graham, G. S., & Denning, P. J. (1971). Protection: principles and practice. In *Proceedings of the November 16-18, 1971, Fall Joint Computer Conference* (pp. 417–429).

Green, M., & Ateniese, G. (2007). Identity-based proxy re-encryption. In J. Katz & M. Yung (Eds.), *Proceedings of Applied Cryptography and Network Security* (Vol. 4521 of LNCS) (pp. 288-306). New York: Springer Verlag.

Ibraimi, L., Tang, Q., Hartel, P., & Jonker, W. (2009). Efficient and provable secure ciphertext-policy attribute-based encryption schemes. In F. Bao, H. Li, & G. Wang (Eds.), *Proceedings of Information Security Practice and Experience* (Vol. 5451 of LNCS) (pp. 1-12). New York: Springer Verlag.

Ivan, A., & Dodis, Y. (2003). Proxy cryptography revisited. In C. Neuman (Ed.), *Proceedings of the Network and Distributed System Security Symposium*. Citeseer.

Jakobsson, M. (1999). On quorum controlled asymmetric proxy re-encryption. In H. Imai & Y. Zheng (Eds.), *Proceedings of Public Key Cryptography* (Vol. 1560 of LNCS) (pp. 112–121). New York: Springer Verlag.

Liang, X., Cao, Z., Lin, H., & Shao, J. (2009). Attribute based proxy re-encryption with delegating capabilities. In W. Li, W. Susilo, & U. Tupakula (Eds.), *Proceedings of the 4th International Symposium on Information, Computer, and Communications Security* (pp. 276-286). New York: ACM.

Mambo, M., & Okamoto, E. (1997). Proxy Cryptosystems: Delegation of the power to decrypt ciphertexts. *IEICE Transactions on Fundamentals of Electronics, Communications and Computer Science, 80*(1), 54–63.

Matsuo, T. (2007). Proxy re-encryption systems for identity-based encryption. In T. Takagi, T. Okamoto, E. Okamoto, & T. Okamoto (Eds.), *Proceedings of Pairing-Based Cryptography - Pairing 2007* (Vol. 4575 of LNCS) (pp. 247-267). New York: Springer Verlag.

Microsoft. (2007). *HealthVault Connection Center.* Retrieved September 15, 2009 from http://www.healthvault.com/

Sahai, A., & Waters, B. (2005). Fuzzy identity-based encryption. In R. Cramer (Ed.), *Proceedings of Eurocrypt 2005* (Vol. 3494) (pp. 457-473). New York: Springer Verlag.

Shamir, A. (1985). Identity-based cryptosystems and signature schemes. In G. R. Blakely & D. Chaum (Eds.) *Proceedings of Crypto 1984 (Vol. 196 of LNCS)* (pp. 47-53). New York: Springer Verlag.

Shoup, V. (2006). Sequences of games: a tool for taming complexity in security proofs. Retrieved October 15, 2009 from http://shoup.net/papers/games.pdf

Tang, P. C., Ash, J. S., Bates, D. W., Overhage, J. M., & Sands, D. Z. (2006). Personal health records: definitions, benefits, and strategies for overcoming barriers to adoption. *Journal of the American Medical Informatics Association, 13*(2), 121–126. doi:10.1197/jamia.M2025

The personal health working group final report. (2004). *Connecting for health.* Retrieved October 2, 2009 from http://www.connectingforhealth.org/resources/wg_eis_final_report_0704.pdf

The US Department of Health and Human Services. (2003). *Summary of the HIPAA privacy rule.* Retrieved October 2, 2009 from http://www.hhs.gov/ocr/privacy/hipaa/understanding/summary/privacysummary.pdf

Wang, L., Cao, Z., Okamoto, T., Miao, Y., & Okamoto, E. (2006). Authorization-limited transformation-free proxy cryptosystems and their security analyses. *IEICE Transactions on Fundamentals of Electronics, Communications and Computer Science,* (1): 106–114. doi:10.1093/ietfec/e89-a.1.106

APPENDIX

A. Review of Pairing

We briefly review the basis of pairing and the related assumptions. More detailed information can be found in the seminal paper (Boneh and Franklin, 2001). A pairing (or, bilinear map) satisfies the following properties:

1. G and G_1 are two multiplicative groups of prime order p;
2. g is a generator of G;
3. $\hat{e}: G \times G \rightarrow G_1$ is an efficiently-computable bilinear map with the following properties:

    Bilinear: for all $u, v \in G$ and $a, b \in Z_p^*$, we have $\hat{e}(u^a, v^b) = \hat{e}(u, v)^{ab}$.

    Non-degenerate: $\hat{e}(g, g) \neq 1$.

As defined in (Boneh and Franklin, 2001), G is said to be a bilinear group if the group action in G can be computed efficiently and if there exists a group G_1 and an efficiently-computable bilinear map $\hat{e}$ as defined above.

The Bilinear Diffie-Hellman (BDH) problem in G is as follows: given $g, g^a, g^b, g^c \in G$ as input, output $\hat{e}(g, g)^{abc} \in G_1$. An algorithm A has advantage ε in solving BDH in G if:

$$\Pr[A(g, g^a, g^b, g^c) = \hat{e}(g, g)^{abc}] \geq \varepsilon.$$

Similarly, we say that an algorithm A has advantage ε in solving the decision BDH problem in G if:

$$|\Pr[A(g, g^a, g^b, g^c, g^{abc}) = 0] - \Pr[A(g, g^a, g^b, g^c, T) = 0]| \geq \varepsilon.$$

here the probability is over the random choice of $a, b, c \in Z_p^*$, the random choice of $T \in G_1$, and the random bits of A (the adversary is a nondeterministic algorithm).

Definition 1. *We say that the (decision) (t, ε)-BDH assumption holds in G if no t-time algorithm has advantage at least ε in solving the (decision) BDH problem in G.*

As in the general group, the Computational Diffie-Hellman (CDH) problem in G is as follows: given $g, g^a, g^b \in G$ as input, output $g^{ab} \in G$. An algorithm A has advantage ε in solving CDH in G if:

$$\Pr[A(g, g^a, g^b) = g^{ab}] \geq \varepsilon.$$

Definition 2. *We say that the (t, ε)-CDH assumption holds in G if no t-time algorithm has advantage at least ε in solving the CDH problem in G.*

Given a security parameter k, a problem (say, BDH) is believed to be intractable if any adversary has only negligible advantage in reasonable time. We usually define a scheme to be secure if any adversary has only a negligible advantage in the underlying security model. The time parameter is usually be ignored.

Definition 3. *The function* $P(k) : Z \to R$ *is said to be negligible if, for every polynomial* $f(k)$, *there exists an integer* N_f *such that* $P(k) \leq \dfrac{1}{f(k)}$ *for all* $k \geq N_f$.

B. Our Construction

In this section we give the construction of the type-and-identity-based proxy re-encryption scheme. In our scheme, the delegator and the delegatee are allowed to be from different domains, which nonetheless share some public parameters.

Suppose that the delegator is registered at KGC_1 in Boneh-Franklin IBE scheme $(\text{Setup}_1, \text{Extract}_1, \text{Encrypt}_1, \text{Decrypt}_1)$ and the delegatee is registered at KGC_2 in Boneh-Franklin IBE scheme $(\text{Setup}_2, \text{Extract}_2, \text{Encrypt}_2, \text{Decrypt}_2)$. The algorithms are defined as follows.

- Setup_1 and Extract_1 are the same as in the Boneh-Franklin scheme, except that Setup_1 outputs an additional hash function $H_2 : \{0,1\}^* \to Z_p^*$. The public parameter is $params_1 = (G, G_1, p, g, H_1, H_2, \hat{e}, pk_1)$, and the master key is $mk_1 = \alpha_1$.

- $\text{Encrypt}_1(m, t, id)$: Given a message m, a type t, and an identifier id, the algorithm outputs the ciphertext $c = (c_1, c_2, c_3)$ where $r \in_R Z_p^*$, $c_1 = g^r$, $c_2 = m \cdot \hat{e}(pk_{id}, pk)^{r \cdot H_2(sk_{id}||t)}$, $c_3 = t$.

- $\text{Decrypt}_1(c, sk_{id})$: Given a ciphertext $c = (c_1, c_2, c_3)$, the algorithm outputs the message
$$m = \frac{c_2}{\hat{e}(sk_{id}, c_1)^{H_2(sk_{id}||c_3)}}$$

Without loss of generality, suppose the delegator holds the identity id_i and the corresponding private key sk_{id_i}. Apart from the delegator, another party cannot run the Encrypt_1 algorithm under the delegator's identity id_i since he does not know sk_{id_i}.

Suppose that the delegatee (with identity id_j) possesses private key sk_{id_j} registered at KGC_2 in the Boneh-Franklin IBE scheme, where the public parameter is $params_2 = (G, G_1, p, g, H_1, \hat{e}, pk_2)$, the master key is $mk_2 = \alpha_2$, and $sk_{id_j} = H_1(id_j)^{\alpha_2}$. For the ease of comparison, we denote the IBE scheme as $(\text{Setup}_2, \text{Extract}_2, \text{Encrypt}_2, \text{Decrypt}_2)$ although these algorithms are identical to those described in Section B.

The Delegation Process

If the delegator wants to delegate his decryption right for messages with type t to the delegatee, the algorithms of the proxy re-encryption scheme are as follows.

$\text{Pextract}(id_i, id_j, t, sk_{id_i})$: Run by the delegator, this algorithm outputs the re-encryption key $rk_{id_i \to id_j}$, where $X \in_R G_1$ and

$$rk_{id_i \to id_j} = (t, sk_{id_i}^{-H_2(sk_{id_i}||t)} \cdot H_1(X), \text{Encrypt}_2(X, id_j)).$$

$\text{Preenc}(c_i, rk_{id_i \to id_j})$: Run by the Proxy, this algorithm, takes a ciphertext $c_i = (c_{i1}, c_{i2}, c_{i3})$ and the re-encryption key $rk_{id_i \to id_j}$ as input where $t = c_{i3}$, and outputs a new ciphertext $c_j = (c_{j1}, c_{j2}, c_{j3})$, where $c_{j1} = c_{i1}$ and

$$c_{j2} = c_{i2} \cdot \hat{e}(c_{i1}, sk_{id_i}^{-H_2(sk_{id_i}||c_{i3})} \cdot H_1(X))$$

$$= m \cdot \hat{e}(g^{\alpha_1}, pk_{id_i}^{rH_2(sk_{id_i}||t)}) \cdot \hat{e}(g^r, sk_{id_i}^{-H_2(sk_{id_i}||t)}) \cdot H_1(X))$$

$$= m \cdot \hat{e}(g^r, H_1(X)),$$

and $c_{j3} = \text{Encrypt}_2(X, id_j)$.

$\text{Decrypt}(c_j, sk_{id_j})$. Given a re-encrypted ciphertext c_j, the delegatee can obtain the plaintext m by computing:

$$m' = \frac{c_{j2}}{\hat{e}(c_{j1}, H_1(\text{Decrypt}_2(c_{j3}, sk_{id_j})))} = \frac{m \cdot \hat{e}(g^r, H_1(X))}{\hat{e}(g^r, H_1(X))} = m.$$

B.1. Security Model

We assume that the Proxy is semi-trusted in the following sense: it will honestly convert the delegator's ciphertexts using the re-encryption key; however, it might act actively to obtain some information about the plaintexts for the delegator and the delegatee. As mentioned in (Chen, 2007), the key escrow problem (TA owns a master key which can be used to decrypt each encrypted data) can be avoided by applying some standard techniques (such as secret sharing) to the underlying scheme, hence, we skip any further discussion in this paper. The delegatee may be curious in the sense that it may try to obtain some information about the plaintexts corresponding to the delegator's ciphertexts which have not been re-encrypted by the Proxy.

As a standard practice, we describe an attack game for modeling the semantic security against an adaptive chosen plaintext attack for the delegator (IND-ID-DR-CPA security) for our scheme. The IND-ID-DR-CPA game is carried out between a challenger and an adversary, where the challenger simulates the protocol execution and answers the queries from the adversary. Note that the allowed queries for the adversary reflect the adversary's capability in practice. Specifically, the game is as follows:

1. **Game setup:** The challenger takes a security parameter k as input, runs the Setup_1 algorithm to generate the public system parameter $params_1$ and the master key mk_1, and runs the Setup_2 algorithm to generate the public system parameter $params_2$ and the master key mk_2.

2. **Phase 1:** The adversary takes $params_1$ and $params_2$ as input and is allowed to issue the following types of queries:

    a. Extract_1 query with any identifier id : The challenger returns the private key sk corresponding to id.

    b. Extract_2 query with any identifier id' : The challenger returns the private key sk' corresponding to id'.

    c. Pextract query with (id, id', t) : The challenger returns the re-encryption key $rk_{id \to id'}$ for the type t.

    d. $\text{Preenc}^\dagger$ query with (m, t, id, id') : The challenger first computes $c = \text{Encrypt}_1(m, t, id)$ and then returns a new ciphertext c' which is obtained by applying the delegation key $rk_{id \to id'}$ to c, where $rk_{id \to id'}$ is issued for type t.

Once the adversary decides that Phase 1 is over, it outputs two equal length plaintexts m_0, m_1, a type t^*, and an identifier id^*. At the end of Phase 1, there are three constraints here:

a. id^* has not been the input to any Extract_1 query.

b. For any id', if (id^*, id', t^*) has been the input to a Pextract query then id' has not been the input to any Extract_2 query.

c. If there is a $\text{Preenc}^\dagger$ query with (m, t, id, id'), then (id, id', t) has not been queried to Pextract

3. **Challenge:** The challenger picks a random bit $b \in \{0, 1\}$ and returns $c^* = \text{Encrypt}_1(m_b, t^*, id^*)$ as the challenge to the adversary.

4. **Phase 2:** The adversary is allowed to continue issuing the same types of queries as in Phase 1. At the end of Phase 2, there are the same constraints as at the end of Phase 1.

5. **Guess (game ending):** The adversary outputs a guess $b' \in \{0, 1\}$.

At the end of the game, the adversary's advantage is defined to be $|\Pr[b' = b] - \frac{1}{2}|$. Compared with the CPA security formalizations in (Ateniese, Fu, Green and Hohenberger, 2006), in our case, we also take into account the categorization of messages for the delegator. The $\text{Preenc}^\dagger$ query reflects the fact that a curious delegatee has access to the the delegator's plaintexts.

B.2. Security Proof

Theorem 1. *For the type-and-identity-based proxy re-encryption scheme described in Section B, any adversary's advantage is negligible.*

Proof sketch. We suppose that the total number of queries issued to H_1 and H_2 is bounded by integer q_1 and q_2, respectively. Suppose an adversary A has the non-negligible advantage ε in the IND-ID-DR-CPA game. The security proof is done through a sequence of games.

Game_0: In this game, B faithfully answers the oracle queries from A. Specifically, B simulates the random oracle H_1 as follows: B maintains a list of vectors, each of them containing a request message, an element of G (the hash-code for this message), and an element of Z_p^*. After receiving a request message, B first checks its list to see whether the request message is already in the list. If the check succeeds, B returns the stored element of G; otherwise, B returns g^y, where y a randomly chosen element of Z_p^*, and stores the new vector in the list. A' simulates the random oracle H_2 as follows: B maintains a list of vectors, each of them containing a request message and an element of Z_p^* (the hash-code for this message). After receiving a request message, B first checks its list to see whether the request message is already in the list. If the check succeeds, B returns the stored element of Z_p^*; otherwise, B returns u which is a randomly chosen element of Z_p^*, and stores the new vector in the list.

Let $\delta_0 = \Pr[b' = b]$, as we assumed at the beginning, $| \delta_0 - \dfrac{1}{2} | = \varepsilon$.

Game_1: In this game, B answers the oracle queries from A as follows.

- **Game setup:** B faithfully simulates the setup phase.
- **Phase 1:** B randomly selects $j \in \{1, 2, \cdots, q_1 + 1\}$. If $j = q_1 + 1$, B faithfully answers the oracle queries from A. If $1 \le j \le q_1$, we assume the j-th input to H_1 is $\tilde{id}$ and B answers the oracle queries from A as follows: Answer the queries to Extract_1, Extract_2, Pextract, and $\text{Preenc}^\dagger$ faithfully, except that B aborts as a failure when $\tilde{id}$ is the input to a Extract_1 query.
- **Challenge:** After receiving (m_0, m_1, t^*, id^*) from the adversary, if one of the following events occurs, B aborts as a failure.
  a. id^* has been issued to H_1 as the i-th query and $i \ne j$,
  b. id^* has not been issued to H_1 and $1 \le j \le q_1$.

Note that, if the adversary does not abort then either $1 \le j \le q_1$ and $id^* = \tilde{id}$ is the input to j-th H_1 query or $j = q_1 + 1$ and id^* has not been the input to any H_1 query. B faithfully returns the challenge.

- **Phase 2:** B answers the oracle queries faithfully.
- **Guess (game ending):** The adversary outputs a guess $b' \in \{0, 1\}$.

The probability that B successfully ends is $\dfrac{1}{q_1 + 1}$, i.e. the probability that B does not abort in its execution is $\dfrac{1}{q_1 + 1}$. Let $\delta_1 = \Pr[b' = b]$ when B successfully ends, in which case $| \delta_1 = \delta_0 |$. Let θ_1 be the probability that B successfully ends and $b' = b$. We have $\theta_1 = \dfrac{\delta_1}{q_1 + 1}$.

$Game_2$: In this game, B simulates the protocol execution and answers the oracle queries from A in the following way.

- ○ **Game setup:** B faithfully simulates the setup phase. Recall that $pk_1 = g^{\alpha_1}$.
- ○ **Phase 1:** B randomly selects $j \in \{1, 2, \cdots, q_1 + 1\}$. If $j = q_1 + 1$, B faithfully answers the oracle queries from A. If $1 \leq j \leq q_1$, B answers j-th query to H_1 with g^β where $\beta \in_R Z_p^*$, and answers the oracle queries from A as follows. Suppose the input of the j-th query to H_1 is $\tilde{id}$.

    a. Answer $Extract_1$ and $Extract_2$ faithfully, except that B aborts as a failure when $\tilde{id}$ is the input to a $Extract_1$ query.

    Pextract query with (id, id', t): If $id = \tilde{id}$, B returns the re-encryption key $rk_{id \to id'}$, where

$$g_{tid'} \in_R G, \; X_{tid'} \in_R G_1, \; rk_{id \to id'} = (t, g_{tid'}, Encrypt_2(X_{tid'}, id')).$$

Otherwise, B answers the query faithfully. If id' has been queried to $Extract_2$, when $X_{tid'}$ is queried to H_1 then B returns $g_{tid'} \cdot h_{tid'}^{-1}$ where $h_{tid'} \in_R G$.

Preenc† query with (m, t, id, id'): If $id = \tilde{id}$, B returns

$$r \in_R Z_p^*, \; X_{tid'} \in_R G_1, \; c' = (g^r, \hat{e}(g^r, H_1(X_{tid'})), Encrypt_2(X_{tid'}, id')).$$

Otherwise, B answers the query faithfully.

- **Challenge:** After receiving (m_0, m_1, t^*, id^*) from the adversary, if one of the following events occurs, B aborts as a failure.

    a. id^* has been issued to H_1 as the i-th query and $i \neq j$,

    b. id^* has not been issued to H_1 and $1 \leq j \leq q_1$.

Note that, if the adversary does not abort then either $1 \leq j \leq q_1$ and $id^* = \tilde{id}$ is the input to j-th H_1 query or $j = q_1 + 1$ and id^* has not been the input to any H_1 query. In the latter case, B sets $H_1(id^*) = g^\beta$ where $\beta \in_R Z_p^*$, and returns $c^* = (c_1^*, c_2^*, c_3^*)$ as the challenge to the adversary, where:

$$b \in_R \{0,1\}, \; r \in_R Z_p^*, \; T \in_R G_1, \; c_1^* = g^r, \; c_2^* = m_b \cdot T, \; c_3^* = t^*.$$

- **Phase 2:** B answers the oracle queries from A as in Phase 1.
- **Guess (game ending):** The adversary outputs a guess $b' \in \{0,1\}$.

Let θ_2 be the probability that B successfully ends and $b' = b$. We have $\theta_2 = \dfrac{1}{2(q_1 + 1)}$ since $T \in_R G_1$. Let E_1 be the event that, for some id' and t, the adversary issues a H_2 query with the input $g^{\alpha_1 \beta} \| t$ or $X_{tid'}$ is issued to H_1 while id' has not been issued to $Extract_2$. Compared with $Game_1$, $Game_2$

differs when E_1 occurs. From the difference lemma (Shoup, 2006), we have $\mid \delta_2 - \delta_1 \mid \leq \varepsilon_2$ which is negligible in the random oracle model based on the BDH assumption. Note that $(\text{Setup}_2, \text{Extract}_2, \text{Encrypt}_2, \text{Decrypt}_2)$ is one-way based on the BDH assumption and BDH implies CDH.

From $\mid \theta_2 - \theta_1 \mid \leq \varepsilon_2$ and $\theta_2 = \dfrac{1}{2(q_1+1)}$, we have $\mid \dfrac{1}{2(q_1+1)} - \theta_1 \mid \leq \varepsilon_2$. In addition, from $\mid \delta_0 - \dfrac{1}{2} \mid = \varepsilon$,

$\mid \delta_1 - \delta_0 \mid \leq \varepsilon_1$ and $\theta_1 = \dfrac{\delta_1}{q_1+1}$, we have $\dfrac{\varepsilon}{q_1+1} \leq \dfrac{\varepsilon_1}{q_1+1} + \varepsilon_2$. Because $\varepsilon_i \ (1 \leq i \leq 2)$ are negligible

and ε is assumed to be non-negligible, we get a contradiction. As a result, the proposed scheme is IND-ID-DR-CPA secure based on the CDH assumption in the random oracle model, given that $(\text{Setup}_2, \text{Extract}_2, \text{Encrypt}_2, \text{Decrypt}_2)$ is one-way.

This work was previously published in International Journal of Computational Models and Algorithms in Medicine, Volume 1, Issue 2, edited by Aryya Gangopadhyay, pp. 1-21, copyright 2010 by IGI Publishing (an imprint of IGI Global).

Chapter 7
Privacy Preserving Integration of Health Care Data

Xiaoyun He
Rutgers University, USA

Basit Shafiq
Rutgers University, USA

Jaideep Vaidya
Rutgers University, USA

Nabil Adam
Rutgers University, USA

Tom White
NY Office of Mental Health & Columbia University, USA

ABSTRACT

For health care related research studies the medical records of patients may need to be retrieved from multiple sites with different regulations on the disclosure of health information. Given the sensitive nature of health care information, privacy is a major concern when patients' health care data is used for research purposes. In this paper, the authors propose approaches for integration and querying of health care data from multiple sources in a secure and privacy preserving manner. In particular, the first approach ensures secure data integration based on unique identifiers, and the second one considers data integration based on quasi identifiers, for which a rule-based framework is proposed for cross-linking data records, including secure character matching.

INTRODUCTION

Health care research studies often involve analysis of huge amount of data collected from various sources including health care providers, pharmacies, insurance companies, government agencies, and research institutions. Given the sensitive nature of health information and the social and legal implications for its disclosure, privacy is a major concern for information sharing in the healthcare domain (Rindfleisch, 1997; Kelman et al., 2002; HIPAA, 2000).

Protecting the privacy of individually identifiable health information is more important when such information is used for clinical or health services related research. The Health Insurance Portability and Accountability Act (HIPAA) privacy rule strictly prohibits sharing of individu-

DOI: 10.4018/978-1-4666-0282-3.ch007

ally identifiable health information with clinical researchers who are not covered entities. The covered entities, as defined in this privacy rule, include health plans, healthcare clearing houses, and healthcare providers that transmit health information electronically in connection with certain defined HIPAA transactions, such as claims or eligibility inquiries (HIPAA, 2000). For research purposes, only de-identified or anonymized health information can be used.

Several National initiatives are addressing the privacy and security concerns raised by HIPAA. The Health Information Security and Privacy Consortium (HISPC) is documenting and reconciling differences in state, local, and federal privacy and security laws with a goal of enabling privacy-protected sharing of data across state lines, and so that those data can be incorporated into a National Health Information Network (NHIN). HISPC must reconcile differences between HIPAA, and numerous state-specific laws regulating sharing of mental health, substance abuse, HIV, and cancer information. In some states, conflicting regulations prevent the sharing of clinical data about mental health and substance abuse within single hospitals, even though many patients have both mental health and substance abuse diagnoses. Successful completion of the HISPC efforts is essential to establish the trust needed to motivate consumers to share their data through the NHIN. In this paper, we present a technique for integrating data across organizations that is of direct relevance to these efforts.

As discussed above, for health care related research studies the medical records of patients may need to be retrieved from multiple sites with different regulations on the disclosure of health information. In absence of the identity information, correlation and integration of such records on a per patient basis in a privacy preserving manner is an important research issue. As an example, consider the following queries related to a research study for determining defective anti-depressant drugs:

Query 1: What percentage of HIV infected patients taking any prescribed anti-depressant medication are diagnosed with acute psychiatric disorder?

Query 2: For each HIV infected patient diagnosed with acute psychiatric disorder find all the prescribed drugs the patient took after being diagnosed with HIV.

The above queries require integrating data from multiple sources including the state health department managing HIV test records, pharmacy databases storing patient records related to prescription drugs, and mental health clinics treating patients with psychiatric disorder. For preserving the privacy of individual records, we need to ensure that the query result do not reveal any individually identifiable information to the querying party. Additionally, during the process of integrating data from multiple sources, none of the sources should be able to learn/infer any information about any of the patients beyond what these sources already know. For instance, the pharmacist should not be able to learn which patients have been tested positive for HIV or which patients are receiving treatment for severe psychiatric disorder.

One of the large challenges in merging data is the lack of a common identifier across data systems. There are numerous commercial applications for creating enterprise master person indexes from distributed databases. Some of these are tolerant of missing, mistyped, or conflicting data. The approach commonly used by Regional Health Information Organizations (RHIOs) is that of RxHub – to only cross-link patients who have exact matches of five elements: first name, last name, birthday, gender, and zip code. RxHub is a third party data aggregator which has contracts with most major pharmacy benefits managers. Hospitals may use RxHub to request all historical pharmacy data from patients by sending those five demographic parameters to RxHub. RxHub queries its data sources to determine whether they have data for the requested patient, and if so, retrieve and organize the data from the various sources, keeping appropriate audit trails.

For now, this paper focuses on the challenges of research use of patient data, and assumes that all data sources either have the same, shared, complete identifier, such as social security number or have quasi identifiers for potential linkage. Thus, assuming that the patients in each source's database are identified by their *social security number* (SSN), the data form multiple sources can be joined on this attribute to answer the above queries. However, this simple joining of data would reveal personally identifiable health information to the querying party as well as to the data sources. Of course, one may trust a third party (like RxHub) to have access to all of the data and perform the join (Kelman et al., 2002). However, this is not sufficient. It would be much better to reduce the trust factor as much as possible. Agarwal et al. (Agrawal et al., 2003) propose an encryption based approach to do information sharing across databases. While the key concepts are similar and it can be used to answer queries like Query 1, the protocol is restricted to only two parties. Also, another problem is that the querying party could actually contribute data, which can lead to severe problems with security if the querying party is malicious. The querying party will also learn the values of all the attributes in the query result. If the query result is computed by joining data from different sources on the SSN field, then the querying party will learn the identity of patients from the query result. The closest work related to ours is the protocol by O'Keefe et al. (2004). Again, there are two problems with their approach. First, it only works for two data sources. More importantly, a malicious querying party can trick the data source and get extra information which is not included in the query result.

In this paper, we propose approaches that allow querying and integration of data from multiple sources in a secure and privacy preserving man-

ner. In particular, the first approach ensures secure data integration based on unique identifiers, and the second one considers data integration based on quasi identifiers, for which we propose a rule-based framework for cross-linking data records, including secure character matching.

The proposed approaches employ cryptography based solutions, whereby all the sensitive values in the query result are encrypted by all the data sources using their own keys. Since the encryption key of a source is not known to any other source or the querying party, therefore it is computationally infeasible for any party to extract the individually identifiable or sensitive information from the query result. Moreover, the proposed approaches do not allow the querying party to retrieve any sensitive or non-sensitive information from sources which is beyond the scope of the query.

PROBLEM DEFINITION

We consider a distributed environment with heterogeneous distribution of data. This means that different sources collect different features of information for the same set of data. As opposed to this, with homogeneous data distribution, different sources collect the same pieces of information about different entities. The second case is easier to deal with since there is no real integration to be done. Therefore we only look at the heterogeneous one. Each source S_i has a relation R_i with attributes $(a_{i1}, a_{i2}, ..., a_{ik})$. We consider two cases. In the first case, we assume that a_{i1} uniquely identifies tuples in the relation R_i, meaning that a_{i1} is the primary key of the relation R_i. Without loss of generality we assume that no other attribute or set of attributes excluding a_{i1} can serve as a candidate key for the relation R_i. The primary key of each relation is the same and the join of two or more relations is always computed on the primary key value, i.e., only those tuples in the relation R_i and R_j can be joined for which $a_{i1} = a_{j1}$. We say that the relation with attributes $(f(a_{i1}), a_{i2}, ..., a_{ik} a_{j2}, ..., a_{jm})$ is a privacy preserving join of relations R_i and R_j if $a_{i1} = a_{j1}$ and it is computationally infeasible for any party including data sources to determine a_{i1} from $f(a_{i1})$. In the second case, we assume that no common identifiers are present across sources and integration has to be done based on quasi-identifiers. By quasi-identifiers, we mean sets of attributes that can together identify a person. For example, name, address, and date of birth can serve as quasi-identifiers.

Given the above two cases, in this paper, we are addressing the problem of computing the privacy preserving join of n relations; whereby a relation R_i $(1 \leq i \leq n)$ is owned by source S_i.

Data Integration

In this section, we present approaches to achieve secure integration of data for the two cases: (1) all data sources have the same unique data identifiers, such as the social security number or health insurance policy number; (2) no common identifiers are present across sources and integration has to be done based on quasi-identifiers.

Data Integration Based on Unique Identifiers

The basic idea of the proposed approach is to use commutative encryption to encrypt all data items in each party's data set. Commutative encryption is an important tool used in many cryptographic protocols. Pohlig-Hellman (1978) is one example of a commutative encryption scheme (based on the discrete logarithm problem). This or any other commutative encryption scheme would work well for our purposes. An encryption algorithm is commutative if the order of encryption does not matter. Thus, for any two encryption keys E_1 and E_2, and any message m, $E_1(E_2(m)) = E_2(E_1(m))$. The same property applies to decryption as well – thus to decrypt a message encrypted by two keys, it is sufficient to decrypt it one key at a time.

The main step is for each source to encrypt its data set with its keys and pass the encrypted data set to the next source. This source again encrypts the received data using its encryption keys and passes the encrypted data to the next source until all sources have encrypted the data. As discussed in the above section, the attributes of a data set can be divided into two: key attribute and non-key attributes. The key attribute of each data set is the same and the join of two or more data sets from different sources is always computed on the values of their key attribute. Since we are using commutative encryption, the encrypted values of the key attribute across different data sets will be equal if and only if their original values are equal. Thus, all the data sets from different sources can be joined on their key attributes which are encrypted by all sources. The encryption prevents any source or querying party from knowing the actual value of the key attribute.

The algorithm for computing the privacy preserving join of data sets from multiple sources consists of three stages: *encryption, joining* and *decryption*. In the following we discuss each of these stages.

1. **Encryption**. In this stage, the joining attribute of each data set is encrypted by all sources. Each source S_i generates two pairs of encryption and decryption keys: (Ek_{i1}, Dk_{i1}) and (Ek_{i2}, Dk_{i2}). For each data set R_i $(1 \leq i \leq n)$, the source S_i encrypts the values of the key attribute and non-key attributes of all tuples in the data set R_i with its keys Ek_{i1} and Ek_{i2} respectively. After this encryption, the source S_i passes the resulting data set $(Ek_{i1}(a_{i1}), Ek_{i2}(a_{i2}), ..., Ek_{i2}(a_{ik}))$ to its right neighbor S_j, where $j = (i+1)$ mod n. The neighbor S_j in turns encrypts the received data set with its encryption keys Ek_{j1} and Ek_{j2}. In addition S_j permutes the tuples in the encrypted data set to prevent the owner of the data set to correlate the encrypted values of the key attribute with their actual values

based on the ordering of tuples in the data set. S_j then forwards the resulting data set to its next neighbor for encryption. This process continues until the data set is encrypted by all the sources. Figure 1(a) illustrates the data flow and message exchange among three sources S_1, S_2, and S_3 for encryption of *prescription drug data* managed by S_1.

2. **Joining**. Once all the data sets are encrypted by all sources, they can be joined on the encrypted value of the key attribute as discussed above. This join can be computed by any source which has all the encrypted data sets. The source computing the join can be specified *a priori* or can be randomly selected. We do not go into the details of selection of the source for joining the encrypted data sets due to the space limitation. Assuming that source for computation of the final join have been selected, each source will forward its local data set which is encrypted by all other sources to the selected source. The selected source then computes the join and sends the resulting data set to the querying party. We will refer to the resulting data set after joining tuples from different data sets on the encrypted value of their key attributes as the *joined data set*. Note that it is computationally infeasible for any source or the querying party to extract the original value of any of the attributes of the joined data set. Figure 1(b) depicts the process of joining of encrypted data from three sources S_1, S_2, and S_3 and forwarding of the integrated dataset with all encrypted values to the querying party.

3. **Decryption**. The joined data set forwarded to the querying party has both key and non key attributes in encrypted form. However, the querying party should be able to retrieve the values of non-key attributes without learning or inferring the actual value of the key attribute in any of the tuples. Therefore, the non-key attribute values in the joined data

set need to be decrypted using the decryption keys of all sources one after the other. Since each source has its own decryption key which is not known to anyone, therefore the decryption of the non key attributes of the joined data set can only occur at each source. As stated earlier, it is sufficient for each party to decrypt these, one followed by the other, to get the actual data. However, the querying party needs to ensure that none of the sources can see the real data.

Therefore, before sending the joined data set for decryption to individual sources, the querying party first encrypts all the attribute values in the data set using its encryption key EKq. This ensures that the actual values of the non-key attributes in the joined data set can be viewed only by the querying party. After encryption, the querying party sends the joined data set to source S_1 which decrypts the non-key attribute of the joined data set using its decryption key DK_{12}. Source S_1 then forwards the resulting data set to S_2 for decryption of the non key attributes using DK_{22}. This process continues until all the sources have applied their decryption keys on the non-key attributes of the received data set. Finally, the data set is sent back to the querying party which applies its decryption key DK_q to retrieve the original values of the non key attributes in the joined data set. Note that during the entire process of decryption, none of the sources can learn the actual value of any of the attributes of the joined data set. Moreover after decryption, the values of the key attribute of the joined data set remain encrypted with the encryption keys of all the sources, and it is computationally infeasible for the querying party to extract the actual values of the key attribute.

The process for decryption of non-key attributes will be similar to the encryption process shown in Figure 1(a), except that instead of applying encryption key on the non-key attributes, each source will now apply its decryption key on these attributes of the joined data set.

Security analysis. The algorithm depicted in Figure 2 computes the join of multiple data sets distributed among different sources without revealing any confidential/private information to the querying party. Note that the querying party cannot be a source for any data set that is integrated with other data sets for query evaluation. If the querying party is one of the sources, then it can infer the actual value of the identity (key) attribute by comparing the values of those non-key attributes that are common between the joined data set and its local data set. For instance, consider Query 2 given in the introduction section. If this query is issued by the pharmacist who has access to the pharmacy database of prescription drugs, then the pharmacist can determine the identity of the patients infected with HIV by comparing the values of the attributes such as Drug Name and Prescription Date that are common between the joined data set (query result) and the prescription drug data set stored in the pharmacy database. Therefore, this algorithm cannot be used to evaluate queries which require joining of vertically partitioned data with the querying party as one of the data source. Another limitation of the proposed algorithm is that it cannot prevent sources from inferring the attribute values if the joined data set corresponding to the query result is too small. In order to avoid this inference of attribute values, the algorithm does not compute the join if the size of any of the input data set is less than certain threshold value r.

Information security against querying party and data sources. Assuming that the querying party does not contribute any of its data set for the join operation and all parties follow the algorithm depicted in Figure 1, then the joined data set generated by the algorithm will be privacy preserving. Specifically, the querying party can view the values of non-key attributes only without learning or inferring the actual values of the key attribute in any of the tuples in the joined data set. Moreover, during the process of hashing,

Figure 1. Graphical illustration of: (a) the data flow for encryption of Prescription Drug Table with three sources; (b) joining of encrypted tables which is sent to the querying party; (c) data flow for decryption of the joined dataset.

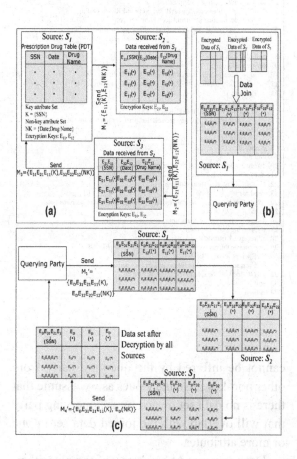

joining, and decryption, no source will learn the actual values of any attribute of any data set that is not owned by that source. In the following, we provide an intuitive reasoning of this claim.

Querying party. In the joined data set, the value of the key attribute in each tuple is encrypted by all sources using their secret keys. Since, these keys are not known to the querying party, it is computationally infeasible for the querying party to learn the actual values of the key attribute from the encrypted values. Also, for any tuple in the joined data set, the value of the key attribute

Figure 2. Privacy-preserving join algorithm

```
Algorithm 1. Securely computing privacy-preserving join
Require: n > 1 sources, each having a local relation Rᵢ.
Require: a querying party QP, that joins the n relations. QP cannot provide any of its
local relations in the joining operation.
Require: threshold r >> 1, used to prevent inference of key attribute values because
of too few tuples in the joined relation
1.   {stage 1 – Hashing}
2.   for all sources Sᵢ {parallel operations} do
3.       if |Rᵢ| < r then broadcast ABORT return ERROR end if
4.       generate the encryption and decryption key pairs (Ek_{i1}, Dk_{i1}) and (Ek_{i2}, Dk_{i2})
5.       M ← EncryptJoiningAttr(Rᵢ, Ek_{i1}) ∪ EncryptOtherAttr(Rᵢ, Ek_{i2})
6.       Permute M
7.       send M to source Sⱼ, where j = (i+1) mod n
8.   end for
9.   for each source Sᵢ, j = 0 … n - 1  do
10.      M' ← receive from source Sᵢ, where i ⊠ (j-1) mod n
11.      M ← EncryptJoiningAttr(M', k_{j1}) ⊠ EncryptOtherAttr(M', k_{j2})
12.      Permute M
13.      p ← (j+1) mod n
14.      if Sₚ is the owner of the relation M'' then
15.          send M'' to S₁ {or any pre-selected party for join computation}
16.      else
17.          send M'' to Sₚ
18.      end if
19.  end for
20.  {stage 2 – Join Computed by S₁ or any pre-selected party}
21.  for j = 0 … n - 1, j ≠ i do
22.      Rⱼʰ ← receive from source Sⱼ
23.  end for
24.  R ← Join R₀ʰ, R₁ʰ,…, R_{n-1}ʰ on the first (joining) attribute of each relation
25.  send R to QP
26.  {stage 3 – Decryption phase initiated by Querying Party}
27.  if Querying Party QP then
28.      receive R from any source
29.      generate the encryption and decryption key pair (Ekₚ, Dkₚ)
30.      Encrypt R with Ekₚ
31.      Each source Sᵢ decrypt R with its key Dk_{i2} one after the other, sending it to QP
32.      QP decrypts the relation received, R with Dkₚ
33.  end if
34.  return
```

cannot be inferred by the querying party from other non-key attribute values as we assume that there is no data set owned by the querying party that will overlap with the joined data set in one or more attributes.

Data sources. At any stage of the algorithm, none of the sources can extract the actual values of any of the attribute in any of the data set owned by other sources because of encryption. Moreover, the requirement that each data set must have at least *r* (>> 1) tuples and the permutation of every data set a source receives for encryption prevent the owner of a data set to correlate the encrypted values of any attribute with their actual values based on the ordering of tuples in the data set.

Data Integration Based on Quasi Identifiers

A major challenge in data integration is the lack of common identifiers that uniquely identify individuals across data sources. There are numerous commercial applications for creating enterprise master person indexes from distributed databases. These applications rely on a trusted third party to link data records from different sources based on the similarity measure of various non-key attributes or quasi identifiers such as name, address, and date of birth. For instance, many Regional Health Information Organizations (RHIOs) request patients' medical history from RxHub (2004) – a third party data aggregator which has contracts with most major pharmacy benefits managers. RxHub queries its data sources to determine whether they have data for the requested patients, and if so, retrieves and organizes the data from the various sources, keeping appropriate audit trails. RxHub cross-links only those patients who have exact matches of five elements: first name, last name, birthday, gender, and zip code. We note here that RxHub in this case serves as a trusted third-party, thus it suffers from the trusted third-party limitations discussed earlier.

A major difficulty in linking records from different sources based on non-key attributes (or quasi-identifiers) is of missing, mistyped, or conflicting values across data sources. Moreover, the sources may store these values in different formats. All these factors and the privacy requirement for healthcare information make the problem of data integration more challenging. To address this challenge, we propose a rule-based record linkage approach that considers matching of the following non-key attributes: name (first name, last name), address, date of birth, and gender. The proposed approach builds on the commutative encryption based technique (discussed earlier) and is tolerant to missing, mistyped, abbreviated, and conflicting data values by supporting approximate matching. The matching criterion is different for different attribute types. Below we explain the rule-based framework for cross-linking data records based on the either exact or approximate matching of attribute types. Next, we discuss how matching is performed for each attribute type, which are needed for the rule-based framework.

1. **Rule specification framework for record linkage.** Any two data records maintained at two different sites may not be linked solely based on the exact or approximate matching of pair-wise non-key attributes. Here, we consider a rule based framework for linking data records distributed across multiple sources. The framework will support specification of rules that defines the criteria for data linkage at the attribute level as well as at the record level. For instance, at the attribute level a rule may define that two name strings are considered as matched if they have at least 80% similarity, i.e., the ratio between the longest common sequences of the two name strings and the longest name string is greater than 0.8 (*Gower* and *Gover* have a similarity measure of 80%). A record level rule specifies the criteria for linking data records based on the matching of one or more attributes. For instance, a record level rule may state that two data records stored at different sites can be linked if the first names match with 70% similarity, the last names match with 90% similarity, and the year of birth matches exactly. In figure 3, we outline the framework for record linking.

Note that, since the criteria for linking data records strongly depends on the underlying application, we shall consult domain experts for creating a comprehensive set of rules for record linkage. These rules can be accessed by users or system administrators, who select the appropriate rules for data retrieval and sharing.

2. **Attribute matching.** Now, we discuss exact and approximate matching for different types of non-key attributes across different data sources.

   ○ **Name matching:** We consider two types of conflicts for name matching: *abbreviation* (e.g., *David Gower* abbreviated as *Dave Gower* in one source and *D. Gower* in some other source), *mistyping* (e.g. *David Gower* in one source and *Davd Gover* in another source).

     ▪ *Abbreviation conflict.* Abbreviation conflicts occur because of the use of nick names or initials by different data sources. Clearly, abbreviation conflicts cannot be resolved by any of the two approximate name matching approaches discussed above in the context of mistyping conflicts. For resolution of abbreviation conflict, we rely on a name ontology which for a given name will provide the corresponding nick names. The nick names along with the name initials will be appended to the original data record as meta-data. For name-matching across data sources, we will again employ the commutative encryption based technique, whereby all the abbreviated names appended as meta-data will be encrypted in addition to the exact name strings. This will allow cross linking of names across different sources in a secure and privacy-preserving manner, where one source may store the full name of an individual, whereas the other source may have the abbreviated name of the same individual.

■ *Mistyping conflict*: For resolving naming conflicts due to mistyping, the following two techniques can be used: secure and private string comparison (Atallah et al., 2003) and encrypted character matching. Note that, in this work, we focus on the latter, for which we propose a secure technique.

' The secure and private string comparison approach, proposed by Atallah et al. (2003), uses weighted edit distance to determine the similarity of two strings. The secure edit distance between two strings is defined as the least-cost set of insertions, deletions, and substitutions required to transform one string into the other. The cost for each individual operation (insertion, deletion, substitution) may not be uniform and may depend on the type of operation as well as on the character on which such operation is performed. For secure computation of the edit distance, the approach relies on the secure two-party protocol for split data with homomorphic encryption system. This protocol ensures that neither party reveals

any information about their strings other than what can be inferred from the edit distance.

On the other hand, our proposed encrypted character matching technique computes the similarity of two strings based on the number of matching characters in a secure manner. This technique is similar to the commutative encryption based data joining technique discussed in the previous section; however in this case, instead of encrypting the entire name string, each individual character of the name string is separately encrypted. The encrypted characters can then be compared for a given set of name strings to determine the similarity measure in terms of the length of the longest common sub-sequence of name strings in the given set. One important feature of the encrypted character matching we present here is to prevent each source learning the other sources' characters that are common to these sources. Figure 4 describes the algorithm of the encrypted character matching.

In the first stage, commutative encryptions are conducted between two sources. After this stage, we may simply exchange the encrypted data among the sources. Then, the common characters among the strings can be discovered. However, this would cause the disclosure of these common characters to the participating sources. To prevent such disclosure, we instead need a round of permutations as described in stage two. But, unless the permutations conducted locally at

Figure 3. Outline of rule framework for record linking

Rule Specification Framework for Record Linking

Require: A rule specifying similarity thresholds $(t_1, t_2, ..., t_m)$ on attributes $(a_1, a_2, ..., a_m)$ respectively

Require: Given two records r_i and r_j from source S_i and S_j respectively

1. {check the corresponding attribute matching based on the next section }
2. **for** all common attributes a_k in r_i and r_j **do**
3.   if (similarity($r_i(a_k)$, $r_j(a_k)$)) does not satisfy t_k)
4.   **return** FAIL
5. **end for**
6. **return** SUCCEED

---

each source are commutative, the character order in each string may not be preserved, leading to the mismatch problem. Nevertheless, such commutative property may not exist in these private permutations. Therefore, we incorporate a set of fresh encryption/decryption into the permutations. Specifically, each party will only see the encrypted character, and the corresponding order of each character from a pair of strings is retained. This is due to the fact that we are able to perform the permutations in the same order on the encrypted string, as evident from line 15 to line 26 in algorithm 2. In this way, we are able to achieve our goal here – conduct character matching while ensuring individual data privacy for each party. That is, each party will not be able to infer any single character in the string that the other parties have. To illustrate the main procedures in Algorithm 2, we give an example as follows.

Example: Source S_1 has a string G_1 that consists of 4 characters a_1, a_2, a_3, a_4, and source S_2 has a string G_2 that consists of 4 characters a_1, a_2, b_3, a_4. After the first stage of encryptions, source S_1 has $E_{11}E_{21}(a_1), E_{12}E_{22}(a_2), E_{13}E_{23}(a_3), E_{14}E_{24}(a_4)$, which we denote as e_1, e_2, e_3, e_4, respectively. Similarly, source S_2 has $E_{21}E_{11}(a_1), E_{22}E_{12}(a_2), E_{23}E_{13}(b_3), E_{24}E_{14}(a_4)$, which we denote as e_1', e_2', e_3', e_4' respectively. Since the encryptions are commutative, we essentially have $e_1 = e_1', e_2 = e_2', e_4 = e_4'$, which would be disclosed to the sources if, at this point, the two sequences (e_1, e_2, e_3, e_4) and (e_1', e_2', e_3', e_4') are directly compared. Therefore, we need another round encryption. Source S_2 does the encryptions $E_2(e_1', e_2', e_3', e_4')$, and send them to source S_1. Source S_1 does the encryptions by E_1 and permutations by F_1, getting $F_1E_1(e_1, e_2, e_3, e_4)$, and $F_1E_1E_2(e_1', e_2', e_3', e_4')$. They are sent to source S_2. Source S_2 does permutations by F_2 and the decryption by D_2, getting $F_2F_1E_1(e_1, e_2, e_3, e_4)$, and $F_2F_1E_1(e_1', e_2', e_3', e_4')$. These two sequences can be compared at any source so as to know whether the corresponding character matches or not.

- **Address matching:** In order to resolve address conflicts due to mistyping or format mismatch, we compare addresses based on geo-codes such as longitude /latitude coordinates or zip code. For geo-code extraction, we can make use of existing GIS services and employ commutative encryption for comparison and cross-linking the extracted geo-codes.

- **Date of birth:** For linking date of birth across different records, we can compare individual fields (year, month, and day) separately. This matching will be ranked based on the number of matching fields, for instance two records that match in both year and month are more likely to be of the same person than the records that only match in the year field. Since, the individual fields are linked based on exact match, the commutative encryption method discussed above can be employed for this purpose.

- **Gender:** We shall consider exact match of the gender attribute for linking data records.

In fact, we also need to have user involvement in the development process for the integration right from the start. As in many other applications, it is better to have a test bed involving users and determining their acceptability. This will facilitate in adjusting the parameters of the solution as well as establish the user acceptability – from the organizational perspective, individual patient perspective, as well as from the researcher perspective. Different interfaces could also be defined and tested within the test bed environment. Once developed, we shall hold workshops and symposia inviting data owners, data users, and industry representatives to demonstrate the scope of our solution and increase its acceptability.

RELATED WORK

The HIPAA privacy law strictly prohibits release of personally identifiable health information of a patient to non-covered entities. Examples of the non-covered entities include medical researchers, administrative staff, and healthcare professionals who are not directly involved in the diagnosis and treatment process of the patient without consent. In order to share protected health information, HIPAA approves two methods for data identification. The first method, called *"safe harbor"*, requires the removal of each of the eighteen identifiers enumerated at Section 164.514(b)(2) of the Privacy Rule (HIPAA, 2000). Data sanitized by removing these identifiers is considered as de-identified, unless the custodian of the data has reason to believe that it would be possible to use the remaining information alone or in combination with other information to identify the subject. In the second method, statistical techniques are employed that provide guarantees, which can be verified by an expert, on the fact that the data has been de-identified to an extent that the risk of privacy loss is small.

Computer science research has demonstrated that the above approaches to de-identification may not be sufficient to protect against data disclosure in the face of auxiliary information (i.e., Samarati & Sweeney, 1998; Bayardo & Agrawal, 2005; Machanavajjhala et al., 2007; Li et al., 2007; Agrawal & Srikant, 1994; Agrawal & Srikant, 2000). For example, a *safe harbor* set of healthcare data may be examined alongside US Census bureau data based on the zip code and date of birth of each patient to determine the owner of each record in the de-identified data set. This is known as a *linking attack*.

A further concern with naïve de-identification, such as the wholesale removal of attributes, is that the attributes in question may be valuable for medical research and the transformed values may actually stem medical analysis and innova-

tion; as correlations and insight may have been blindly removed.

An initial approach to address the problems in the context of data sharing was outlined by Samarati and Sweeney (1998) in their paper on k-anonymity. In a k-anonymized data set, each record is indistinguishable from at least $k-1$ other records. The process of k-anonymization involves data suppression (deleting cell values or entire tuples) and cell-value generalization (replacing specific values with more generals ones). A larger value of k provides greater privacy protection, but less specific data. K-anonymization was designed to avoid linkage attacks, while preserving the integrity of the de-identified data. However, k-anonymity and its enhanced variants (Machanavajjhala et al., 2007; Li et al., 2007) do not address the issue of data integration at the individual patient level because of the introduction of noise/error during the anonymization process.

Our proposed work supports secure and privacy-preserving integration, querying, and analysis of distributed data without employing trusted third parties. To address the limitation of anonymization and de-identification techniques for data integration, we utilize cryptographic techniques to protect privacy. In this area, Lindell and Pinkas (2002) were the first to propose a cryptography based technique for the construction of decision trees.

All of the cryptographic work falls under the theoretical framework of Secure Multiparty Computation. Yao first postulated the two-party comparison problem (Yao's Millionaire Protocol) and developed a provably secure solution (Yao, 1986). This was extended to multiparty computations by Goldreich et al. (1987). They developed a framework for secure multiparty computation, and in (Goldreich, 2004) proved that computing a function privately is equivalent to computing it securely. The key result in this field is that any function can be computed securely. Thus, the generic circuit evaluation technique can be used to solve our current problem.

Figure 4. Secure character matching algorithm

Algorithm 2. Secure character matching

Require: A pair of strings G_i and G_j with maximum length L.

Require: G_i is owned by source S_i and G_j is owned by a different source S_j

1. {stage 1 – a round of encryptions}
2. At source S_i (resp., S_j):
3.   generate the encryption keys $(E_{i1}, E_{i2}, ..., E_{iL})$ (resp., $(E_{j1}, E_{j2}, ..., E_{jL})$)
4.   **for** each character $G_i[k]$ (resp., $G_j[k]$) in string G_i (resp., G_j) **do**
5. $EG_i[k] \leftarrow Encrypt(E_{ik}, G_i[k])$ (resp., $EG_j[k] \leftarrow Encrypt(E_{jk}, G_j[k])$)
6.   send $EG_i[k]$ (resp., $EG_j[k]$) to source S_j (resp., S_i)
7.   **end for**
8.   **for** each character $EG_j[k]$ (resp., $EG_i[k]$) in string EG_j (resp., EG_i) **do**
9. $EG_j[k] \leftarrow Encrypt(E_{ik}, EG_j[k])$ (resp., $EG_i[k] \leftarrow Encrypt(E_{ik}, G_i[k])$)
10.   send $EG_j[k]$ (resp., $EG_i[k]$) to source S_j (resp., S_i)
11.   **end for**
12.
13. {after stage 1, source S_i (resp., S_j) receives its own encrypted string EG_i (resp., EG_j)}
14. {stage 2 – encryption and permutation}
15. Source S_i (resp., S_j) generates a set of encryption/decryption keys (E_i, D_i) (resp., (E_j, D_j))
16. At S_j: $EG_j^{~j}[k] \leftarrow Encrypt(E_j, EG_j[k])$, where $k=1..L$
17.   Send string $EG_j^{~j}$ to S_i
18. At S_i: $EG_i^{~i}[k] \leftarrow Encrypt(E_i, EG_i[k])$
19. $EG_j^{~ji}[k] \leftarrow Encrypt(E_i, EG_j^{~j}[k])$
20.   Permute $EG_i^{~i}$ and $EG_j^{~ji}$ using permutation F_i
21.   Send the permuted string $F_i(EG_i^{~i})$ and $F_i(EG_j^{~ji})$ to source S_j
22. At S_j: $F_i(EG_j^{~i}[k]) \leftarrow Decrypt(D_j, F_i(EG_j^{~ji}[k]))$
23.   Permute $F_i(EG_i^{~i})$ and $F_i(EG_j^{~i})$ using permutation F_j
24.   Send string $F_j(F_i(EG_i^{~i}))$ and $F_j(F_i(EG_j^{~i}))$ to S_i
25. At S_i: $F_j(F_i(EG_i[k])) \leftarrow Decrypt(D_i, F_j(F_i(EG_i^{~i}[k])))$
26. $F_j(F_i(EG_j[k])) \leftarrow Decrypt(D_i, F_j(F_i(EG_j^{~i}[k])))$
27.
28. The matching step of $F_j(F_i(EG_i))$ and $F_j(F_i(EG_j))$ can be done at any source
29. **return**

CONCLUSION

In this paper, we propose approaches that allow joining of vertically partitioned data in a secure and privacy preserving manner. In particular, the first approach ensures secure data integration based on unique identifiers, and the second one considers data integration based on quasi identifiers, for which we propose a rule-based framework for cross-linking data records, including secure character matching. The proposed approaches employ cryptography based solutions, whereby the attribute values of all the qualifying data sets from every source is encrypted by all the sources using their own keys. Since the algorithms use commutative encryption, the encrypted values of the key attribute across different data sets will be equal if and only if their original values are equal. Thus, all the data sets from different sources can be joined on their key attributes which are encrypted by all sources. The encryption prevents any source or querying party from extracting the individually identifiable or sensitive information from the joined data set.

The main contribution of this work is to present a protocol for data integration that would not require a trusted intermediary to do all joining. Having a standards-based, high through-put communication channels among all joining parties in a federated system in necessary for this to work efficiently. In the future, we plan to efficiently incorporate additional record linkage techniques into our work and also support privacy-preserving record de-duplication.

REFERENCES

Agrawal, R., Evmfimievski, A., & Srikant, R. (2003). Information sharing across private databases. In *Proceedings of ACM SIGMOD International Conference on Management of Data*, San Diego, California.

Agrawal, R., & Srikant, R. (1994). Fast algorithms for mining association rules. In *Proceedings of the 20th International Conference on Very Large Data Bases (VLDB)* (pp. 487-499). Santiago, Chile.

Agrawal, R., & Srikant, R. (2000). Privacy-preserving data mining. In *Proceedings of the 2000 ACM SIGMOD Conference on Management of Data* (pp. 439-450).

Atallah, M. J., Kerschbaum, F., & Du, K. (2003). Secure and private sequence comparisons. In *Proceedings 2d. ACM Workshop on Privacy in the Electronic Society (WPES)* (pp. 39-44). Washington, DC.

Bartschat, W. E. A. (2006). Surveying the rhio landscape. a description of current rhio models with a focus on patient identi‾cation. *Journal of American Health Information Management Association*, 77(1), 64A–64D.

Bayardo, R. J., & Agrawal, R. (2005). Data privacy through optimal k-anonymization. In *ICDE '05: Proceedings of the 21st International Conference on Data Engineering* (pp. 217-228) Washington, DC: IEEE Press.

Clifton, C., Doan, A., Elmagarmid, A., Kantarcioglu, M., Schadow, G., Suciu, D., & Vaidya, J. (2004). Privacy preserving data integration and sharing. In *Proceedings of The 9th ACM SIGMOD Workshop on Research Issues in Data Mining and Knowledge Discovery (DMKD'2004)*.

Goldreich, O. (2004). *The Foundations of Cryptography* (Vol. 2), chapter General Cryptographic Protocols. Cambridge, UK: Cambridge University Press.

Goldreich, O., Micali, S., & Wigderson, A. (1987). How to play any mental game - a completeness theorem for protocols with honest majority. In *Proccedings of the 19th ACM Symposium on the Theory of Computing* (pp. 218-229).

Hewitt, J., & O'Connor, M. (2002). Connecting care through EMPIs. *Journal of American Health Information Management Association*, 73(10).

HIPAA. (2000). The health insurance portability and accountability act of 1996. Technical Report Federal Register 65 FR 82462, Department of Health and Human Services, Office of the Secretary.

Kelman, C., Bass, A., & Holman, C. (2002). Research use of linked health data - a best practice protocol. *Australian and New Zealand Journal of Public Health*, 26, 251–255.

Li, N., Li, T., & Venkatasubramanian, S. (2007). T-closeness: Privacy beyond k-anonymity and l-diversity. In *Proceedings of the ICDE* (pp. 106-115).

Lindell, Y., & Pinkas, B. (2002). Privacy preserving data mining. *Journal of Cryptology*, 15(3), 177–206. doi:doi:10.1007/s00145-001-0019-2

Machanavajjhala, A., Kifer, D., Gehrke, J., & Venkitasubramaniam, M. (2007). L-diversity: Privacy beyond k-anonymity. *ACM Trans. Knowl. Discov. Data*, 1(1), 3. doi:doi:10.1145/1217299.1217302

O'Keefe, C. M., Yung, M., Gu, L., & Baxter, R. (2004). Privacy-preserving data linkage protocols. In *WPES '04: Proceedings of the 2004 ACM workshop on Privacy in the electronic society* (pp. 94-102). New York: ACM.

Pohlig, S. C., & Hellman, M. E. (1978). An improved algorithm for computing logarithms over GF(p) and its cryptographic significance. *IEEE Transactions on Information Theory*, 24, 106–110. doi:doi:10.1109/TIT.1978.1055817

Rindfleisch, T. C. (1997). Privacy, information technology, and health care. *Communications of the ACM*, *40*(8), 92–100. doi:doi:10.1145/257874.257896

RxHub. (2004). The opportunity and challenge of RxHub meds. RxHub White Paper.

Samarati, P., & Sweeney, L. (1998). Protecting privacy when disclosing information: *k*-anonymity and its enforcement through generalization and suppression. In *Proceedings of the IEEE Symposium on Research in Security and Privacy*, Oakland, CA.

Vaidya, J., & Clifton, C. (2003). *Leveraging the "multi" in secure multi-party computation*. Paper Presented at the Workshop on Privacy in the Electronic Society held in association with the 10th ACM Conference on Computer and Communications Security.

Yao, A. C. (1986). How to generate and exchange secrets. In *Proceedings of the 27th IEEE Symposium on Foundations of Computer Science* (pp. 162-167). Washington, DC: IEEE.

This work was previously published in International Journal of Computational Models and Algorithms in Medicine, Volume 1, Issue 2, edited by Aryya Gangopadhyay, pp. 22-36, copyright 2010 by IGI Publishing (an imprint of IGI Global).

Chapter 8
Regulatory Compliance and the Correlation to Privacy Protection in Healthcare

Tyrone Grandison
IBM Almaden Research Center, USA

Rafae Bhatti
Oracle Corporation, USA

ABSTRACT

Recent government-led efforts and industry-sponsored privacy initiatives in the healthcare sector have received heightened publicity. The current set of privacy legislation mandates that all parties involved in the delivery of care specify and publish privacy policies regarding the use and disclosure of personal health information. The authors' study of actual healthcare privacy policies indicates that the vague representations in published privacy policies are not strongly correlated with adequate privacy protection for the patient. This phenomenon is not due to a lack of available technology to enforce privacy policies, but rather to the will of the healthcare entities to enforce strong privacy protections and their interpretation of minimum compliance obligations. Using available information systems and data mining techniques, this article describes an infrastructure for privacy protection based on the idea of policy refinement to allow the transition from the current state of perceived to be privacy-preserving systems to actually privacy-preserving systems.

INTRODUCTION

In the healthcare industry, privacy concerns are among the main inhibitors to the deployment and use of electronic records systems. In the last decade, the increase in the number of data breaches (Privacy Rights Clearinghouse, 2009) has led to an increase in the number of companies who are concerned about data and brand protection, which has translated into increased spending on healthcare privacy compliance efforts. In the United States, the Health Insurance Portability and Accountability Act[1] (U.S. Department of Health and Human Services, 1996), the new security and privacy requirements imposed by the Health Information Technology for Economic and Clini-

DOI: 10.4018/978-1-4666-0282-3.ch008

cal Health Act[2] (U.S., 2009) and the changes to HIPAA mandated by the American Reinvestment and Recovery Act[3] (U.S.A., 2009) are normally assumed to provide the baseline for privacy compliance for healthcare entities.

As healthcare organizations implement the required privacy policies, what remains to be ascertained is the impact these policies have on the improvement of privacy practices. More specifically, we address the question: *How well does the use of privacy policies translate into good privacy practices?* The *use of privacy policies* refers to the specification, notification and enforcement of policy; while *privacy practices* refer to the processes and mechanisms (i.e. technological and otherwise) that enable the safe handling of sensitive information.

The answer to our question lies in the design and enforceability of the policy itself. As we will reveal, a policy may be designed to cover all the relevant provisions of the regulation, and yet may still be vague enough to afford very little privacy protection to the patient. We will discuss this further in a later section. Concerns about the inadequate state of privacy protection despite the enactment of data protection regulations have long existed in mainstream media (Pear, 2009). In addition to design issues, studies also indicate that the enforcement of policies governing the use of protected patient information in current healthcare information systems is also lax and that policy is often bypassed or subverted during regular operation (Rostad & Edsburg, 2006).

This scenario makes it possible to purport compliance with privacy regulations, while engendering a false sense of security (or more aptly, a false sense of privacy) among patients. It makes the existence of a policy, in the first place, insignificant; as it does not precisely represent the company's true stance on data protection. Also, this undermines the notion of empowering the patient, as his consent to a policy is no longer a genuine reflection of the company's privacy practices. In an electronic health records environment, this co-

nundrum highlights the need for privacy enhancing technology. No prior work has investigated how stated privacy policies measure up to the levels of protection required to truly ensure the safety of patient data, and whether the current system can be elevated from one that purports regulatory compliance to one that really safeguards the privacy of healthcare data. Our goal is to contribute to the solution of this pressing need.

We believe that it is possible, and desirable, to define appropriate mechanisms to ensure that privacy protection moves from the adherence to minimum standards to a level that truly reflects good privacy protection for patients. In this paper, we first evaluate the current *HIPPA-inspired* privacy practices against the needs of the patient and then present a privacy management architecture called PRIMA that enables refinement of privacy policies based on actual practices of the organization. *Policy refinement* helps mitigate the stated conundrum because it allows one to (i) improve the design of the policies in order to elevate the level of privacy protection afforded to the patient, and (ii) better align the policies with actual privacy practices of the organization.

The rest of the paper is organized as follows. First, we summarize the base constructs for a discussion on healthcare privacy in the United States. Then, we describe our survey of actual privacy policies used by healthcare organizations and assess them. This is followed by a description of infrastructure for privacy protection that is based on this notion of *policy refinement*, which enables improved privacy practices in healthcare. Finally, we conclude with a synopsis of the insight gained from this work.

BACKGROUND

Several data protection regulations have surfaced around the globe (Wong, 2009) over the last few decades that directly impact healthcare privacy. Among these are the Personal Information Protection and Electronic Documents Act[4] (Office of the Privacy Commissioner of Canada, 2000), the Personal Data Protection Law (Japanese Ministry of Internal Affairs, Communications Information, & Communications Policy, 2003), and laws enacted pursuant to the European Union Directive on Data Protection. In the United States, a combination of federal laws, state laws, and common law, i.e. tort and contract, requirements define the bounds of privacy protection. In the past few years, HIPAA compliance has become the measure of adequate privacy protection for the healthcare sector. This is becoming more relevant with the recent reports encouraging a transition to a secure, private, interoperable electronic health infrastructure (U.S., 2009; HIMSS, 2009; U.S. PITAC, 2004).

To ground our discussion, the rest of this section will focus specifically on privacy protection in healthcare sector as mandated by the HIPAA Privacy Rule (U.S. Department of Health and Human Services, 1996), and the amendments and additions mandated by HITECH (U.S., 2009) and ARRA (U.S.A., 2009).

The Legal Requirements

As a pre-requisite to summarizing the requirements of the HIPAA Privacy Rule, we must define fundamental terms used. *Covered entities* refer to health plans, health care providers and health care clearinghouses. *Protected Health Information (PHI)* refers to all individually identifiable health information held or transmitted by a covered entity or its business associate, electronically, on paper, or orally. Appendix A presents the allowable disclosures under HIPAA and highlights in greater detail the provisions of the HIPAA Privacy Rule. Here, we present the high-level overviews of the five key principles of the HIPAA Privacy Rule assertions:

1. **Notification:** Patients should receive a notice of a covered entity's privacy practices.

2. **Authorization and consent:** Written authorization is required for disclosures not permitted under the Privacy Rule.

3. **Limited use and disclosure:** Covered entities must use or disclose the *minimum necessary* PHI for a specific purpose and ensure the development and implementation of policies and procedures governing access and use.

4. **Auditing and accounting:** Patients have the right to an accounting of all disclosures of their PHI for non-allowed HIPAA operations.

5. **Access:** Patients have the right, under most circumstances, to access the covered entity's designated record set. Covered entities must amend information that is inaccurate or incomplete.

The HITECH Act (U.S., 2009) augmented HIPAA by 1) strengthening the enforcement risk, e.g. increasing penalties for HIPAA violations, 2) creating a breach notification requirement for the healthcare industry, 3) extending the coverage of the HIPAA requirements to business associates, 4) re-enforcing the audit and authorization rights of patients, and 5) prohibiting the sale of an individual's health information without their authorization.

In addition to solidifying provisions in HITECH, ARRA (U.S.A., 2009) further clarified and refined issues that were previously deemed nebulous, e.g. restrictions on healthcare information sharing for self-pay scenarios, limited data sets, minimum necessary, marketing provisions, etc.

As both HITECH (U.S., 2009) and ARRA (U.S.A., 2009) are fairly recent and most organizations have not had time to updated their policies to reflect the new mandates, in order to have a fair and standard platform our analysis is based on the original HIPAA Privacy Rule mandates. For the rest of this text, reference to *policy* is to a *technical privacy policy artifact* and not to a *legislative policy artifact*. However, the assumption is made that technical policy should be a mechanism to support and instantiate legislative policy.

The first step in enabling privacy compliance, under HIPAA, is defining the entity's privacy policy rules such as which users may use or disclose data, for what purposes will it be used, under what conditions and who will be the end consumers of this data (i.e. the recipients).

P3P and Privacy Policies

Platform for Privacy Preference (P3P) (Cranor et. al., 2002) defines a standard XML format for a computer-readable privacy policy called a P3P policy. A P3P policy includes elements that describe the kinds of data a web site collects, the purposes for which data is used, potential data recipients, data retention policies, information on resolving privacy-related disputes, an indication as to whether a site allows individuals to gain access to their own data, and other information (Byers et. al., 2003). The purposes for which data may be used are typically divided into categories such as current (for which information is being directly supplied), develop (site administration), admin (website improvement), pseudo-analysis or individual analysis (user profiling and customization), telemarketing, and users are provided with the option to consent to the disclosure of their personal information for an indicated purpose. User can supply their preferences using the P3P Preference Exchange Language[5] (Byers et. al., 2003). In other words, privacy preferences encoded as rules in APPEL can be used to evaluate a P3P policy against the preferences of the user. Many tools, such as the Privacy Bird engine (Byers et. al., 2003), exist to allow such an analysis.

The adoption and significance attributed to P3P varies across the market segments and many researchers have also pointed out weaknesses in, and extensions to, P3P (Karjoth et. al., 2002; Schunter et. al., 2002; Li et. al., 2003). However, P3P is now considered a well-accepted and well-adopted standard in electronic commerce (Byers et.

al., 2003) and is used by a majority of websites to make customers aware of the policy of a company regarding the protection of their privacy.

HEALTHCARE PRIVACY POLICIES SURVEY

In order to answer our initial question, we commissioned a study of patients, gave them a survey based on the five HIPAA Privacy principles articulated above and collated their expectations with regards to each category. We then conducted a survey of the healthcare privacy policies, which were selected from twenty healthcare companies on Thomson Reuters Top 100 Hospitals list. For each policy, we analyzed it against both the regulation and patient expectations.

Before we proceed, we must further clarify our use of the term *privacy policy*. A typical covered entity in our survey provided an electronic copy of its *HIPAA Notice of Privacy Practices*, as required by regulation. This document specifies how the organization maintains the privacy of members' medical information. An electronic copy of this notice is posted on their websites. Most organizations in our survey also posted a separate *Website Privacy Policy*, which only applies to information collected, used and or disclosed through the company's website. For our purposes, we use the term *policy* or *privacy policy* to mean the virtual combination of both. This ensures that our survey results are valid for the entire electronic healthcare experience.

Generally, the surveyed companies structured their policies to convey information on the following areas: *Collection of Information, Information Types, Information Use* and *Changes to Information*. There were slight differences in terminology amongst the policies, but the higher-level concepts were equivalent. We found the policies to be very clear in articulating the information that will be collected. This information falls into one of three classes: 1) *Protected Health Information*, which includes name, address, social security number, email address, licensure, certifications, education and employment history, etc. and is normally assumed critical for the delivery of care and the company's normal business functions, 2) *Derived Information*, which includes individual access history and usage patterns, which is gathered through *cookies* in order to improve their site and allow personalization or customization, and 3) *Aggregate Information*, which is statistical information, consolidated from IP addresses, computer information and locations (amongst other things), for promotion and marketing.

In the following sections, we examine the trends in the policy statements made by the organizations in our survey, in the light of HIPAA privacy provisions.

Notification, Authorization and Consent

At the start of their policies, the healthcare companies either stated (1) that they do not collect personal information from web page visitors, but do collect web usage statistics in the aggregate form and if one wishes to register with them, then personal information will be collected or (2) that by accessing the companies' web pages you have consented to their privacy policy. Both cases lead to a situation where the patient is assumed to have implicitly consented to the privacy policy through the action of browsing the companies' web pages. We note that this does not satisfy the notification requirement in the HIPAA Privacy Rule necessary to use or disclose PHI.

We also noticed that none of the websites actually published a policy in P3P, or any similar privacy language, and only the natural language version is available online for manual review. The fact that no P3P policy is available on the Website precludes us from performing automated interpretation and analysis. Further, the intentional ambiguity in the regulation and its natural language representation mean that they cannot be directly

translated in a machine-readable form, like P3P. In this regard, healthcare is behind other sectors (e.g., online retail), where posting P3P policies on their website is now common practice. Admittedly, the privacy requirements in healthcare are more complex.

Another particularly alarming trend that was observed in our survey related to the communication of policy updates to the patients. From their policies, fifteen of the twenty of the organizations were content with simply updating the policy on the website, and making it the responsibility of the user to check for policy changes. It is a general theme that privacy policy changes are communicated with very little concern for the patient. The five companies that stated otherwise indicated they would alert the patient (via post, email, etc.) in case of a policy update. Again, we note that this type of notification is generally insufficient to revise policies for previously collected PHI under HIPAA.

Analysis

Current practices around issuing a notice and obtaining consent are not sufficient unless they provide the patient an opportunity to clearly and easily understand the policy and negotiate any objectionable provisions. This will continue to be a manually intensive task unless the policies are presented to the patient in a format that not only highlights the key segments in the policy, but also allows reasonable modifications to be made by the patient at his/her discretion. The use of P3P and APPEL technology, for example, may facilitate this task. Though recent studies have shown that privacy policies are unreadable by their target audience, irrespective of their format, (McDonald et. al., 2009) and that less than 26% of Internet users read privacy policies (Jensen et. al., 2005), we assert that the codification of policy would enable computer to analyze them and visualize potential problems, perhaps based on a specification of the user's concerns or *hot buttons*.

Unfortunately, HIPAA does not require that the notice be issued in P3P or similar machine-readable format that would facilitate automatic interpretation or analysis. It only goes as far as saying that the notice should be placed in "a clear and prominent location" (U.S. Department of Health and Human Services, 1996, pp. 89), which is completely consistent with the regulation's goal of *technology neutrality*. However, more positive impact would be achieved if some guidance was provided with respect to using the most current and expedient communication mechanisms, e.g., emails and instant messaging. Overall, we observed that industry practices regarding privacy policy notification and changes fell short of the spirit of the HIPAA requirements by failing to obtain patient acknowledgments.

Limited Use and Disclosure

On all websites surveyed, use and disclosure of information are associated with a purpose and specific purposes are defined for information. However, we found that all the organizations have defined very broad and all encompassing purposes, which may be used to exploit exceptions in the HIPAA privacy rules. For example, all the policies mention collecting information for the purpose of *administering healthcare*. They settled for a granularity so coarse that it could subsume a huge category of uses and disclosures of information. As a result, a whole host of activities, which the patient may not be in agreement with, could be interpreted as included within these purposes.

For disclosures to third parties and affiliates, it is common to see the phrase "we require the third parties to comply with policy" in privacy policies. However, there are two significant hurdles here. Firstly, a proposition to either *comply with policy* or to have *use limited by policy* is only meaningful if the policy is not broadly defined and implicitly inclusive of a wide range of business functions. Secondly, apart from *business associate contracts* with the third parties that perform services, requir-

ing PHI, for them, there are no guarantees of the actual enforcement of policy on the third party. Ideally, covered entities will proactively monitor these third parties to assure that they comply with the business associate agreements. However, the policies make no mention of the (general) terms and ramifications of such agreements.

None of the privacy policies surveyed provides a fine-grained list of roles or employee categories that have the authorizations to view specific categories of patient data. For internal use, the collected information is available to all *members of medical staff*. This is the only requirement for being an *authorized* employee. Nowhere are the precise conditions for being *authorized* stated, nor is there any criteria specified under which any exception-based accesses may be granted (such as in *break the glass* scenarios). Overall, the counsel or consent of the patient is not incorporated in assigning more specific access privileges to employees.

Analysis

While HIPAA requires organizations to obtain unambiguous authorization of the patient before use or disclosure of information for a purpose other than what it was collected for, and recommends adoption of the principle of *minimum necessary* disclosure, there exist exceptions in HIPAA to allow organizations to design policies with broadly defined purposes, and still remain regulatory compliant. This concern has also been highlighted in the public media (Pear, 2009). For instance, while *marketing* is identified as a purpose that requires authorization, various sub-categories are defined, such as *communications for treatment of patient*, that are exempt from the rule, making it possible to disclose patient data for marketing under the assumed purpose. Therefore, it may be assumed that the levels of disclosure post-HIPAA will not necessarily shrink, and in fact a data disclosure previously considered a breach may now fall within the folds of the policy to which the patient has consented. Anton et al. (2007) observe a similar phenomenon, where disclosures increased post-HIPAA.

Although HIPAA requires an organization to develop and implement internal policies and procedures for controlled access to patient information, this requirement is not re-enforced by requiring the use of stringent technical mechanisms. In other words, this requirement may simply be fulfilled by organizations using the minimal set of access controls, and employee training programs. For instance, while researchers (Anderson, 1996) and medical professionals (IHE, 2006) have clearly articulated the need for fine-grained access control for patient health records, all organizations in our survey are legally compliant even though they simply chose to give an umbrella authorization to all of their employees under the cover of *members of medical staff*. While an argument can be made for unhindered access to electronic healthcare resources so as to not impede the clinical workflow, the ethically responsible organizations should still do their level best to adopt the principle of *minimum necessary* use and (voluntarily) implement access controls at a finer granularity. We note that in the multi-vendor ecosystem of the American healthcare, most of the vendors have heavy investment in their existing tools and the economic motivation to move to these fine-grain systems may be low.

Additionally, even within organizations that implement finer-grained access control through the use of mechanisms such as role-based access control (RBAC), an over-use of exception-based accesses has been reported in a recent study (Rostad & Edsburg, 2006). While such accesses are usually meant to be exercised in emergencies, the study revealed that they are increasingly being utilized in non-emergency tasks. This effectively means that even in the presence of fine-grained access controls, the frequency with which exceptions (i.e., bypassing of the access control) are utilized can effectively render that system equivalent to one with umbrella authorizations.

Audit and Accounting

The privacy policies of all organizations advise that patients can obtain audit records for information disclosures. All policies mention that protected health information may be disclosed to government and regulatory authorities for compliance with law. Although not explicitly stated on the websites, the literature from the medical community (Anderson, 1996; Blobel, 2004) suggests that most organizations advocate the use of audit trails of all actions pertaining to patient medical records to meet the audit reporting and accounting requirement. Our experience with clients indicates that audit trails do not record all the necessary context information, such as purpose and recipient amongst other attributes. More alarmingly was the tendency of corporate executives to turn off audit systems because of the storage and performance burden incurred when they ran.

Analysis

The fact that current healthcare audit systems do not capture the required context information in order to provide an accounting means that they do not currently meet this requirement. Even though HIPAA requires organizations to account for all activity (including data disclosures) and provide detailed reporting for audit purposes, fulfilling this requirement by itself would still not be effective in improving levels of privacy protection unless measures are taken to compensate for shortcomings in the data disclosure and access rules in the privacy policy.

When the purpose or authorization is not established at a fine granularity before any disclosure or access is allowed, the burden falls on the audit mechanism to be able to capture any action that may actually constitute as a violation of the policy. Additionally, when an exception-based mechanism is in place that allows users to override normal access controls, the need for audit-based controls is further accentuated.

While an argument can be made that the deterrent factor of audits is more suited to the healthcare sector because of the critical nature of the services provided, it should certainly not become an excuse for failing to do better.

Access

The privacy policies posted on all the websites in our survey indicated that patients have the right to access or update their personal information maintained by the company through phone or email or an online account.

Analysis

Meeting this requirement may not translate to adequate privacy protection for patient. There are several reasons for this. First, the ability of a patient to access or update personal information maintained by the organization provides no measure of how much information is actually protected unless the patient is also in control of the use and disclosure rules, and, based on our preceding discussion, this is not the case. Second, navigating the processes of information access and update can be simple or laborious for the patient depending on the organization. As per the access policy of all organizations, only personal information, such as name and address, can be accessed and updated online. To access or change medical data on the patient maintained by the organization, a written request is required and it can take up to 60 days to receive a paper copy of one's medical record.

Further Observations

From our analysis, the language used in the privacy policies appears to be unnecessarily convoluted. This is corroborated by other researchers in the field (Hochhauser, 2001; Graber et al., 2002) for healthcare and finance. Given this, it will likely not be understandable by the average patient. Also, the language used in all these policies was clearly ambiguous. For example, one policy in the study

states *"...will not sell, license or transmit to anyone any personal information that members or practitioners provide to us online. We may disclose information obtained online to our partners involved in administering or providing services for our health benefits plans"*. These are possibly two seemingly contradictory, yet consistent statements that seem to have a nullifying effect on each other. This observation is supported by work in the medical informatics community (Ball et al., 2007) and the computer science community (Anton et al., 2007). Additionally, the policies downplayed the privacy risk involved (Pollach, 2007).

Secondly, the use of P3P was restricted only to cookies and exists in their abbreviated form. This raises an interesting issue. In addition to the information explicitly identified as PHI, three companies also classified cookies as PHI, whereas the remainder did not. If a policy clearly states that cookies are not PHI, then the act of attaching a P3P policy to them becomes meaningless, since non-PHI legally does not fall within the scope of a privacy policy. In the case of attaching a P3P policy to a non-PHI cookie, the act only makes sense if the cookie acts as a housing agent and the policy is used in the validation of all forms submitted via the healthcare company's pages, which was not what we observed.

Finally, the use of *machine-readable policies*, e.g., specified using P3P, on healthcare websites and generally in healthcare information systems, is currently unsatisfactory. In fact, none of the organizations in our survey has a P3P version of their notice of privacy practices available on the website. The benefits of better policy design and analysis that a machine-readable policy is envisioned to provide can be manifested in the healthcare sector when the notices of privacy practices are actually posted and utilized in this form on the healthcare organization's website and in their systems. At its core, the use of machine-readable policies will force entities to define less ambiguous privacy policies, which would be a huge victory for patients.

Summary

The overall message from our survey was that even though the privacy policies cover enough ground to enable healthcare organizations to arguably claim *regulatory compliance*, they are not adequate to communicate understandable privacy practices to the patient or provide adequate privacy safeguards. We believe that, while using artifacts such as broadly defined purposes, exception-based accesses and umbrella authorizations may still allow the organizations to claim regulatory compliance, organizations should strive to do better. It is only a matter of time before gaining patient confidence and trust with regards to privacy concerns plays a more significant role.

We alluded to the fact that the levels of privacy protection achieved by a policy depend on its design and enforceability. We observe that the design of a HIPAA-inspired policy hinges primarily on the limited use and disclosure provision, which enables the proactive, fine-grained protection of personal health information. We address how the state of the art can be improved for this provision in the next section.

PRIVACY MANAGEMENT ARCHITECTURE

The goal of PRIMA (PRIvacy Management Architecture) (Bhatti & Grandison, 2007) is to enable the design of policies with better limited use and disclosure rules. Given the significant investment in healthcare infrastructure and compliance, a key design requirement for privacy-enhancing technology that seeks to bridge the disparity between law and practice is that healthcare information systems must be transformed, with the least possible impact, to an enhanced state of protection.

The task of privacy management in the healthcare industry is complicated by the methods of healthcare services delivery. The clinical workflow in healthcare organizations is fundamentally dif- ferent from the business process workflow in commercial organizations because of the tremendous amount of human involvement at every step of the way. While it is possible to introduce privacy controls such as auditing and access control between transactions in a business process workflow without compromising its integrity, the same cannot be said about clinical workflows.

For example, a physician routinely takes notes on a piece of paper, and then hands it over to a nurse or other medical staff to input it into the computer system. Whether or not the nurse or medical staff is authorized to view private notes of the doctor becomes a secondary concern in the interest of carrying out the clinical workflow (i.e. delivering care), which would otherwise be impeded if the physician is burdened with the task of typing in the information himself. Similar situations exist when a new patient is admitted to a ward, or is brought to the emergency department, and the *on duty* assistant needs to take (possibly sensitive) notes or retrieve personal information about the patient. Therefore, there is an even stronger requirement for privacy technology that is used in healthcare workflows. This requirement is to ensure that privacy controls are seamlessly embedded into the clinical workflow without impeding the delivery of care.

The problem addressed by PRIMA is how to improve the design of use and disclosure rules in the policy by leveraging the audit results of actual access and disclosure instances, and analyzing those instances that were not explicitly covered by the existing rules in the policy, i.e. accesses allowed through the use of exception mechanism. Improving the policy increases its *coverage*, which is the ratio of the number of accesses and disclosures addressed by the policy to the total number of access and disclosure instances that were recorded in the system, including exceptions. This is particularly important because progress in the specification of privacy policy may not be a pressing national issue, but the need to ensure that the policy embodies what is being done is very pressing for healthcare. Thus, we view this process of policy refinement to increase policy coverage as a critical phase for innovation in health information systems.

There are four main concepts underlying PRIMA (Figure 1). *Stakeholders policies* define the privacy policies of the involved parties. We acknowledge that the patient is the ultimate stakeholder. However, in this context, we expand its scope to include practitioners, payers, etc. *Privacy controls* are the technology components that embody the requirements that need to be enforced in the clinical workflow. *Deployment* is the process that integrates or embeds the privacy controls into the clinical workflow. *Refinement* is the process of continually refining the definition of privacy controls based on audit analysis. In the following section, we discuss each of these concepts in greater detail.

Stake Holder Policies

The multiple stakeholders in a clinical workflow (patient, physician, medical staff, insurance, pharmacy, etc.) may have their own rules and preferences regarding the use and disclosure of protected patient information. These policies need to be studied in order to be able to specify the privacy policy that applies to the clinical workflow. This can be viewed as a bottom-up approach to policy specification. We expect that a comprehension of the domain and environment will lead to more informed initial policy.

Privacy Controls

The privacy controls of the system in question are based on the privacy policy designed in the previous step. This PRIMA module determines the components, which are to be integrated into the workflow, that enforce the policy specifications. For example, if Juanita disallows the disclosure of her medical record to a medical staff *B* for

Figure 1. System architecture

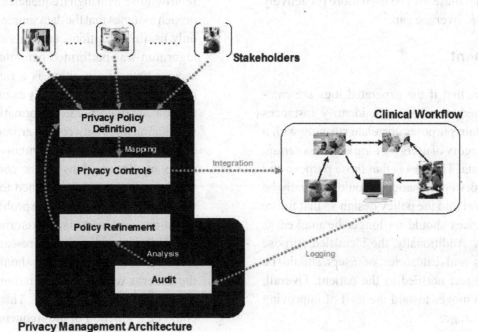

purpose *Y*, such a rule demands that information retrieved by *B* from the medical database needs to be controlled.

Deployment

The goal of the PRIMA deployment module is to provide a staged deployment of privacy controls by integrating them within the clinical workflow without impeding normal clinical activity. Our survey uncovered that current practice typically allows data access and disclosure against broadly defined purposes and umbrella authorizations as defined in the policy; and enables the subversion of disclosure controls so that care can be delivered, i.e. allows exception-based access control. Here is a stereotypical example. When *Chiaki*, who is a medical practitioner at Jenkins Community Hospital, requests a record *R* for a patient *P* for purpose *X* that *Chiaki* does not have explicit authorization to view, the system normally provides the information and creates an entry in the audit log that exception access was given. Today, these logs are only used when someone raises a red flag about the improper disclosure of their data. We propose that these logs be used more proactively to close the coverage gap.

Refinement

We purport that if the generated logs are carefully studied, then one can identify instances where certain purposes correlate strongly with a certain category of users wishing to access certain kinds of data. The idea is that those purpose and user category combinations should gradually be incorporated into the policy design so that future such instances should no longer be marked as exceptions. Additionally, the identified purpose definitions and categories of users should be advertised and notified to the patient. Overall, the system moves toward the goal of improving policy coverage.

The Framework for Refinement The audit logs of a covered entity may contain different kinds of information. There may be data on attempts to break into the system, i.e. possible violations or data breaches, or information that represents undocumented, informal clinical practice. Thus, the process of distilling useful facts from the logs requires multiple steps:

1. **Prune:** This is an optional phase, depending on the extract algorithm used to find informal clinical practice patterns in the log. The overall goal is to reduce the number of artifacts that must be examined in the extract phase by separating, as much as possible, useful exceptions from violations. This is an area that requires further examination from the research community.

2. **Extract:** In this phase, an algorithm is applied to the data source to extract patterns that could possibly be incorporated into the policy. There are two types of algorithms that could be used here. The first is a simple matching algorithm that looks for the number of occurrences of term combinations and returns those with high frequencies. This approach assumes that the data source contains only useful exceptions, and thus a pruning algorithm was performed beforehand. The second type of algorithm is a richer data mining algorithm that not only examines the text, but also incorporates information about the relationships between the artifacts being examined. This class of algorithms does not make any assumptions on the contents of the data source and is assumed to contain functionality that reduces the probability of violations appearing in the returned result set. This is another fertile research area. Both classes of algorithms should return the patterns with associated ratings, which indicate the level of usefulness. This measure could be a function of the frequency of the pattern amongst other things. It should also

be noted that extraction algorithms must be tailored to the environment in which they are deployed.

3. **Filter:** Not all the patterns produced from the extraction phase will be appropriate for inclusion into policy; and eventually into the clinical workflow. In fact, some patterns may represent behavior that needs to be stopped. In this phase, either a human is asked which patterns are worthy of inclusion or a program is designed that automatically includes patterns into the policy based on threshold values for the usefulness measure. Even though refinement is an ongoing process, we assume that there has to be a training period, where a reasonable amount of information is collected in the audit log. This training period is totally dependent on the particular healthcare entity deploying the system.

Bhatti & Grandison (2007) provide a use case scenario that demonstrates how PRIMA would enable enhanced privacy protection. The ultimate value of PRIMA lies in its ability to utilize information in the way medical practitioners use data to inform improvements in the policy design, and in the fact that it helps to reduce the number of exceptions over time; since they can become policy rules. As a result, the limited use and disclosure rules, as refined using PRIMA, enable improved privacy protection for the patient. Other technology that would empower patient privacy with regards to the limited use and disclosure provision of HIPAA are: 1) support for fine-grained, purpose-based disclosure controls, 2) support for electronic patient designation of representatives, 3) conflict resolution technology to address multiple policies, state and federal laws, organizational directives, etc., and 4) support for sophisticated data retention and recovery policies. Appendix B contains our thoughts on the key technology needed to enable the other HIPAA Privacy Rule provisions.

CONCLUSION

In this paper, we examined policies from 20 healthcare companies and analyzed the trends with respect to the HIPAA Privacy provisions and to patient privacy expectations. Our survey reveals that the healthcare industry is in need of improved practices. Current practice allows companies to claim compliance with regulation, but fell short of what patients expect with regards to their privacy. We then focused on a particular problem that currently exists in healthcare companies and presented a solution, based on policy refinement, that enables better design of policy by leveraging information from the clinical workflow.

REFERENCES

Anderson, R. (1996). A security policy model for clinical information systems. In Proceedings of the IEEE Symposium on Security and Privacy. Oakland, CA: IEEE Press.

Anton, I., Eart, J. B., Vail, M. W., Jain, N., Gheen, C. N., & Frink, J. M. (2007). HIPAA's effect on web site privacy policies. IEEE Security and Privacy, 5(1), 45–52. doi:10.1109/MSP.2007.7doi:10.1109/MSP.2007.7

Ball, M. J., Smith, C., & Bakalar, R. S. (2007). Personal Health Records: Empowering Consumers. *Journal of Healthcare Information Management, 21*(1).

Bhatti, R., & Grandison, T. (2007). Towards Improved Privacy Policy Coverage in Healthcare Using Policy Refinement. In *Proceedings of the 4th VLDB Workshop on Secure Data Management*. Vienna, Austria: Springer Verlag.

Blobel, B. (2004). Authorisation and Access Control for Electronic Health Record systems. *International Journal of Medical Informatics, 73*(3), 251–257. doi:10.1016/j.ijmedinf.2003.11.018

Byers, S., Cranor, L. F., & Kormann, D. (2003). Automated Analysis of P3P-enabled web sites. In *proceedings of the International Conference on Electronic Commerce* (pp. 326-338). Pittsburgh, Philadelphia, USA: ACM Press.

Cranor, L., Langheinrich, M., Marchiori, M., Presler-Marshall, M., & Reagle, J. (2002). The Platform for Privacy Preferences 1.0 specifications. *W3C Recommendation*. Retrieved November 27, 2009 from http://www.w3.org/TR/P3P/

Graber, M. A., D'Alessandro, D. M., & Johnson-West, J. (2002). Reading level of privacy policies on internet health web sites. *Journal of Family Practice*.

HIMSS. (2009). *Privacy and Security Toolkit*. Retrieved November 27, 2009 from http://www.himss.org/CPRIToolkit/html/4.11.html

Hochhauser, M. (2001). *Lost in the fine print: Readability of financial privacy notices*. Retrieved November 27, 2009 from http://www.privacy-rights.org/ar/GLB-Reading.htm

IHE. (2006*). The Patient Care Coordination Technical Framework: Basic Patient Privacy Consents, Supplement 2005-2006*. Retrieved November 27, 2009 from http://www.ihe.net/Technical_Framework/upload/IHE_PCC_TF_BPPC_Basic_Patient_Privacy_Consents_20060810.pdf

Japanese Ministry of Internal Affairs, Communications Information, and Communications Policy. (2003). *Personal data protection law*. Retrieved November 27, 2009 from http://www.kantei.go.jp/jp/it/privacy/houseika/hourituan/index.html

Jensen, C., Potts, C., & Jensen, C. (2005). Privacy practices of Internet users: Self reports versus observed behaviour. *International Journal of Human-Computer Studies, 63*, 203–227. doi:10.1016/j.ijhcs.2005.04.019

Karjoth, G., Schunter, M., & Waidner, M. (2002). Platform for Enterprise Privacy Practices: Privacy-enabled management of customer data. In *Proceedings of the International Workshop on Privacy Enhancing Technologies*. San Francisco, California, USA: Springer Verlag.

Li, N., Yu, T., & Anton, A. I. (2003). *A Semantics-based Approach to Privacy Languages* (Tech. Rep.). Center of Education and Research in Information Assurance and Security. Retrieved November 27, 2009 from http://www4.ncsu.edu/~tyu/pubs/p3p-csse06.pdf

McDonald, A., Reeder, R., Kelley, P., & Cranor, L. (2009). Comparative Study of Online Privacy Policies and Formats. In *Proceedings of the Annual Privacy Enhancing Technology Symposium (PETS) (LNCS Vol. 5672)*. Seattle, Washington, USA.

Office of the Privacy Commissioner of Canada. (2000). *Personal Information Protection and Electronic Documents Act (PIPEDA)*. Retrieved November 27, 2009 from http://www.priv.gc.ca/legislation/02_06_01_e.cfm

Pear, R. (in press). Warnings over privacy of us health network. *New York Times*.

Pollach. (2007). What's wrong with online privacy policies? *Communications of the ACM, 30*(2), 103-108.

Privacy Rights Clearinghouse. (2009). *A chronology of data breaches*. Retrieved November 27, 2009 from http://www.privacyrights.org/ar/ChronDataBreaches.htm

Rostad, L., & Edsburg, O. (2006). A study of access control requirements for healthcare systems based on audit trails from access logs. In *proceedings of the Annual Computer Security Applications Conference* (pp. 175-186). Miami Beach, Florida, USA: IEEE Computer Society.

Schunter, M., Herreweghen, E. V., & Waidner, M. (2002). Expressive Privacy Promises how to improve the Platform for Privacy Preferences (P3P). In *Proceedings of the W3C Workshop on Future of P3P*. Dulles, Virginia, USA. Retrieved November 27, 2009 from http://www.w3.org/2002/p3p-ws/pp/ibm-zuerich.pdf

U.S. (2009). Health *Information Technology for Economic and Clinical Health (HITECH) Act*. Retrieved November 27, 2009 from http://waysandmeans.house.gov/media/pdf/110/hit2.pdf

U.S. Department of Health and Human Services. (1996). *Health Insurance Portability and Accountability (HIPAA) Act*. Retrieved November 27, 2009 from http://www.hhs.gov/ocr/privacy/hipaa/administrative/privacyrule/adminsimpregtext.pdf

U.S. President's Information Technology Advisory Committee (PITAC). (2004). *Revolutionizing Health Care Through Information Technology*. Retrieved November 27, 2009 from http://www.nitrd.gov/pitac/reports/index.html

U.S.A. (2009). *American Recovery and Reinvestment Act (ARRA)*. Retrieved November 27, 2009 from http://frwebgate.access.gpo.gov/cgi-bin/getdoc.cgi?dbname=111_cong_bills&docid=f:h1enr.pdf

Wong, R. (2009). *An overview of data protection laws around the world*. Retrieved November 27, 2009 from http://pages.britishlibrary.net/rwong/dpa.html

ENDNOTES

[1] The Health Insurance Portability and Accountability Act is commonly referred to as HIPAA.

[2] The Health Information Technology for Economic and Clinical Health Act is commonly referred to as HITECH

[3] The American Reinvestment and Recovery Act is commonly referred to as ARRA.

[4] The Personal Information Protection and Electronic Documents Act is commonly referred to as PIPEDA

[5] P3P Preference Exchange Language is commonly referred to as APPEL

APPENDIX A: HIPAA PROVISIONS AND ALLOWED USES/DISCLOSURES

Provisions

The five key principles of the HIPAA Privacy Rule are:

1. **Notif ication:** Each covered entity must provide all patients with a notice of its privacy practices, describing the ways in which the covered entity may use and disclose protected health information. It must notify patients of their rights under the law, the covered entity's duties regarding PHI, and their right to complain to the Department of Health and Human Services (HHS) and the covered entity.
2. **Authorization and consent:** Covered Entities must obtain written authorization from the patient for disclosures that are not for treatment, payment, or health care operations or otherwise permitted by the Privacy Rule. For instance, a covered entity must obtain written patient authorization prior to disclosing any personal health information for marketing purposes subject to limited exceptions.
3. **Limited use and disclosure:** Covered Entities must make reasonable efforts to use, disclose, and request only the minimum amount of protected health information necessary to accomplish the intended purpose (known as the *minimum necessary* principle). They also must develop and implement policies and procedures that restrict access and uses of protected health information based upon the specific roles of the members of their workforce.
4. **Auditing and accounting:** Patients have the right to an accounting of all disclosures of their protected health information by a covered entity the covered entity's business associates for a maximum of six years past. The covered entity does not have to account for disclosures: (a) for treatment, payment, or health care operations; (b) to the patient or its representative; (c) to individual's involved in patient's health care or payment; (d) pursuant to authorization; (e) of a limited data set; (f) for national security or intelligence purposes; (g) for inmates in lawful custody; (h) incident to otherwise permitted uses or disclosures.
5. **Access:** Patients have the right, under most circumstances, to access the covered entity's designated record set, which contains medical, billing, and other information used to make decisions about that individual patient upon patient request. Covered entities must amend information that is inaccurate or incomplete.

Allowed Uses and Disclosures

Under the HIPAA Privacy Rule, PHI can be used or disclosed:

1. To the individual,
2. For treatment, payment, or health care operations,
3. When patients are given the opportunity to agree or object, i.e. in the creation of patient directories, etc.,
4. When it is incident to an otherwise permitted use or disclosures,
5. When it is in the public interest and benefit activities, e.g. law enforcement, public health activities, domestic violence, health oversight activities, judicial/administrative proceedings, law enforcement, threat to health or safety, IRB-approved research, and
6. When a *limited data set* is used for research, public health, or health care operations.

Generally, there are no restrictions on the use or disclosure of de-identified information, which is defined as information with no identifiers. Under HIPAA, an acceptable level of de-identification has been reached under the following conditions:

1. **Limited data set:** The covered entity has removed a list of sixteen () direct identifiers (named in the Privacy Rule) and a data use agreement is in place.
2. **Safe harbour:** Removal of base 16 identifiers plus (1) all geographic identifiers except first three digits of zip code (if more than 20,000 people); (2) all elements of dates except year; (3) any other unique identifying number, characteristic, or code, except as permitted for re-identification purposes provided certain conditions are met.
3. **Alternate de-identification method:**A person with appropriate knowledge of generally accepted statistical and scientific methods determines there is a very small risk that the information could be used, alone or in combination with other available information, to identify the data subject; and the covered entity documents the methods and results of this determination.

APPENDIX B: RECOMMENDATIONS

Technology developed to address the recommendations below should be designed with two imperatives in mind: 1) solutions must be efficient, in terms of system resources required and execution timescales, and 2) solutions must be transparent, i.e. allow for seamless and non-intrusive inclusion into existing healthcare infrastructure and workflows.

1. **Notification:** Emerging healthcare solutions should address how one tracks and triggers (technology) events that lead to notification and how one ensures receipt and includes the receipt of notification into the electronic system.
2. **Authorization and consent:** Current posted notices of privacy practices and policies do not facilitate automated analysis. The first step in enabling this is the creation of systems and mechanisms for the electronic representation of patient authorizations and consents. Going a step further, one needs to identify the appropriate granularity for authorizations and consents and develop tools that collect and proactively use these authorizations and consents in healthcare information systems.
3. **Auditing and accountability:** Auditing technology for all healthcare activity (i.e. disclosures, modifications, etc.) is sorely needed. The audit results must be presented in order of relevance and summarized to be meaningful to the person issuing the audit. Technology for ensuring tamper-resistance of audit logs and the development of new audit structures and mechanisms that have small storage footprints and performance impact is critical. Enhanced functionality on top of audit logs should be defined to ensure better data quality, analyze behavior and provide other valuable insight.
4. **Access:** Patients need technology that enables the secure access and download of their electronic health record.

These are a few of higher-level technology contributions that can be made to foster better healthcare privacy practices.

This work was previously published in International Journal of Computational Models and Algorithms in Medicine, Volume 1, Issue 2, edited by Aryya Gangopadhyay, pp. 37-52, copyright 2010 by IGI Publishing (an imprint of IGI Global).

Chapter 9
Computer Aided Detection and Recognition of Lesions in Ultrasound Breast Images

Moi Hoon Yap
Loughborough University, UK

Eran Edirisinghe
Loughborough University, UK

Helmut Bez
Loughborough University, UK

ABSTRACT

The authors extend their previous work on Ultrasound (US) image lesion detection and segmentation, to classification, proposing a complete end-to-end solution for automatic Ultrasound Computer Aided Detection (US CAD). Carried out is a comprehensive analysis to determine the best classifier-feature set combination that works optimally in US imaging. In particular the use of nineteen features categorised into three groups (shape, texture and edge), ten classifiers and 22 feature selection approaches are used in the analysis. From the overall performance, the classifier RBFNetworks defined by the WEKA pattern recognition tool set, with a feature set comprising of the area to perimeter ratio, solidity, elongation, roundness, standard deviation, two Fourier related and a fractal related texture measures out-performed other combinations of feature-classifiers, with an achievement of predicted A_z value of 0.948. Next analyzed is the use of a number of different metrics in performance analysis and provide an insight to future improvements and extension.

INTRODUCTION

Early detection of cancer plays a vital role in reducing mortality rates. Therefore many countries have established screening programmes where citizen groups who are at higher risk of developing cancer are routinely monitored (National Health Service, 2008; Smith et al., 2003). For example, in the United Kingdom, screening is currently carried out using analogue films, with a rather small number of centres trialling computed radiology and full field digital mammographic screening.

DOI: 10.4018/978-1-4666-0282-3.ch009

It is planned that by 2010 every screening centre will have at least one digital mammography unit. Therefore in the near future digital images and their computer aided analysis are likely to play a major role in screening, detection and treatment of cancer.

At present there are a number of research groups worldwide who are investigating breast sonograms. The main focus is to create automated, ultrasound, Computer Aided Diagnosis (CAD) systems with high sensitivity, specificity and consistency. Despite these efforts CAD of ultrasound images still remains an area with many open research problems that needs solutions. In this paper we identify a key open research problem in ultrasound imaging which is thoroughly investigated in order to develop a new method of ultrasound image processing for extracting relevant tissue structure information that will help differentiate between normal and malignant tissues. The ultimate goal is to provide fast and reliable tools for the early detection of malignant tissues in ultrasound images.

The current practical use of a typical US CAD system can be illustrated as in figure 1. The input of a CAD system consists of a rectangular region of interests, manually selected by a radiologist. The output provides a statistical analysis that can aid the radiologist in the final decision making, i.e., the malignancy and/or type of cancer.

The above approach (Figure 1) to CAD of breast ultrasound images has a limitation in that no aid is provided to the radiologist who selects the Region of Interest (ROI) of the lesions. Modern computer vision approaches can be used for fully automatic initial lesion detection, which can then be used as an aid to the decision making process of the radiologist, thus improving the accuracy of their performance. Further at this initial stage the need of a radiologist can be completely eliminated by allowing for a higher degree of false positives which can later be removed by further CAD or the presence of a radiologist at the final decision making stage. Thus in this paper we aim to use our previous work in initial lesion detection and segmentation to remove the need of a radiologist at the initial lesion detection stage and then propose a novel approach for the selection of lesion features and feature based lesion classification to automatically determine the lesion type. In particular within the research context of this paper we aim to develop a framework for the selection of best feature-classifier combinations in US breast imaging. To the authors knowledge such an attempt has previously not been published in relevant literature.

The aims of our research are: (i) to automate the Region of Interest (ROI) selection and (ii) to improve the segmentation and classification algorithms. Figure 2 illustrates the above aims. It is important to note that both above automations will improve the information provided to the radiologist to aid in decision making (at the ROI cropping and final decision making stages,

Figure 1. Existing US CAD approach

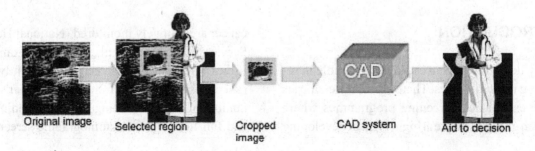

refer to Figure 1), improving the overall accuracy of the CAD system and reducing human error.

For clarity of presentation this paper has been divided into 5 sub-sections. Apart from this section which provides the reader an introduction to the problem domain and setting out the objectives of the proposed research, State-of-the-art US CAD Systems section introduces a detailed review of the state-if-the-art in US CAD system research. Method section proposes the proposed end-to-end solution to US CAD, with particular emphasis given to the recognition stage. Experimental results and analysis section provides details of experimental design, results and a comprehensive analysis. Finally Conclusions section provides the conclusions with an insight to possibilities of further research.

STATE-OF-THE-ART US CAD SYSTEMS

This section presents a summary of a comprehensive literature survey on existing Computer Aided Diagnostic systems, i.e. systems that provide a complete solution to the detection and recognition/classification problem of US images.

Some early researchers implemented and utilised texture analysis and neural network for the purpose. In 1999, Chen, D. R. et al. (1999) proposed an alternative CAD system, which was tested on a US database containing 140 pathologically proved tumours, i.e., 88 benign and 52 carcinomas. Initially the ROI is manually extracted by the physician. The texture information of the ROI is subsequently extracted, and a neural network classifier with autocorrelation features is used to classify the tumour. The reported accuracy of the system was 95.0%, with sensitivity 98%, specificity 93%, positive predictive value 89%, and negative predictive value 99%. Further in year 2000, they studied the texture analysis of breast tumours on sonograms (Chen, D. R. et al., 2000). A total of 1020 images from 255 patients were used in the experiment. The ROI images were initially identified by the physician. Subsequently, a neural network model, using 24 autocorrelation texture features, was used in the classification of tumours. The area under the ROC curve (A_z) for the model was reported to be 0.9840±0.0072.

Figure 2. The aims of proposed research (a) automate the ROI selection, (b) improve the segmentation and classification algorithms

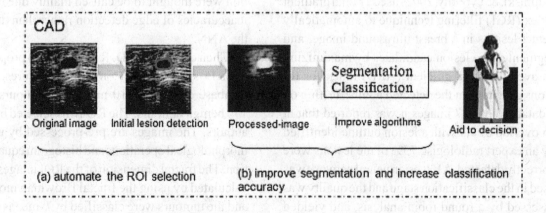

In 2002 Chen et al. (Chen, D. R., Chang, Kuo, Chen, & Huang, 2002) proposed a further novel CAD system. Initially the ROI is manually selected by the physician. This is followed by a segmentation algorithm based on wavelet transforms. Three features, namely, variance contrast, autocorrelation contrast, and distribution distortion of wavelet coefficients were extracted from the ROI images. These features were subsequently used in a multilayered perceptron (MLP) neural network, which is trained by an error back-propagation algorithm with momentum. The authors reported that A_z for the proposed system was 0.9396±0.0183, with sensitivity is 98.77%, specificity is 81.37%, positive prediction value is 72.73%, and negative predictive value is 99.24%.

Horsch et al. (Horsch, Giger, Venta, & Vyborny, 2002) presented a CAD method for the detection of breast lesions in ultrasound images that is based on the automatic segmentation of lesions and the automatic extraction of four features related to lesion shape, margin, texture, and posterior acoustic behaviour. The database used consisted of 400 cases (94 malignant lesions, 124 complex cysts, and 182 benign solid lesions). The use of linear discriminate analysis as a classification method of breast lesions was investigated. An average A_z value of 0.87 was reported in the task of distinguishing malignant from benign lesions.

Drukker et al. (2002) (Drukker, Giger, Horsh, Kupinski, & Vyborny, 2002) used a radial gradient index (RGI) filtering technique to automatically detect lesions in a breast ultrasound image, and segmented the lesion candidates by maximizing an average radial gradient (ARD) index for regions grown from the detected points. Testing on a database of 757 images it was reported that at an overlap of 0.4 with a lesion outline identified by an expert radiologist, 75% of the lesions were correctly detected. A Bayesian neural network was used in the classification stage and the quality was assessed by a round robin analysis, and yielded an A_z value of 0.84, with 94% sensitivity at 0.48 false-positive per image.

Chen et al. (C. M. Chen et al., 2003) proposed a CAD system by setting independent features (i.e., feature extraction) and using a ANN. The database contained 2 sets of images, first set with 160 images, and second set with 111 images. Seven morphological features were used, and a multilayer feed-forward neural network was used as the classifier. The A_z reported for the ROC curve was 0.950±0.005, overall.

Joo et al. (Joo, Yang, Moon, & Kim, 2004) proposed a CAD algorithm by using multiple ultrasound features and a ANN. The test database consisted 584 histological confirmed cases. The ROIs of images were manually selected by expert radiologists. Median filtering was initially applied to the ROI images and a simple segmentation consisting of contrast enhancement and thresholding segmentation, were subsequently applied. The reported accuracy of the system was 91.4%, sensitivity: 92.3% (131/142), and specificity: 90.7% (136/150). Further experimental results were reported during which the cut-off level of the thresholding segmentation was adjusted. It was shown that this resulted in an increase in accuracy (99.3% (141/142) and 100% (142/142)) but resulted in a decrease of sensitivity (53.3% (136/150) and 7.3% (11/150) respectively). In the above work, even though a simple segmentation approach was adopted, high level of classification accuracy was achieved. The errors in classification were thought to be caused mainly due to the inaccuracies of edge detection rather than due to the ANN.

Chen et al. (Chen, D. R. et al., 2005) proposed a CAD system based on fractal features. The database contained 110 malignant tumours and 140 benign tumours. The ROI was selected by the authors. The images are pre-processed by using morphological operations and histogram equalization. The fractal dimension of the ROI images was calculated by using the fractal Brownian motion, and the tumours were classified by k-means classification methods. The reported ROC area index A_z was 0.9218.

In the latter phase of the research, Support Vector Machine (SVM) gained popularity and most researchers have gradually implementing SVM in classification stage. In 2005, Chang et al. (Chang, Wu, Moon, & Chen, 2005) proposed a CAD system with automated ultrasound segmentation and morphology based diagnosis of solid breast tumours. The database consisted of 90 malignant tumours and 120 benign tumours. The ROIs were pre-selected by a radiologist. Anisotropic diffusion filtering was used to pre-process the images, followed by the level set method of segmentation introduced by the authors. Support Vector Machine (SVM) based on six morphological features is used to classify the tumours. They reported results were: accuracy 90.95%, sensitivity 88.89%, specificity 92.5%, positive predictive value 89.89%, and negative predictive value 91.74%.

Huang et al. 2005 (Huang & Chen, 2005) evaluated two pathologically proven ultrasonic databases, DB1, which contained 140 images, and DB2, which contained 250 images. The ROIs of the images were selected by a physician. Textural features were used in SVM based classification of tumours. The ROC indexes reported for DB1 and DB2 are 0.9695±0.0150 and 0.9552±0.0161 respectively.

In the most recent work in classification of lesions, i.e., Huang et al. 2008 (Huang et al., 2008), 118 breast lesions were evaluated out of which 34 were malignant and 84 were benign. The ROI were manually selected by a physician. 19 morphological features from the extracted contour were obtained and PCA was used to find the independent features. A SVM classifier was finally used in the classification. The reported A_z value when using all morphological features and the when using only the lower-dimensional principal vector were, 0.91 and 0.90, respectively.

Classification algorithms also play a key role in US CAD systems. A number of approaches for classification of lesions have been investigated in literature. However the determining the best classifier for a given CAD system not only depends on the general accuracy of the classifier selected, but also on the nature of the dataset (e.g., US, mammographic) and the feature set used in classification. To this effect in the classification of US images there is a significant research gap in identifying the best feature set – classifier combinations that can directly impact in improving the accuracy, sensitivity and specificity of CAD systems. Addressing this issue we present a detail study using, different feature sets, feature selection approaches and classifiers in identifying the best feature set – classifier combinations for US CAD systems. To our knowledge this is the first detailed investigation carried out in this respect.

METHOD: PROPOSED CAD SYSTEM

Figure 3 illustrated that the proposed CAD system comprises four key stages, namely, Stage-1: initial ROI detection, Stage-2: lesion boundary identification, Stage-3: feature detection and Stage-4: classification based on selected feature sets. In our previous research we have proposed effective approaches to ROI detection (initial lesion detection) (Yap, Edirisinghe, & Bez, 2008) and lesion boundary identification (Yap, Edirisinghe, & Bez, 2007), i.e. stages 1 and 2. Within our present research context we incorporate these two stages with further novel stages of feature detection and classification, to produce a novel CAD system, the performance of which is evaluated and compared with other state-of-the-art CAD systems in experimental results and analysis section.

Initial Lesion Detection, Segmentation and Boundary Detection

Figure 3 illustrates the detailed block diagram of stages 1 (Yap et al., 2008) and 2 (Yap et al., 2007).

Stage 1 is to obtain the position of the region of interest, i.e., initial lesion detection, thereby acting as an aid and reducing the region labelling time

Figure 3. Architecture of Stage-1 and Stage-2

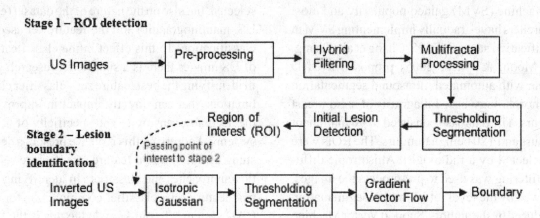

of a radiologist in a typical diagnostic procedure. It consists of a number of sub-stages that include histogram equalisation, hybrid filtering, multifractal analysis, thresholding segmentation, and a rule-based approach to remove false positives. Histogram equalisation results in a re-distribution of pixel values in the image evenly into pixel value bins (i.e., equal sized ranges) within the range 0-255, thereby guaranteeing the homogeneity of images taken by different scanning devices and examined by different radiologists. In the hybrid filtering stage we combine two filter types with complementary advantages towards noise reduction and edge preservation, i.e. we combine the strength of *Nonlinear Diffusion* filtering to produce edge-sensitive speckle reduction, with *Linear* filtering (Gaussian blur) to eliminate over segmentation. The hybrid filtering stage is followed by a multifractal analysis stage that is capable of improving the contrast against ROI boundaries by generally making the dark regions darker and the light regions lighter. Finally a thresholding stage is used to segment the Regions of Interest (ROI) and a rule based approach that assumes that the captured ultrasound image would have its ROIs

located more around the central region of the image is used to remove false ROI detections. Figure 4 illustrates the output of each sub-stage for quick reference purposes. We refer the readers interested in the details of the above initial lesion detection algorithm to (M. H. Yap, et al., 2008), in which the performance has been compared with that of the best known algorithm for ROI detection, and proven to be better.

In stage 2 (Yap et al., 2007), we obtain an initial estimate of the contour of the tumour by using an Isotropic Gaussian function, and further enhance it by using a special type of snake, namely, Gradient Vector Flow (GVF) (Xu & Prince, 1998). In obtaining the initial estimate of the contour the image is first inverted and then multiplied by an Isotropic Gaussian function to incorporate the lesion shape into the creation of partition between the lesion and external areas. This stage is followed by a simple segmentation step which uses a single threshold value to obtain an initial estimate to the contour segmented ROI. The subsequent use of the GVF based active contour model results in the movement of the estimated boundary closer to the real. The spe-

Figure 4. Illustration of the operation of the sub stages of the intial lesion dectection algorithm (a) the original image. Image after, (b) pre-processing (histogram equalization) (c) hybrid filtering (d) multi-fractal processing (e) thresholding segmentation (f) and labelling of region of interest (ROI).

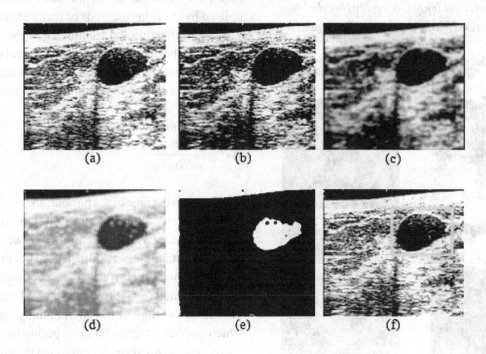

cific use of GVF allows a better convergence to the real boundary in cases where the initial boundary detected will be substantially further away from the real and in the presence of boundary concavities. The outputs of the sub-processes of the two sub-stages are illustrated in Figure 5 and Figure 6.

We refer readers interested in the details of the sub-processes/stages above to our previous work of (Yap et al., 2007), in which the approach is compared with a number of state-of-the-art lesion boundary detection algorithms, proving improved segmentation accuracy.

Classification

A preliminary study carried out by us (Yap, Edirisinghe, & Bez, 2009) on two popular appearance based approaches to US lesion classification, namely PCA (Principle Component Analysis) and LDA (Linear Discriminant Analysis), proved

that PCA achieved a success rate of 0.55, whilst 2D-LDA achieved a success rate of 0.50. These results indicate that appearance based approaches are inefficient in the classifications of US lesions. In contrast due to the added resiliency shown to noise, feature based approaches are more reliable in lesion classification and have hence been used as the primary classification approach in many state-of-the-art US-CAD systems. Hence, in our present research context we adopt this approach. Further we carry out a comprehensive study to determine the feature-classifier combination that performs best on the test US image database used. To this effect we analyse the performance of a large selection of popular classifiers and feature sets.

Feature based approaches to image classification generally consists of two stages, namely, feature extraction and feature classification. Often when the number of features extracted is very high, an additional intermediate stage of feature selection is used.

Figure 5. Outputs at various stages of the initial boundary detection sub-stage of stage 2: (a) Inverted image, (b) after applying Isotropic Gaussian on the inverted image, (c) after thresholding segmentation and (d) the detected lesion boundary

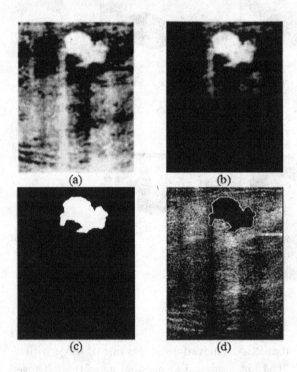

(a)

(b)

(c)

(d)

Features Extraction Approaches

Features can generally be used as a concise representation of an image. In particular feature extraction in ultrasound images is a challenging task due to the speckle noise. For ease of discussion and analysis, we classify the typical features of an ultrasound image into three groups, namely, shape, texture and edge descriptors. These categories are detailed in the following sub-sections.

Shape Descriptors

Shape analysis has been widely utilised in computer vision and has been intensively developed over the past decades in both theoretical and applied domains (Russ, 2007). Due to the fact that most US image lesions vary in shape according

to their type (e.g., cyst, malignant etc.); various shape descriptors have been used in their classification. This section discusses the shape descriptors utilised by previous methods of feature based US lesion classification and a number of further shape descriptors that have been utilised in general within other computer vision applications (Costa & Cesar, 2000) with potential applicability in US imaging:

Area to Perimeter ratio (AP):

$$AP = \frac{area}{perimeter},$$

where area is the area of the tumour, and perimeter is the perimeter of the tumour. Tumour perimeter and tumour area are dependent on size of a tumour. Hence as a standalone feature, it does not provide useful information. However, the aspect ratio of the area to perimeter will provide useful information as a malignant tumour has an irregular boundary, which implies a higher value in perimeter.

A Convex Hull provides important information about the description of a shape. Figure 7 illustrates the shapes of the lesions that correspond to their convex hulls.

From the above analysis, the convexity and solidity of the lesions can be calculated as follows:

$$Solidity: Solidity = \frac{area}{convex\ area},$$

where *area* is the area of the tumour region, and *convex area* is the area of the convex hull. It is clearly shown that the malignant tumours (as in Figure 7 (c) and (d)) have a larger convex hull area as compared to the benign tumours (as in Figure 7 (a) and (b)).

$$Convexity: Convexity = \frac{convex\ perimeter}{perimeter},$$

where the *major axis* is the line passing through the foci, centre and vertices of the ellipse, and

Figure 6. Outputs at various stages of the final boundary detection sub-stage of stage-2: (a), (d) Original image (b), (e) Initial boundary detected by the Isotropic Gaussian (c), (f) Final enhanced boundary obtained by applying gradient vector flow approach

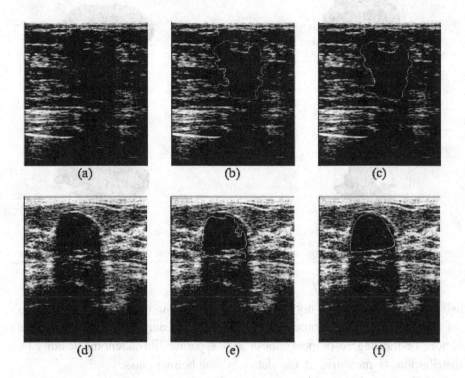

minor axis is a line through the centre of an ellipse which is perpendicular to the major axis, as illustrated after Figure 8 in Figure 9.

$$Compactness: Compactness = \frac{\sqrt{4\pi \times area}}{major\ axis},$$

where *area* is the area of the tumour, and *major axis* as defined in Figure 9.

Roundness:

$$Roundness = \frac{4 \times area}{\pi \times Max\_Diameter^2},$$

where *area* denotes the area of the tumour, and *Max_Diameter* denotes the length of the *major axis*. Figure 10 illustrates the roundness values for malignant and benign tumours. Note that a benign tumour has a higher roundness value as compared to a malignant tumour.

Texture Descriptors

Texture descriptors can be used to differentiate between lesions having differences in internal texture. Figure 12 illustrates that texture within tumours vary from benign to malignant types.

The texture can be represented in the form of four central moments and by entropy of a pixel value distribution:

- **Mean/average intensity:** This refers to the first central moment, i.e., the average intensity of the lesion, in gray-scale.
- **Standard deviation:** This refers to the second central moment, i.e., a measure of the sparsity of the pixel value intensity within a lesion.
- **Skewness:** This refers to the third central moment, i.e., a measure of the degree of asymmetry of the pixel value distribution.

Figure 7. Lesions and convex hull (a), (b) benign tumours, (c), (d) malignant tumours

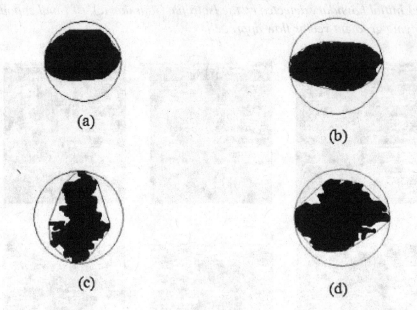

(a)

(b)

(c)

(d)

- **Kurtosis:** This refers to the normalised form of the fourth central moment of a distribution, or the degree of peakedness of a distribution. It measures if the data are peaked or flat relative to a normal distribution.

Minimum cross entropy (MCE): The cross entropy of a probability distribution q with respect to a prior distribution p is defined by

$$H(q, p) = \sum_j q_j \log \frac{q_j}{p_j}$$

The idea of *MCE* is to choose the distribution *q* that has the least cross entropy, with respect to the given prior *p*(Ojala, Pietikainen, & Maenpaa, 2002). In classifying benign tumours from malignant tumours, a particular challenge met is that typically the pixel intensity value distribution of a fibroadenoma lesion is close in resemblance to pixel intensity value distribution of a normal lesion. Therefore if a normal lesion acts as the prior distribution *p*, it is expected that fibroadenoma lesions will have the least *MCE*

as compared to the *MCE*s that results from other types of diagnosis. Hence, *MCE* may be used to separate fibroadenoma lesions from lesions of the benign class.

Edge Descriptors

Polar coordinate analysis, Fourier descriptors, and fractal analysis are widely used in literature as edge descriptors. The following sections define these parameters and summarises their potential use in classification.

- **Polar coordinate analysis:** The edge irregularity can be measured using polar coordinate analysis. However, our observations of the characteristic features of datasets revealed that while some lesions can be analysed perfectly (as in Figure 13 (a)) some cannot be analysed by polar coordinate analysis as they consist of multiple edge points on a given diagonal (as in Figure 13 (b)).
- **Fourier descriptor:** Fourier descriptors are commonly used in pattern recognition

Figure 8. The bounding rectangle

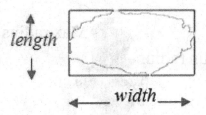

Figure 9. The major axis and minor axis

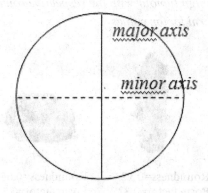

applications due to their invariance to the starting point of the boundary and rotation (Costa & Cesar, 2000). Figure 14 illustrates the possibility of using Fourier descriptors in differentiating malignant tumours from benign tumours. The Fourier descriptors of a lesion boundary are presented by an array of complex numbers which correspond to the pixels of the object boundary if the image is placed in the complex plane. Fourier descriptors are calculated by combining Fourier transform coefficients of the complex array (Costa & Cesar, 2000). It is noted that using a lower number of Fourier descriptors, the general shape can be described (figure 14 (a) and figure 14 (b), 10 descriptors). The detail information of the shape is described by using the high frequency components of the series (as shown in figure 14(a) and figure 14(b), 50 descriptors). For consistency, in our preliminary experiments the boundaries are re-sampled to the same size, i.e., 100 descriptors are obtained for each. Note that in our experiments the descriptor *Fourier1* (see Experimental results and Analysis section) represents the summation of the coefficients of real numbers while descriptor *Fourier2* represents the summation of the coefficients of the imaginary numbers. As it is expected that malignant tumours, with irregular edges, produce higher values in high frequency domain as compared

to benign tumours, the above summations can be used for differentiating benign/malignant tumours.

- **Fractal dimension:** Fractal dimension (Barnsley et al., 1988) can be used to describe the roughness of the edges. Note that in our experiments, the descriptor, *Fractal1* (see Experimental results and analysis section) represents the mean of the fractal dimension, while *Fractal2* represents the standard deviation of the fractal dimension.

Lesion Classification

There are many choices for an appropriate lesion classifier in US imaging, ranging from Bayesian classifiers to neural networks. The performance of a classifier is dependent not only on its general accuracy but also on the dataset and the features used for classification. To further investigate the performance of different classifiers, experiments with different combinations of feature-sets are conducted. We use WEKA (The Waikato Environment for Knowledge Analysis) (Witten & Frank, 2005), the popular, open source, Java based data mining tool in our experimentation. WEKA is a collection of implementations of popular machine learning algorithms for data mining tasks (Witten & Frank, 2005) which includes the implementa-

Figure 10. The shape of a: (a) malignant tumour, (b) benign tumour with the respective roundness and form factor values

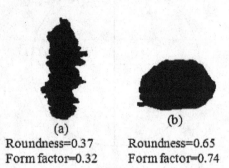

Roundness=0.37   Roundness=0.65
Form factor=0.32   Form factor=0.74

Figure 11. Maximum and minimum radii

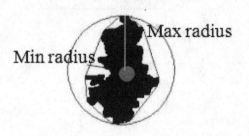

tion of a number of different classifiers. It is still in active development (version 3.5.8) at present.

Due to their general popularity in a wide range of other applications, ten classifiers were chosen for investigation, namely, Bayesian Network (BayesNet), Naïve Bayesian Network (Naïve-Bayes), Support Vector Machine (SVM), Multi Layer Perceptron (MLP), Radial basis function networks (RBF Networks), Bagging, Adaptive Boosting (AdaBoost), LogitBoost, Random Tree, and Random Forest. Note that in our investigations, the default parameters of WEKA have been used. A summary of explanations of each of the above classifiers can be presented as follows:

- **BayesNet:** Bayesian approach is based on the probability theory (Witten & Frank, 2005). Given the probability distribution, a Bayes Classifier can achieve optimal results.
- **NaiveBayes:** The Naïve Bayes classifier is a simple probabilistic classifier based on applying Bayes' theorem with strong (naïve) assumptions of independence (John & Langley, 1995). It is also known as an "independent feature model". For further reading, readers are referred to (John & Langley, 1995).
- **SVM:** The support vector machines (SVMs) were introduced by Vapnik

(Vapnik, 1995) and are based on statistical learning theory. In pattern classification applications, it has been proved that SVMs provide better generalized performance than the traditional techniques, such as neural networks (Witten & Frank, 2005). The benefits of SVMs include, rapid and excellent classification capability (Huang et al., 2008) and the ability to generalize in high-dimensional spaces. Hence it is widely accepted as an excellent choice in classification. In addition, the task of classifying malignant tumours from benign tumours can be defined as a binary classification problem. According to (Vapnik, 1995), SVM is powerful in solving binary classification problems.

- **MLP:** MLP is a type of artificial neural network that uses back propagation to classify instances. We refer readers to (Witten & Frank, 2005) for further reading.
- **RBFNetwork:** WEKA includes an implementation of a normalized Gaussian radial basis function network (RBFNetwork). It uses the *k*-means clustering algorithm to provide the basis functions and learns via either a logistic regression (discrete class problems) or a linear regression (numeric class problems). We refer readers to (Witten & Frank, 2005) for further details.
- **Bagging:** Bagging also known as bootstrap aggregating, is a meta-algorithm to improve machine learning of classification

Figure 12. Texture within contours of the detected lesions (a) malignant (b) fibroadenoma (c) cysts

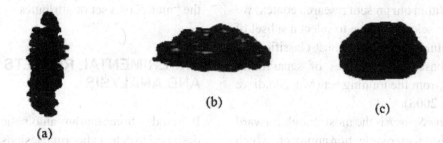

and regression models in terms of stability and classification accuracy (Breiman, 1996). We refer readers to (Breiman, 1996) for further details.

- **AdaBoost:** AdaBoost is a boosting method based on Freund et al.'s (Freund, 1999) original work. This meta-classifier is adaptive in the sense that subsequent classifiers built are tweaked in favour of those instances misclassified by previous classifiers (Freund, 1999).
- **LogitBoost:** LogitBoost is a boosting algorithm formulated by Friedman et al. (Friedman, Hastle, & Tibshirani, 2000). It casts the AdaBooast algorithm into a statistical framework.
- **Random tree:** With k random features at each node, a Random tree is a tree drawn at random from a set of possible trees (Witten & Frank, 2005). In this context, "at random" means each tree in the set of trees has an equal chance of being sampled. Random

trees can be generated efficiently and the combination of large sets of Random trees generally leads to accurate models.

- **Random forest:** A Random Forest (Breiman, 2001) is a meta-learner that comprises of many individual trees. They are designed to operate quickly over large datasets and to be diverse by using random samples to build each tree in the forest. For further reading refer to (Breiman, 2001).

Feature Selection

Although a large number of features can be derived from an image, not all will be suitable for classification. The relevant features for accurate classification will depend on the data set and also of the classifier used. Irrelevant features may increase the possibility of the number of outliers and can hence reduce the overall accuracy of the classifier to be used. Hence, it is important to filter out the irrelevant features, or remove

Figure 13. Analysing edges using polar co-ordinates (a) single point (b) multiple points

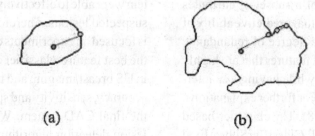

the features that reduce the accuracy of a given classifier. Within our present research context we use a feature selection stage to select a subset of relevant features to build a robust classification procedure based on measures of separability constructed from the training set (Mu, Nandi, & Rangayyan, 2008).

Exhaustive Search is the most straightforward and the earliest feature selection approach, which investigates all possible combinations of subsets. However as the number of subsets grow, *Exhaustive Search* becomes impractical. *Best First* (Witten & Frank, 2005) searches the space of attribute subsets by greedy hill-climbing (Witten & Frank, 2005) augmented with a backtracking facility. *Linear Forward Selection* is an extension of *Best First*, which takes a restricted number of k attributes into account. For further reading, refer to (Guetlein, 2006). *Genetic Search* performs a search using a simple genetic algorithm described in Goldberg (Goldberg, 1989). *Greedy Stepwise* (Witten & Frank, 2005) algorithm performs a greedy forward or backward search through the space of attribute subsets. *Greedy stepwise* algorithm can move either forward or backward through the search space, while *Best First* algorithm has the option to consider both at any given point in the search. However the *Greedy stepwise* algorithm is faster but tends to generate errors.

The WEKA tool has implementations of a range of feature selection methods including the above. We used these implementations for our experimentation. WEKA consists of implementations of further feature selection algorithms that includes the following: Correlation-based Feature Subset Selection (CfsSubsetEval class in WEKA) evaluates the relevance of a subset of attributes by considering the individual predictive ability of each feature along with a degree of redundancy between them. Subsets of features that are highly correlated with the class while having low inter-correlation are preferred. For further explanations, please refer to (Hall, 1998). The classifier-based feature selector, named ClassifierSubsetEval

(Hall, 1998) in WEKA, uses a classifier to estimate the "merit" of a set of attributes.

EXPERIMENTAL RESULTS AND ANALYSIS

It should be noted that any automatic system that is designed to detect abnormal lesions in ultrasound images should be finally verified/compared with the judgment of a medical expert/radiologist. The test images used in this research are obtained from a professionally compiled Breast Ultrasound CD (Prapavesis, et al., 2001), which consists of explanations and verifications from several qualified expert Radiologists. A total of 174 images from the Breast Ultrasound CD were selected for the experiments. Of the 174 images, 50 were malignant, and 104 were benign. Each image has been manually processed by an expert radiologist and the extreme points of the suspected lesions have been marked with 'crosses'. We use this information for evaluation of the performance of our CAD system. Further in line with experiments conducted in relevant literature (Chen, D. R. et al., 2005; Drukker et al., 2002; Huang et al., 2008), in our experiments, the dataset is divided equally into a training set and a testing set. The training set is used to build the classifier models, while the testing set is used for evaluation of the models.

In our previous work (Yap et al., 2007; Yap et al., 2008) we evaluated the performance of stages-1 and 2 in comparison to the performance of key state-of-the-art initial lesion detection and lesion boundary detection algorithms. It was proven that the stage-1 and stage-2 of the proposed CAD system were able to effectively detect the boundary of suspected lesions. Therefore our present analysis is focused on experiments carried out to determine the best feature-classifier combination to be used in US breast imaging and to determine the overall accuracy, sensitivity and specificity obtainable by the final CAD system. We have used the initial lesion detection algorithms of (Yap et al., 2008)

Figure 14. Fourier descriptors for a (a) benign tumour and a (b) malignant tumour, and their corresponding reconstructions of edges using different numbers of descriptors/coefficients

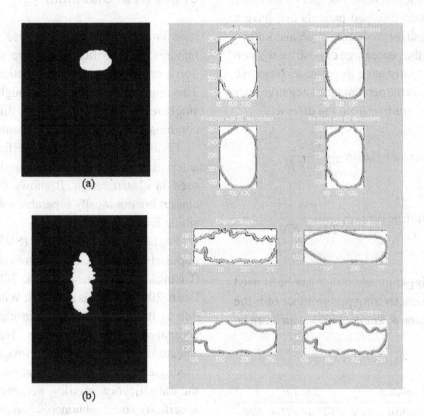

and the lesion boundary detection algorithm of (Yap et al., 2007) in all experiments as stage-1 and stage-2 of the US CAD pipeline.

Performance Measures

The measurements used to evaluate the performance includes accuracy, sensitivity, specificity, positive predictive value (PPV), negative predictive value (NPV) and the predicted A_z value, as implemented by the software tool WEKA. The measure of accuracy is defined as the percentage of correct classifications obtained, which is not suitable as a sole performance measurement measure in lesion classification as for e.g. terms such as false positives can play an important role in the suitability of a classification algorithm.

In order to use a single measurement for comparison, most of the medical research works

have used A_z value. However though A_z value is a better single measure of performance as compared to using *accuracy*, due to the prediction approach adopted by WEKA to calculate the A_z value, our experiments revealed that its use is far from being perfect. For binary classifiers, a number of authors of previous literature have used the *success rate* as a single performance metric. It is defined as:

$$success\ rate = \frac{TP + TN}{TP + FP + TN + FN}$$

where, TP (true positives), TN (true negatives), FP (false positives) and FN (false negatives) are defined as:

There are two types of errors in medical diagnosis: *false-negative (FN)* and *false positive (FP)* findings. *True positive fraction (TPF)* or *sensitivity* is the percentage of diseased patients that have a positive test. *Sensitivity* is also known as *recall*. *True negative fraction (TNF)* or *specificity* is the percentage of non-diseased patients that have a negative test. Positive predictive value, also known as *precision*, is the percentage of positive tests on patients that actually have the disease. Negative predictive value is the percentage of negative tests on patients who are free from the disease.

$$Positive\ predictive\ value = \frac{TP}{TP + FP}$$

$$Negative\ predictive\ value = \frac{TN}{TN + FN}.$$

A further single measure that has been used popularly in characterizing performance of is the F-measure (Witten & Frank, 2005), which can be defined as:

F-measure =
$$\frac{2 \times recall \times precision}{recall + precision} = \frac{2 \times TP}{2 \times TP + FP + FN}.$$

Due to the fact that a number of different single performance metrics have been used in previous literature for performance characterisation, in this research we use all popular measures with the aim of identifying the best metrics for evaluating algorithms tested on ultrasound images.

For clarity of presentation the performance is analysed as follows: Performance Evaluation of the SVM Classifier analyses the use of different performance metrics defined above when using SVM as the classifier and different selections of feature descriptors. Performance Evaluation of Other Classifiers continues to analyse the remaining classifiers as defined and implemented by the WEKA tool. Comparison of Feature Selection Methods analyses different feature selection algorithms as defined and implemented by the WEKA software tool.

Performance Evaluation of the SVM Classifier

It is important to study the use of individual features in classification before the classification is conducted using combinations of features. This approach will provide a rough idea on how single features perform and how different feature combinations may therefore potentially perform.

Figure 15 illustrates the performance characteristics when a number of single features are used in classification. It shows that the lesion classes are not ideally separable using any of the single features.

Support Vector Machines (SVM) have been popularly used as a classifier in existing literature (Chang, Wu, Moon, & Chen, 2003; Huang & Chen, 2005; Huang et al., 2008; Wikipedia, 2008) due to its general accuracy in classification as compared to other classifiers. Hence we have selected it as the classifier to investigate the use of single features in classification. In Figure 16 the classification metrics, accuracy, sensitivity, specificity and A_z obtained when using individual features (note: all are shape descriptors as defined in *Shape Descriptors* subsection) with SVM as the classifier, is tabulated. It shows that the feature *convexity*, provides the best separability to the classes as it consistently gives a clear maxima (or minima) for different measures tested. Note the use of additional metrics, positive predictive value (PPV) and negative predictive value (NPV).

A further experiment was performed to evaluate the performance of SVM based classification when all shape, texture and edge descriptors are used as individual, but separate groups. Figure 17 tabulates the results. An important observation is that the use of shape descriptors consistently performed best with all metrics used for performance evaluation.

A further observation is that the use of only the shape descriptors is not more efficient than the use of all features. This provides a hint as to

Figure 15. Analysis of the use of individual features in classification. The blue and red areas represent malignant and benign classes, respectively. The x-axes represent the value of each parameter represented in feature extraction. The y-axis represents the number of cases. Note that for accurate classification one should be able to select a specific threshold where the malignant and benign tumours are separable with the least amount of outliers. The graph representing convexity is the best in this regard. Note that the bottom-right graph is only an indication of number of malignant (i.e., 25) and number of benign (i.e., 62) cases.

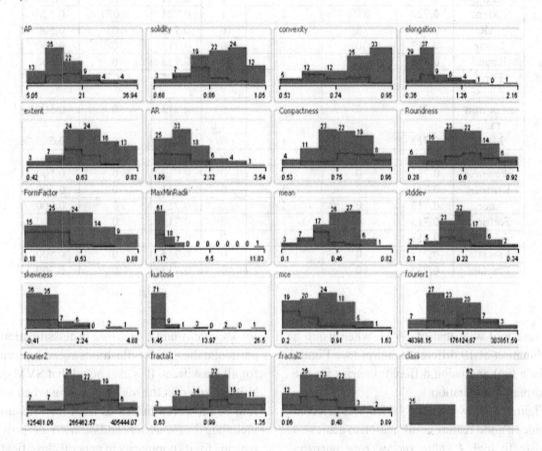

the fact that optimal feature combination may consist of shape descriptors plus a number of other non-shape descriptors. This implies that feature selection is crucial in obtaining the optimal performance of any classification algorithm.

Performance Evaluation of Other Classifiers

This section compares the performance of other popular classifiers implemented within the WEKA

Disease/ Test result	Disease present	Disease absent	Total
Positive	True positive (TP)	False positive (FP)	TP+FP
Negative	False negative (FN)	True negative (TN)	FN+TN
	TP+FN	FP+TN	

Figure 16. Summary of statistics in using a single feature in SVM based classification

Features	Success rate	Sensitivity	Specificity	PPV	NPV	F-measure	A_z
AP	0.713	0	1	0	0.713	0	0.500
Solidity	0.839	0.52	0.968	0.867	0.833	0.650	0.744
Convexity	0.862	0.6	0.968	0.882	0.857	0.714	0.784
Elongation	0.724	0.04	1	1	0.721	0.077	0.520
Extent	0.724	0.04	1	1	0.721	0.077	0.520
AR	0.713	0	1	0	0.713	0	0.500
Comp	0.713	0	1	0	0.713	0	0.500
Round	0.713	0	1	0	0.713	0	0.500
Form Factor	0.724	0.04	1	1	0.721	0.077	0.520
Max/min radii	0.713	0	1	0	0.713	0	0.500
Mean	0.713	0	1	0	0.713	0	0.500
Std dev	0.713	0	1	0	0.713	0	0.500
Skewness	0.713	0	1	0	0.713	0	0.500
Kurtosis	0.713	0	1	0	0.713	0	0.500
mce	0.713	0	1	0	0.713	0	0.500
Fourier1	0.713	0	1	0	0.713	0	0.500
Fourier2	0.713	0	1	0	0.713	0	0.500
Fractal1	0.713	0	1	0	0.713	0	0.500
Fractal2	0.713	0	1	0	0.713	0	0.500

software tool with that of SVM, when using a combination of 19 different features (see Figure 16 for a list) and using different metrics for the performance evaluation.

Figure 18 shows that the 19 features selected provides a good feature combination to achieve a consistently high A_z value, *success rate, sensitiv-* *ity, specificity* and *F-measure* in classification. In particular the A_z value illustrates a clear high value for all classifiers. It is also noted that SVM classifier resulted in the highest reading when using four of the seven measures used for evaluation, including the *F-measure* and *success rate*, proving reasons for its popularity in general classification

Figure 17. Effect of using different groups of features in SVM based lesion classification

Features	Success rate	Sensitivity	Specificity	PPV	NPV	F-measure	A_z
All features	0.931	0.840	0.968	0.913	0.938	0.875	0.904
Shape descriptors	0.931	0.800	0.984	0.952	0.924	0.870	0.892
Texture descriptors	0.851	0.680	0.919	0.773	0.877	0.723	0.800
Edge descriptors	0.712	0	1	0	0.713	0	0.500

Figure 18. Summary of statistics for different classifiers implemented within WEKA when using all of the 19 features

Classifier	Success rate	Sensitivity	Specificity	PPV	NPV	F-measure	A_z
BayesNet	0.851	0.880	0.839	0.688	0.945	0.772	0.914
NaiveBayes	0.897	0.880	0.903	0.786	0.949	0.830	0.944
SVM	0.931	0.840	0.968	0.913	0.938	0.875	0.904
MLP	0.897	0.720	0.968	0.900	0.896	0.800	0.944
RBFNetwork	0.908	0.880	0.919	0.815	0.950	0.846	0.955
Bagging	0.839	0.720	0.887	0.720	0.887	0.720	0.899
AdaBoost	0.885	0.720	0.952	0.857	0.894	0.783	0.940
LogitBoost	0.885	0.800	0.919	0.800	0.919	0.800	0.891
Random Tree	0.839	0.760	0.871	0.704	0.900	0.731	0.815
Random Forest	0.862	0.800	0.887	0.741	0.917	0.769	0.926

tasks. The results tabulated in Figure 18 proves that classification can be reliably performed using the combination of features.

In the following section, we analyse the performance of different classifiers when using all features belonging to different groups namely, shape, texture and edge feature groups. The purpose of this study is investigating towards the possibility of identifying the optimum feature set for different classifiers.

Figure 19 compares the performance of different classifiers when using all shape based feature descriptors. The results show that the RBFNetwork has the highest *success rate* (i.e., 0.931), *sensitivity*, *specificity* and *F-measure*. SVM performs best when using *success rate* as a metric.

Figure 19. Summary of statistics for different classifiers when using all shape features

Classifier	Success rate	Sensitivity	Specificity	PPV	NPV	F-measure	A_z
BayesNet	0.839	0.84	0.839	0.677	0.929	0.750	0.894
NaiveBayes	0.897	0.88	0.903	0.786	0.949	0.830	0.942
SVM	0.931	0.8	0.984	0.952	0.924	0.870	0.892
MLP	0.897	0.8	0.935	0.833	0.921	0.816	0.928
RBFNetwork	0.931	0.92	0.935	0.852	0.967	0.885	0.926
Bagging	0.862	0.76	0.903	0.76	0.903	0.760	0.898
AdaBoost	0.851	0.76	0.887	0.731	0.902	0.745	0.913
LogitBoost	0.874	0.84	0.887	0.75	0.932	0.792	0.935
Random Tree	0.931	0.84	0.968	0.913	0.938	0.875	0.904
Random Forest	0.828	0.68	0.887	0.708	0.873	0.694	0.901

Figure 20. Summary of statistics for different classifiers when using all texture features

Classifier	Success rate	Sensitivity	Specificity	PPV	NPV	F-measure	A_z
BayesNet	0.747	0.76	0.742	0.543	0.885	0.633	0.795
NaiveBayes	0.724	0.880	0.661	0.512	0.932	0.647	0.861
SVM	0.851	0.680	0.919	0.773	0.877	0.723	0.800
MultiLayer Perceptron	0.793	0.76	0.806	0.613	0.893	0.679	0.870
RBFNetwork	0.747	0.680	0.774	0.548	0.857	0.607	0.825
Bagging	0.701	0.800	0.661	0.488	0.891	0.606	0.834
AdaBoost	0.759	0.680	0.790	0.567	0.860	0.618	0.714
LogitBoost	0.632	0.480	0.694	0.387	0.768	0.429	0.718
Random Tree	0.644	0.480	0.710	0.400	0.772	0.436	0.595
Random Forest	0.770	0.720	0.790	0.581	0.875	0.643	0.777

Figure 20 compares the performance of different classifiers when using all texture based feature descriptors. Results show that SVM performs best when using *success rate*, *specificity* and *F-measure*. However overall, the combination of texture features performs worse as compared to the combination of shape features, indicating that shape descriptors will play a more important role in lesion classification tasks as compared to texture based features. This is further discussed in next section under feature selection.

Figure 21 compares the performance of different classifiers when using all edge based feature descriptors. The results illustrate that none of the classifiers performs consistently well when using different metrics and the overall performance is significantly poor as compared to using all of shape or all of texture features. This implies that a combination of edge features will not provide

Figure 21. Summary of statistics for different classifiers when using all edge features

Classifier	Success rate	Sensitivity	Specificity	PPV	NPV	F-measure	A_z
BayesNet	0.828	0.440	0.984	0.917	0.813	0.595	0.768
NaiveBayes	0.793	0.600	0.871	0.652	0.844	0.625	0.829
SVM	0.716	0	1	0	0.713	0	0.500
MLP	0.793	0.400	0.952	0.769	0.797	0.526	0.788
RBFNetwork	0.793	0.440	0.935	0.733	0.806	0.550	0.759
Bagging	0.816	0.400	0.984	0.909	0.803	0.556	0.814
AdaBoost	0.805	0.520	0.919	0.722	0.826	0.605	0.806
LogitBoost	0.770	0.480	0.887	0.632	0.809	0.545	0.785
Random Tree	0.713	0.640	0.742	0.500	0.836	0.561	0.691
Random Forest	0.713	0.480	0.806	0.500	0.794	0.490	0.732

Figure 22. Features and their corresponding numbers

Features	Numbering
AP	1
Solidity	2
Convexity	3
Elongation	4
Extent	5
AR	6
Comp	7
Round	8
Form Factor	9
Max/min radii	10
Mean	11
Std dev	12
Skewness	13
Kurtosis	14
mce	15
Fourier1	16
Fourier2	17
Fractal1	18
Fractal2	19

a viable solution for feature classification. However there may be individual edge features that may help improve the classification when used within an ensemble of other shape and texture based features. This is the focus of investigations carried out in the following section.

Comparison of Feature Selection Methods

To obtain more reliable results, a detailed experiment on the use of well-known feature selection algorithms (*Best First, LFS, Genetic Search*, and *Greedy Stepwise*) was conducted.

Figure 22 summarises the feature combinations selected when different feature selection algorithms implemented within WEKA were used. For the ease of representation, we used a number to represent each feature. Figure 22 illustrates the features with their corresponding numbers.

For example, from Figure 23 it is seen that the feature selection technique, CfsSubsetEval, picked up a feature subset that consists of features, 2 (solidity), 4(elongation), 9(form factor), 11(mean)

and 12(standard deviation) as the best fitting set of features for subsequent classification.

Figure 24 shows the comparison of statistics by using the subset chosen by CfsSubsetEval, which proves that feature selection has lead to an improvement in classification. RBFNetwork performed the best among the classifiers with a *success rate* of 0.920, *sensitivity* of 0.840, *specificity* of 0.952, and *F-measure* of 0.857.

Further performance evaluations under combinations of different features were conducted. It was observed that although the reduction of features resulted in a reduction of complexity, the feature reduction cannot be carried out without limits. In certain cases removal of certain features resulted in an improved performance of classification. However in general the purpose of reducing the features is to find a trade-off between complexity and the cost. In medical analysis, the *sensitivity* and *specificity* is far more important than complexity issue. Although the complexity of a machine is affordable, reduction of *sensitivity* and *specificity* is not acceptable due to the nature of application and impact on human life.

Figure 23. Feature sets selected by different feature selection algorithms implemented within WEKA

Feature Selection Method	1	2	3	4	5	6	7	8	9	10	11	12	13	14	15	16	17	18	19
CfsSubsetEval		√		√					√		√	√							
ClassifierSubsetEval																			
BayesNet, Best First		√		√							√								
BayesNet, LFS		√		√							√								
BayesNet, Genetic Search				√	√											√			
BayesNet, Greedy Stepwise		√		√							√								
NaiveBayes, BestFirst	√	√						√				√					√		
NaiveBayes, LFS	√	√						√				√					√		
NaiveBayes, Genetic Search	√			√	√				√			√			√				
NaiveBayes, Greedy Stepwise	√	√						√											
SVM, Best First		√	√	√								√			√				
SVM, LFS		√	√	√								√			√				
SVM, Genetic Search		√	√	√					√			√	√		√		√		
SVM, Greedy Stepwise		√	√	√								√			√				
MLP, Best First	√	√	√	√															√
MLP, LFS		√	√	√					√						√				
MLP, Genetic Search	√			√			√			√	√	√			√	√	√	√	
MLP, Greedy Stepwise	√	√	√	√															√
RBFNet, Best First	√	√		√			√					√				√	√	√	
RBFNet, LFS	√	√		√				√				√				√	√	√	
RBFNet, Genetic Search	√			√		√			√			√	√			√	√	√	
RBFNet, Greedy Stepwise		√		√													√		
Bagging, Best First		√						√											√
Bagging, LFS		√						√											√
Bagging, Genetic Search	√		√	√								√			√	√	√		
Bagging, Greedy Stepwise		√						√										√	
AdaBoost, Best First	√	√	√									√							√
AdaBoost, LFS		√					√		√	√				√		√			
AdaBoost, Genetic Search	√	√		√							√	√		√			√	√	
AdaBoost, Greedy Stepwise	√	√																	√
LogitBoost, Best First	√	√	√	√					√										√
LogitBoost, LFS	√	√	√	√					√										√
LogitBoost, Genetic Search				√	√				√		√	√		√				√	√
LogitBoost, Greedy Stepwise		√		√															
RandomTree, Best First	√																		
RandomTree, LFS												√							
RandomTree, Genetic Search					√			√											√
RandomTree, Greedy Stepwise	√																		
RandomForest, Best First				√															
RandomForest, LFS										√									
RandomForest, Genetic Search					√			√											√
RandomForest, Greedy Stepwise				√															

Figures 25 to 31 summarise the statistical results of classification when using features selected by CfsClassifierSubset in conjunction with each classifier. It is observed that the RBFNetwork with Best First feature selection approach or RBFNetwork with LFS feature selection approach (Figure 28) resulted in an improved performance and produced reliable results with a *success rate* of 0.943, *sensitivity* of 0.88, *specificity* of 0.968, and *F-measure* of 0.898. By using 8 features

Figure 24. A comparison of statistics when features 2,4,9,11,12 (CfsSubsetEval selection) are used by different classifiers

Classifier	Success rate	Sensitivity	Specificity	PPV	NPV	F-measure	A$_z$
BayesNet	0.897	0.800	0.935	0.833	0.921	0.816	0.894
NaiveBayes	0.897	0.880	0.903	0.786	0.949	0.830	0.930
SVM	0.912	0.760	0.986	0.950	0.910	0.844	0.872
MLP	0.908	0.800	0.952	0.870	0.922	0.833	0.937
RBFNetwork	0.920	0.840	0.952	0.875	0.937	0.857	0.925
Bagging	0.862	0.720	0.919	0.783	0.891	0.750	0.911
AdaBoost	0.851	0.840	0.855	0.700	0.930	0.764	0.897
LogitBoost	0.885	0.880	0.887	0.759	0.948	0.815	0.940
Random Tree	0.782	0.720	0.806	0.600	0.877	0.655	0.763
Random Forest	0.874	0.800	0.903	0.769	0.918	0.784	0.941

Figure 25. Results for BayesNet with selected feature sets

Feature Selection Method	Success rate	Sensitivity	Specificity	PPV	NPV	F-measure	A$_z$
Best First LFS Greedy Stepwise (2,4,11)	0.885	0.760	0.935	0.826	0.906	0.792	0.886
Genetic Search (4,5,15)	0.874	0.800	0.903	0.769	0.918	0.784	0.898

Figure 26. Results for NaiveBayes with selected feature sets

Feature Selection Method	Success rate	Sensitivity	Specificity	PPV	NPV	F-measure	A$_z$
Best First LFS (1,2,8,12,17)	0.874	0.800	0.903	0.769	0.918	0.784	0.926
Genetic Search (1,4,5,9,12,15)	0.874	0.88	0.871	0.733	.0947	0.800	0.934
Greedy Stepwise (1,2,8)	0.874	0.80	0.903	0.769	0.918	0.784	0.928

Figure 27. Results for SVM with selected feature sets

Feature Selection Method	Success rate	Sensitivity	Specificity	PPV	NPV	F-measure	A$_z$
Best First LFS Greedy Stepwise (2,3,4,12,15)	0.908	0.800	0.952	0.870	0.922	0.833	0.876
Genetic Search (3,4,5,9,12,13, 15,17)	0.908	0.76	0.968	0.905	0.909	0.826	0.864

Figure 28. Results for MLP with selected feature sets

Feature Selection Method	Success rate	Sensitivity	Specificity	PPV	NPV	F-measure	A$_z$
Best First Greedy Stepwise (1,2,3,4,19)	0.897	0.760	0.952	0.864	0.908	0.809	0.951
LFS (2,3,4,9,15)	0.920	0.760	0.984	0.950	0.910	0.844	0.931
Genetic Search (1,4,7,10,11,12 ,15,16,17,18)	0.885	0.800	0.919	0.800	0.919	0.800	0.915

Figure 29. Results for RBGNetwork with selected feature sets

Feature Selection Method	Success rate	Sensitivity	Specificity	PPV	NPV	F-measure	A$_z$
Best First (1,2,4,7,12,16, 17,18)	0.943	0.880	0.968	0.917	0.952	0.898	0.939
LFS (1,2,4,8,12,16, 17,18)	0.943	0.880	0.968	0.917	0.952	0.898	0.948
Genetic Search (1,4,6,9,12,13, 16,17,18)	0.908	0.840	0.935	0.840	0.935	0.840	0.942
Greedy Stepwise (2,4,17)	0.885	0.800	0.919	0.800	0.919	0.800	0.947

Figure 30. Resulst for AdaBoost with selected feature sets

Feature Selection Method	Success rate	Sensitivity	Specificity	PPV	NPV	F-measure	A_z
Best First (1,2,3,12,19)	0.897	0.720	0.968	0.900	0.896	0.800	0.884
LFS (2,7,9,11,15,17)	0.828	0.720	0.871	0.692	0.885	0.706	0.875
Genetic Search (1,2,4,11,12,14,17,18)	0.874	0.72	0.935	0.818	0.892	0.766	0.889
Greedy Stepwise (1,2,19)	0.828	0.640	0.903	0.727	0.862	0.681	0.873

(1,2,4,7,12,16,17,18) or (1,2,4,8,12,16,17,18), RBFNetwork performed best with reduced complexity. On the other hand, single feature selection by using Random Tree and Random Forest approaches are not reliable as indicated by the results tabulated in Figure 30.

CONCLUSION

We have proposed an end-to-end approach to fully automatic US image lesion detection and recognition. The lesion recognition stage comprising of initial detection of ROI and lesion boundary identification/segmentation were carried out with the use of two previous approaches we have proposed. Thus the focus of this paper has been on a thorough investigation of the best possible approaches to lesion type recognition.

Figure 31. Results for Random Forest with selected feature sets

Feature Selection Method	Success rate	Sensitivity	Specificity	PPV	NPV	F-measure	A_z
Best First Greedy Stepwise (4)	0.701	0.640	0.726	0.485	0.833	0.552	0.770
LFS (10)	0.678	0.400	0.790	0.435	0.766	0.417	0.588
Genetic Search (5,8,19)	0.816	0.640	0.887	0.696	0.859	0.667	0.852

A number of feature based approaches to classification were investigated. The use of different types of features, divided into three groups, shape based, texture based and edge based, that can be used in classification was investigated. Experimental results concluded that in general, shape based features are the most reliable for classification of lesion type; while edge based features are the least reliable. Further investigations revealed that different feature combinations perform best when used in conjunction with different classifiers.

The major novel contribution of this research is the evaluation of the use of ten different feature-based classifiers and experimentally determining the optimum feature set for each classifier. To authors knowledge such a comprehensive analysis has not been carried out previously. From the overall performance, RBFNetwork with feature set {1 (area to perimeter ratio), 2 (solidity), 4 (elongation), 8 (roundness), 12 (standard deviation), 16 (fourier1), 17 (fourier2), 18(fractal1)} out-performed other combinations of feature-classifier, with an achievement of predicated A_z value of 0.948. Within the selected dataset, the feature based classifiers performed reasonably well, but there is still scope for testing with large datasets, inspired by the data mining principle, "the larger the training set, the better the classifier model"(Witten & Frank, 2005).

Images with no abnormalities are not captured or stored by Sonographers during a typical diagnostic process, as the interest is only in the capture of abnormal lesions. Consequently, it is common to find an acute shortage of normal images in a typical test database. To overcome this problem, close collaborative work with hospitals and clinics is needed. With a well balanced, larger training set, a better classification model can be achieved, leading to an improved tolerance and consistency in classification.

ACKNOWLEDGMENT

The authors would like to thank Prapavesis et al. (2001) for providing the ultrasound images. This research was supported by Department of Computer Science, Loughborough University, under a research scholarship awarded to Moi Hoon Yap.

REFERENCES

Barnsley, M. F., Devaney, R. L., Mandlebrot, B. B., Peitgen, H., Saupe, D., & Voss, R. F. (1988). *The Science of Fractal Images*. New York: Springer-Verlag. doi:10.1007/978-1-4612-3784-6

Breiman, L. (1996). Bagging Predictors. *Machine Learning*, 24(2), 123–140. doi:10.1007/BF00058655

Breiman, L. (2001). Random Forests. *Machine Learning*, 45(1), 5–32. doi:10.1023/A:1010933404324

Chang, R. F., Wu, W. J., Moon, W. K., & Chen, D. R. (2003). Improvement in breast tumor discrimination by support vector machines and speckle-emphasis texture analysis. *Ultrasound in Medicine & Biology, 29*(5), 679–686. PubMed doi:10.1016/S0301-5629(02)00788-3

Chang, R. F., Wu, W. J., Moon, W. K., & Chen, D. R. (2005). Automatic ultrasound segmentation and morphology based diagnosis of solid breast tumors. *Breast Cancer Research and Treatment, 89*(2), 179–185. PubMed doi:10.1007/s10549-004-2043-z

Chen, C. M., Chou, Y. H., Han, K. C., Hung, G. S., Tiu, C. M., Chiou, H. J., et al. (2003). Breast lesions on sonograms: computer-aided diagnosis with nearly setting-independent features and artificial neural networks. *Radiology, 226*(2), 504–514. PubMed doi:10.1148/radiol.2262011843

Chen, D. R., Chang, R. F., Chen, C. J., Ho, M. F., Kuo, S. J., Chen, S. T., et al. (2005). Classification of breast ultrasound images using fractal feature. *Clinical Imaging, 29*(4), 235–245. PubMed doi:10.1016/j.clinimag.2004.11.024

Chen, D. R., Chang, R. F., & Huang, Y. L. (1999). Computer-aided diagnosis applied to US of solid breast nodules by using neural networks. *Radiology, 213*, 407–412.

Chen, D. R., Chang, R. F., Huang, Y. L., Chou, Y. H., Tiu, C. M., & Tsai, P. P. (2000). Texture analysis of breast tumors on sonograms. *Seminars in Ultrasound, CT, and MR, 21*(4), 308–316. PubMed doi:10.1016/S0887-2171(00)90025-8

Chen, D. R., Chang, R. F., Kuo, W. J., Chen, M. C., & Huang, Y. L. (2002). Diagnosis of breast tumors with sonographic texture analysis using wavelet transform and neural networks. *Ultrasound in Medicine & Biology, 28*(10), 1301–1310. PubMed doi:10.1016/S0301-5629(02)00620-8

Costa, L. D. F. D., & Cesar, R. M. (2000). *Shape analysis and classification: theory and practise* (1st ed.). Boca Raton, FL: CRC Press Inc.

Drukker, K., Giger, M. L., Horsh, K., Kupinski, M. A., & Vyborny, C. J. (2002). Computerized lesion detection on breast ultrasound. *Medical Physics, 29*(7), 1438–1446. PubMed doi:10.1118/1.1485995

Freund, Y. S., R. E. (1999). A short introduction to boosting. *Journal of Japanese Society for Artificial Intelligence, 14*(5), 771–780.

Friedman, J., Hastle, T., & Tibshirani, R. (2000). Additive logistic regression: a statistical view of boosting. *Annals of Statistics, 28*(2), 337–407. doi:10.1214/aos/1016218223

Goldberg, D. E. (1989). *Genetic algorithms in search, optimization & machine learning*. Reading, MA: Addison Wesley.

Guetlein, M. (2006). Large scale attribute selection using wrappers.

Hall, M. A. (1998). *Correlation-based feature subset selection for machine learning*. Unpublished dissertation/thesis, University of Waikato, Hamilton, New Zealand.

Horsch, K., Giger, M. L., Venta, L. A., & Vyborny, C. J. (2002). Computerized diagnosis of breast lesions on ultrasound. *Medical Physics, 29*(2), 157–164. PubMed doi:10.1118/1.1429239

Huang, Y. L., & Chen, D. R. (2005). Support vector machines in sonography application to decision making in the diagnosis of breast cancer. *Journal of Clinical Imaging, 29*, 179–184. doi:10.1016/j.clinimag.2004.08.002

Huang, Y. L., Chen, D. R., Jiang, Y. R., Kuo, S. J., Wu, H. K., & Moon, W. K. (2008). Computer-aided diagnosis using morphological features for classifying breast lesions on ultrasound. *Ultrasound Obstet. Gynecol.*

John, G. H., & Pat Langley, P. (1995, 1995). *Estimating continuous distributions in Bayesian classifiers.* Paper presented at the Proceedings of the Eleventh Conference on Uncertainty in Artificial Intelligence, San Mateo, CA.

Joo, S., Yang, Y. S., Moon, W. K., & Kim, H. C. (2004). Computer-aided diagnosis of solid breast nodules: use of an artificial neural network based on multiple sonographic features. *IEEE Transactions on Medical Imaging, 23*(10), 1292–1300. PubMed doi:10.1109/TMI.2004.834617

Mu, T., Nandi, A. K., & Rangayyan, R. M. (2008). Classification of breast masses using selected shape, edge-sharpness, and texture features with linear and kernel-based classifiers. *Journal of Digital Imaging, 21*(2), 153–169. PubMed doi:10.1007/s10278-007-9102-z

National Health Service. (2008). *National Health Service Breast Screening Programme* (*Vol. 2008*). U. K.

Ojala, T., Pietikainen, M., & Maenpaa, T. (2002). Multiresolution gray-scale and rotation invariant texture classification with local binary patterns. *IEEE Transactions on Pattern Analysis and Machine Intelligence, 24*(7), 971–987. doi:10.1109/TPAMI.2002.1017623

Platt, J., Scholkopf, B., Burges, C., & Smola, A. (1999). Fast training of support vector machines using sequential minimal optimization. In Anonymous, (Ed.), *Advances in Kernel Methods - Support Vector Learning*. Cambridge, MA: MIT Press.

Prapavesis, S. T., Fornage, B. D., Weismann, C. F., Palko, A., & Zoumpoulis, P. (2001). *Breast ultrasound and US-guided interventional techniques*. Thessaloniki, Greece.

Russ, J. C. (2007). *The image processing handbook* (5th ed.). Boca Raton, Fla: CRC Press.

Smith, R. A., Saslow, D., Sawyer, K. A., Burke, W., Costanza, M. E., Evans, W. P., et al. (2003). American Cancer Society guidelines for breast cancer screening: update 2003. *CA: a Cancer Journal for Clinicians, 53*(3), 141–169. PubMed doi:10.3322/canjclin.53.3.141

Vapnik, V. (1995). *The nature of statistical learning theory*. New York: Springer-Verlag.

Wikipedia (2008). Support vector machine: MediaWiki.

Witten, I. H., & Frank, E. (2005). *Data mining - Practical machine learning tools and techniques*. United States of America: Morgan Kaufmann, Elsevier.

Xu, C., & Prince, J. L. (1998). Generalized gradient vector flow external forces for active contours. *Signal Processing, 71*, 131–139. doi:10.1016/S0165-1684(98)00140-6

Yap, M. H., Edirisinghe, E. A., & Bez, B. E. (2007, Feb 2007). *Fully automated lesion boundary detection in ultrasound breast images*. Paper presented at the SPIE Medical Imaging Conference, San Diego, CA.

Yap, M. H., Edirisinghe, E. A., & Bez, H. E. (2008). A novel algorithm for initial lesion detection in ultrasound breast images. *Journal of Applied Clinical Medical Physics, 9*(4), 181–199. doi:10.1120/jacmp.v9i4.2741

Yap, M. H., Edirisinghe, E. A., & Bez, H. E. (2009). *A comparative study in ultrasound breast imaging classification*. Paper presented at the SPIE Medical Imaging.

This work was previously published in International Journal of Computational Models and Algorithms in Medicine, Volume 1, Issue 2, edited by Aryya Gangopadhyay, pp. 53-81, copyright 2010 by IGI Publishing (an imprint of IGI Global).

Chapter 10
An Effective Streams Clustering Method for Biomedical Signals

Pimwadee Chaovalit
National Science and Technology Development Agency, Thailand

ABSTRACT

In the healthcare industry, the ability to monitor patients via biomedical signals assists healthcare professionals in detecting early signs of conditions such as blocked arteries and abnormal heart rhythms. Using data clustering, it is possible to interpret these signals to look for patterns that may indicate emerging or developing conditions. This can be accomplished by basing monitoring systems on a fast clustering algorithm that processes fast-paced streams of raw data effectively. This paper presents a clustering method, POD-Clus, which can be useful in computer-aided diagnosis. The proposed method clusters data streams in linear time and outperforms a competing algorithm in capturing changes of clusters in data streams.

INTRODUCTION

Recently, the healthcare industry has generated massive amounts of signal data to aid with physicians' diagnoses. Examples of different types of biomedical signals data include ECG (Electrocardiogram), EEG (Electroencephalogram), and PCG (Phonocardiogram) signals. These signals share some common characteristics as follows. They are being collected at an extremely fast pace. For example, an ECG sampling rate can range from 100 Hz to more than 1000 Hz (Bragge, Tarvainen, & Karjalainen, 2004). They are potentially "unbounded" (Lu & Huang, 2005) for the fact that

their sequences of observation values are possibly open-ended. For instance, EEG data, which are used to monitor brain waves for diagnosing epilepsy or sleep patterns, can be recorded for days (Sun & Sclabassi, 1999). These streams of data collected from sensors and other equipments can be referred to in general as "data streams".

An automatic monitoring device such as a digital ECG is used in monitoring heart-related conditions. An ECG can have up to 10 wires to collect a heart's electrical signal, providing up to 12 or even 15 "angles" of how a heart functions (Cowley, 2006). The heart's electrical activities are monitored via the electrical signals from various

DOI: 10.4018/978-1-4666-0282-3.ch010

designated places on the body. Wires are often placed on a patient's limbs and chest, capturing signals of tissue muscle contractions which relate to the heart's pumping motion. As these heart's electrical data are continuously gathered at the rate of 100 – 1,000 samples per second (Bragge et al., 2004), a 5-minute recording of ECG can produce up to 10 time series (from 10 wires), each with 300,000 samples, leading to 3,000,000 data points. This is an enormous amount of data to handle.

Various conditions can be revealed from the analysis of abnormal heartbeats. For example, the height of waves can be used to diagnose tissue death caused by blocked blood supply. Retrieving and analyzing these large amounts of data in a timely manner for quick diagnosis are challenging, as constantly arriving data may cause the data to become too large to either transmit over a network (Sun & Sclabassi, 1999) or fit in the main memory of the device. Hence, processing on data streams has to happen online and incrementally while data streams arrive, instead of offline and in batches.

There exists a need for effective data streams mining techniques that can handle such data streams efficiently. This paper presents a study on *data streams clustering*, which can be incorporated into computer-aided analysis and used by physicians to cluster biomedical signals for diagnosis. By grouping biomedical signals into homogeneous clusters, we learn about data characteristics which may indicate emerging or developing conditions. Results obtained from clustering biomedical signals can then be developed into classification models or predictive models useful in healthcare diagnoses. We propose a novel method called POD-Clus (Probability and Distribution-based Clustering) with significant improvements on clustering results as compared to the competing algorithm for data streams clustering.

BACKGROUND

A data stream is a fast-arriving, transient sequence of data values. Data streams' characteristics (Domingos & Hulten, 2000; Gama, Rodrigues, & Aguilar-Ruiz, 2007) are summarized as follows:

1. Data usually coming in at a detailed level
2. Streaming data arriving at a fast pace
3. Potentially unbounded observations of data
4. Possibly limited storage and memory resources for processing data streams
   a. As high-volume and high-speed data streams challenge data miners to shift data mining paradigm from mining in batches to mining incrementally. Employing the "incremental" approach allows data miners to avoid an expensive processing of potentially large-sized data at the end of the streams by processing data in a small amount at a time. The criteria for a capable data streams clustering method include (Babcock, Babu, Datar, Motwani, & Widom, 2002; Barbará, 2002; Domingos & Hulten, 2001; Golab & Özsu, 2003):
      - Recursive updating of clustering results: The clustering result and clustering models should continually and recursively incorporate the incoming data. Researchers also need to assure that the results from the recursive updates should be as close as possible to the results that can be obtained from batch clustering.
      - Building and updating clustering models in one pass: The high-speed and high-volume nature of data streams prohibit multiple re-scans of all the data, because the amount of computa-

tion required will be excessive. Thus, incremental clustering methods are limited to ideally one view of data. Once the data has been viewed and processed, the viewed data items can be discarded.

- Using small time per data record: The processing of these systems also needs to take a smaller constant time than the rate in which data are arriving, in order to keep up with the speed of data.
- Using linear processing time: A data streams clustering system will see unbounded streams of data. The processing time per record should be constant, thereby ensuring a linear runtime of the algorithm. Otherwise the overall runtime can grow exponentially to the increasing volume of data.
- Handling concept drift: A concept drift happens when the overall formation of data points changes, possibly affecting the number of clusters. A streams clustering method has a real challenge of adapting the clustering models to always reflect the transient nature of data, because it cannot view future data before the start of the clustering process.
- Having available answers or models at any time: As data streams are unbounded, answers from the clustering algorithms need to be available to users anytime. The answers should also be new and should take into account the most recently viewed data instances.

Literature Review

The above requirements have shaped research directions in the data streams clustering field. In the past decade, research efforts have resulted in various data streams clustering algorithms reviewed below in chronological order of publishing. We pay attention to how the incremental clustering is achieved, what type of clustering mechanism is employed, whether the algorithm handles cluster evolution, and if so, how. We also make note of another recently important concept, data fading, which suggests that old data items should be given less importance for clustering.

STREAM (Guha, Meyerson, Mishra, Motwani, & O'Callaghan, 2003) is one of the earliest algorithms in data streams clustering. This Stanford-originated algorithm generates k cluster centers by running a k-medians algorithm over data, when k represents the number of clusters. STREAM then maintains k-centers in memory and discards local data points. The k-centers are grouped into larger clusters. With this scheme, clusters are built incrementally and hierarchically with a single pass on data. STREAM focuses on providing a solution to clustering data points with guarantees of constant-factor approximation to optimal results with an efficient memory usage. However, STREAM neither clusters data streams with different types of cluster evolution, nor considers the fading of data points. As STREAM bases its clustering mechanism on the k-medians clustering, k (the number of clusters) needs to be provided from user input, and cannot change.

CluStream (Aggarwal, Han, Wang, & Yu, 2003) consists of online and offline components. The online component incrementally updates micro-clusters and their summary information. The micro-clusters information is stored in snapshots in a pyramidal framework of time, which enables users to later select their desired time window to group micro-clusters into bigger clusters. The offline component clusters the micro-clusters using their summary information. CluStream relies on the k-means clustering algorithm as its clustering mechanism for both online and offline components. CluStream supports cluster evolution analysis by allowing users to compare the distribution of clusters at the beginning and at the ending of a specified time horizon. The clusters added or deleted from the beginning of the time period reveal the appearance or disappearance of clusters. However, the concept of data fading is not applied in CluStream.

HPStream (Aggarwal, Han, Wang, & Yu, 2004) focuses on clustering high-dimensional data streams. The algorithm performs dimension subset selection by projecting on the original high-dimensional data. It incrementally updates a set of summary data called *Fading Cluster Structure (FCS)* which incorporates the fading of outdated data points into the algorithm. HPStream starts by initializing original clusters which include all dimensions. Based on those clusters, dimensions are projected and new cluster centroids are calculated. Dimension projection and centroid calculation are alternated and repeated until clusters converge. For incoming data streams, HPStream finds the closest cluster for each data point by calculating centroid-to-point distances for only the projected dimensions. The cluster evolution is handled through heuristics. If the new data point lies outside the natural radius of the assigned cluster, a new cluster needs to be formed. Clusters can also disappear in two ways: when the total number of clusters produced by HPStream exceeds the maximum number of clusters and when none of the dimensions are projected for a cluster. HPStream also implements the k-means clustering algorithm as its initialization process. Thus, it might experience the well-known drawbacks of k-means: an arbitrary k, and the random seed selection.

The E-Stream algorithm (Udommanetanakit, Rakthanmanon, & Waiyamai, 2007) incrementally updates data points into cluster representations called *Fading Cluster Structure with Histogram (FCH)*, which contains an *FCS* similar to that of HPStream and an α-bin histogram. In E-Stream,

each data point is assigned to the closest cluster among active clusters. An active cluster is a cluster with a high enough weight and therefore is able to assemble new data points, whereas an inactive cluster is a cluster whose data points have faded away when applying a decay function causing its weight to decline to a number beyond threshold. E-Stream tackles various types of cluster evolutions. At each time interval, E-Stream fades all clusters, and then checks for any possible cluster splitting using histogram analysis. A cluster is split when a statistically significant valley is found in at least one dimension of its histogram. Next, E-Stream checks for any possible cluster merging by analyzing pairwise cluster distances. If a cluster-to-cluster distance falls below a threshold, these clusters will be merged as it indicates an overlap of the two clusters. E-stream also merges clusters when the number of clusters exceeds the maximum number of clusters. Furthermore, E-Stream creates a new cluster if the distance of the new data point to its closest cluster is above a radius threshold.

D-Stream (Chen & Tu, 2007) aims to find arbitrarily-shaped clusters and is free from the parameter k which is required by k-means based clustering methods. Clusters are assumed to have dense grids inside and sparser grids outside. D-Stream is composed of online and offline components. The online component incrementally maps incoming data onto a density-based grid structure, while the offline component computes all grids' densities. D-Stream also incorporates the fading concept, which allows clusters to disappear by classifying grids as: *Dense*, *Sparse*, and *Transitional* according to their average densities. The fading concept is vital for D-Stream's grid management, allowing D-Stream to use less memory by deleting grids that do not have enough density. D-Stream handles the cluster evolution by merging clusters whenever possible by way of connecting neighboring grids and by splitting clusters when sporadic grids are removed causing a cluster to become separated.

METHODOLOGY

The paper provides a theoretical framework which addresses data streams clustering. The framework is developed using the requirements of data streams clustering technique as a guide and improves on existing data streams clustering techniques. Practically, the paper introduces a clustering method that does the following:

- Yields superior, high-quality clustering results
- Produces results in an efficient manner
- Handles cluster evolution, that includes:
  - Migrating of data points among clusters
  - Creating of new clusters, either when a new cluster splits from an existing cluster or when a new cluster emerges
  - Dissolving of existing clusters, either when a cluster merges with another cluster or when a cluster vanishes
- Handles outliers

Problem Formalization

The methodology focuses on clustering transient data streams, which is considered a form of incremental clustering for its growing time dimension. Another viewpoint exists in which the number of data sources producing data streams can grow (Yang, 2003). The latter viewpoint is not the main focus of this paper, although a slight modification of our approach can achieve the latter viewpoint.

Under the generic method of data streams clustering, we propose the algorithms by different classes: the clustering without cluster evolution and with cluster evolution. In order to provide corresponding comparisons to the related work, first we developed the clustering approach without the cluster evolution capability. Then, the approach is enhanced with an ability to detect and adapt the clustering model to changes in cluster formations.

The POD-Clus algorithms are developed within these different classes.

We define important concepts under the scope of this paper as follows.

- **Definition 1:** [*Data Streams*] Let us consider a set of data streams $DS = \{S_1, S_2, ..., S_n\}$, where S_i is a data stream obtained from data source i, and n is the number of data streams in DS. Furthermore, $S_i = \{s_{i1}, s_{i2}, ..., s_{it}\}$, where s_{ij} is the recorded value of S_i at time j.
- **Definition 2:** [*Clustering Data Streams*] Let us consider a set of clusters $C = \{C_1, C_2, ..., C_k\}$, where C_x is a cluster, and k is the number of clusters in C. Given a DS, all non-outlier data points s_{ij} belong to some cluster C_x such that $\{\forall s_{ij} \in S_i \; \exists C_x \mid s_{ij} \in C_x\}$. It is also possible that there exists another data point s_{ih} such that $\{s_{ih}, s_{ij} \in S_i\}$, however $s_{ih} \in C_m$ where $m \neq x$.
- **Definition 3:** [*Clustering Data Streams without Cluster Evolution*] Suppose there is a set of clusters C, whose centroids are denoted by c, and k is the number of clusters in C. Without cluster evolution, k remains constant while c changes over time. A clustering result consists of a mapping of $(DS \rightarrow C)$ in which all s_{ij} are mapped to C_x.
- **Definition 4:** [*Clustering Data Streams with Cluster Evolution*] Suppose there is a set of clusters C, whose centroids are denoted by c, and k is the number of clusters in C. With cluster evolution, both k and c can change over time. A clustering result consists of a mapping of $(DS \rightarrow C)$ in which some s_{ij} are mapped to C_x. There may be a mapping of $(DS \rightarrow O)$ in which some s_{ij} are mapped to O_y. O is a set of outlier groups, when $O_y, y = 1..l$ is an outlier group, and l is the number of outlier groups. Each s_{ij} is assigned to either a member of the set of clusters or a member of the set of outliers. The assignment is collectively exhaustive

and mutually exclusive such that $S_i \in C \cup O$ $\forall i$; $s_{ij} \in C \cup O \; \forall i, \forall j$; and $C \cap O = \emptyset$.

With all concepts defined, two different classes emerge under the generic method for data streams clustering, and they are:

1. Clustering data streams without cluster evolution, using Definitions 2 and 3
2. Clustering data streams with cluster evolution, using Definitions 2 and 4

Data Streams Clustering Framework

This section outlines how data streams clustering can be accomplished to meet the requirements below:

a. The system requires only one scan of data.
b. The system updates new data observations to the previously mined model.
c. The system makes available the answers of the clustering problem to users at anytime.
d. The system spends a small amount of processing time per data observation.
e. The system uses a small (preferably fixed) amount of memory.
f. The system is able to handle cluster evolutions.

The essentials of time series clustering comprise three components: 1) the clustering algorithms, 2) the distance measures, and 3) the evaluation criteria on clustering results (Liao, 2005), illustrated in Figure 1 (left). To perform any clustering, all of these components are defined and selected.

The framework of data streams clustering is adjusted from these basics. In Figure 1 (right), an additional process block, which assists in data streams clustering, is inserted between data streams and the clustering process. The block views data only once and then incrementally

updates only crucial pieces of information for the clustering model.

Clustering algorithms then perform clustering using the minimal information at hand. Since the distance functions are often computed from summary information of data, collecting only a minimal amount of information (also known as sufficient statistics) is usually adequate for the calculation of clustering algorithms. Therefore, this framework enables the clustering techniques to obtain good quality clustering results in an incremental manner.

POD-Clus Algorithm

This section presents the proposed algorithm for data streams clustering: POD-Clus. POD-Clus is an algorithm which handles the challenges pre-

Figure 1. The data streams clustering framework (right) in comparison to the time series clustering framework (left)

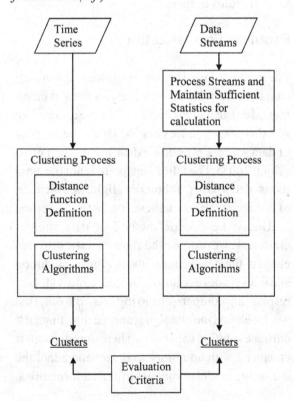

sented by data streams clustering. It incrementally updates clustering results, makes the clustering results available at anytime, requires only one pass of data, and processes streams of data using a small constant time. POD-Clus overcomes the challenges of clustering data streams by:

- Maintaining cluster synopses and discarding detailed information of individual data points. The synopsis is cluster information which is described by multivariate normal distribution.
- Assigning n data points to k clusters. Given $k \ll n$, this operation is much more efficient than a pairwise similarity comparison of n. While the time complexity of the pairwise similarity comparison is $O(n^2)$, the cluster assignment process in POD-Clus has the time complexity of $O(kn)$.
- Recursively updating current clusters when new data is available. The time complexity for this process is $O(n)$.

In short, POD-Clus assigns data points to their respective clusters by probability by tracking cluster synopses. The methods and algorithms of POD-Clus will be described in two parts: *without cluster evolution* and *with cluster evolution*, respectively.

Incremental Data Streams Clustering without Cluster Evolution

Main Idea

The methodology starts with the assumption that some initial cluster formation exists at time T_0. Any existing clustering algorithms may be used to perform the initial clustering. This is a realistic assumption in real-life situations such as monitoring patients' heart rates, where heart conditions can be initially clustered based on similarity measures. In addition, we assume that there are a fixed number (M) of data sources that

are sending readings at a given periodic interval. Even though the incoming data streams can continue indefinitely, without loss of generality, we assume that N number of data points will be transmitted from time T_1 to T_N. When the data at T_1 arrives, the method calculates the probability that it belongs to any of the existing clusters and is assigned to the cluster with the highest probability. Given a set of k clusters, we collect the mean (m), standard deviation (σ), and number of points (n) for each cluster. For a multi-dimensional dataset where each data point contains observations from D dimensions, we collect the mean (m) for each data dimension and the covariance matrix (S) for each cluster. We refer to the above collection as "cluster synopsis". After a cluster is modified, the corresponding cluster synopsis is updated.

Cluster Synopsis Maintenance

Cluster synopses are updated as follows. Let n_C, m_C, and $\sigma_C (S_C)$ be the number of data points within a cluster C, the mean of C, and the standard deviation (the covariance matrix) of C. After a new data point x^{new} has been added, the new n_C, m_C, and $\sigma_C (S_C)$ are updated by the equations (1)-(6).

$$n^{new}{}_C = n^{old}{}_C + 1 \tag{1}$$

$$\mu^{new}_C = \frac{n^{old}_C \mu^{old}_C + x^{new}}{n^{new}_C} \tag{2}$$

$$\sigma^{new}_C = \sqrt{\frac{((n^{old}_C - 1)\sigma^{old2}_C + n^{old}_C \mu^{old}_C + x^{new2}) - n^{new}_C \mu^{new2}_C}{n^{new}_C - 1}} \tag{3}$$

The first term of the numerator in the equation (3) updates the summation of the square of all data points in the cluster C. The second term updates the square of data mean in C multiplied by the number of new data points. Thus, the equation

(3) equates a simplified version of calculating an estimated standard deviation of the population.

$$\mu^{shift} = n_C^{old} \left(\mu_C^{old} - \mu_C^{new} \right) \left(\mu_C^{old} - \mu_C^{new} \right)^T$$

(4)

$$\text{cov}\_ x^{new} = \left(x^{new} - \mu_C^{new} \right) \left(x^{new} - \mu_C^{new} \right)^T$$

(5)

$$\Sigma_C^{new} = \frac{(n_C^{old} - 1)\Sigma_C^{old} + \mu^{shift} + \text{cov}\_ x^{new}}{n_C^{new} - 1}$$

(6)

From the equation (6), the update of the co-variance matrix S_C involves weighting the old covariance matrix (the first term of the numerator) by the old number of data points, shifting the centers of the cluster C (the second term of the numerator), and calculating covariance of the new data point x^{new} (the third term of the numerator). All components are added and then weighted by the new number of data points to create a new covariance matrix.

The basic idea of this algorithm is to assign new data points to the closest cluster using the calculated probabilistic values of x^{new} belonging to clusters 1 to k. We utilize the normal (Gaussian) distribution probability density function for both one-dimensional and multi-dimensional data. For an incoming data point (x^{new}) and a cluster synopsis of the cluster C (m_C, σ_C), we calculate the probability of data membership using the probability density function for one-dimensional data by:

$$y_C = p(x^{new} \mid \mu_C, \sigma_C) = \frac{1}{\sigma_C \sqrt{2\pi}} e^{\frac{-(x^{new} - \mu_C)^2}{2\sigma_C^2}}$$

(7)

Similarly, we calculate the probability of data membership using the probability density function for multi-dimensional data of D dimensions for an incoming data point (x^{new}) and a cluster synopsis (m_C, S_C) by:

$$y_C = p(x^{new} \mid \mu_C, \Sigma_C) = \frac{1}{\sqrt{(2\pi)^D |\Sigma_C|}} e^{-\frac{1}{2}\left((x^{new} - \mu_C)^T \Sigma_C^{-1} (x^{new} - \mu_C) \right)}$$

(8)

The POD-Clus Algorithm

This section describes our proposed data streams clustering algorithm in detail. The POD-Clus algorithm for *clustering data streams without cluster evolution* is explained using a pseudo-code. Let us define the notations used in our pseudo-code as (Figure 2):

- x^{new}: a novel data point
- k: the total number of clusters
- (m_C, S_C): a cluster synopsis of the cluster C
- n_C: the number of data points within the cluster C
- y_C: a probabilistic value that x^{new} belongs to the cluster C
- j: the cluster j among C = 1..k which yields the highest y_C
- DS: a set of data streams with M data sources, N time points
- Label(DS,C): a set of mapping from every data point within DS to C

The main POD-Clus algorithm starts by considering the next data point in DS in line 2. From lines 3 to 5, the probabilistic values that this data point belongs to each of the clusters 1 to k are evaluated using the functions given above in the equation (7) or (8). In line 6, all probabilistic

Figure 2. Algorithm POD-Clus

The POD-Clus Algorithm	
Input:	DS, (μ_C, Σ_C), and n_C, when C = 1..k
Output:	Label(DS,C), $(\mu^{new}_C, \Sigma^{new}_C)$, and n^{new}_C, when C = 1..k

```
1    repeat
2         x^new = the next data point in DS
3         for C = 1..k
4              y_C = p(x^new |(μ_C, Σ_C))
5         end for
6         j = arg max(y_C)
                  c
7         Label(DS,C) for x^new = j
8         update μ_j, Σ_j
9         n_j = n_j + 1
10   until end-of-file
11   wait for new data
```

values y_c are compared and the cluster with the highest probabilistic value (the cluster j) is considered the closest cluster to the data point x^{new}. Therefore, x^{new} is mapped to the cluster j in line 7. In line 8, the cluster synopsis of cluster j (m_j, S_j) is updated following the equations (1)-(6), and the number of time points is added by 1 in line 9. This process is repeated M*N times for M*N data points within the dataset DS.

Complexity Analysis

From the algorithm POD-Clus, the steps from lines 2 to 9 repeat *n* times, when *n* is the total number of data points. Thus, the main algorithm has a time complexity of O(*n*). For each data point x^{new}, the algorithm calculates the probability that x^{new} belongs to C in line 4. This step requires the computation of O(*k*) for each data point and hence O(*kn*) in total, where *k* is the total number of clusters. Overall, POD-Clus has the time complexity of O(*n*). The space required to store all cluster synopses is O(*k*), as POD-Clus stores only the cluster synopses in memory and discards the detailed data observations.

On the Normality Assumption

Since we model clusters using a normal distribution, the data is assumed to be normally distributed. This section explains why the normality assumption is a reasonable assumption for this study.

A structure of a data stream set DS can be viewed as:

$$\begin{bmatrix} t_{11} & t_{12} & \cdots & t_{1m} \\ t_{21} & t_{22} & \cdots & t_{2m} \\ \cdots & \cdots & \cdots & \cdots \\ t_{n1} & t_{n2} & \cdots & t_{nm} \end{bmatrix}$$

when t_{ij} is a data item value. Each row of t_{ij} represents data from an independent stream source. An example is data from an ECG sensor that is different from other ECG sensors. Moreover, data points are clustered regardless of their sources, thereby removing any dependency among data points within the same source. As a result, t_{ij} and t_{kl} ($i \neq k$ and $j \neq l$) are independent random variables.

Normal distribution has been found to be a good approximation for a vast number of datasets. Even if the underlying distribution of original data is non-normal, the central limit theorem states that as the sample size increases, the distribution of data approaches normal distribution (Thompson & Tapia, 1990). Since we propose a data stream clustering method designed to handle fast-paced streams of data, the method will likely view sufficiently large samples of data. Consequently, assuming data by normal distribution is reasonable. For the worst-case scenario where initial data is found to be non-normal, a Galton transformation can be used to transform non-normal data to normal data (Thompson & Tapia, 1990).

For the reasons shown above, the assumption of normality is appropriate for the scope of this paper.

Incremental Data Streams Clustering with Cluster Evolution

The POD-Clus algorithm is now extended to handle cluster evolution by exploiting the collection of cluster synopses maintained by POD-Clus. We developed a heuristic-based approach to detect and handle cluster evolution.

Types of Cluster Evolution

Cluster evolution consists of four main types, as illustrated by Figure 3. *Cluster appearance* happens when a new cluster is formed by new incoming data points. *Cluster splitting* occurs when data points within a cluster start to move apart, creating multiple distinct clusters. *Cluster disappearance* takes place when data points are no longer associated with a particular cluster, causing that cluster to disappear. *Cluster merging* occurs when data points from two clusters move towards each other until they overlap significantly.

The POD-Clus Algorithm and Other Algorithms for Cluster Evolution

We present the pseudo-code of the POD-Clus algorithm in Figure 4. We use the following notations in our pseudo-code:

- x^{new}: a novel data point
- k: the total number of clusters
- (m_C, S_C): a cluster synopsis of the cluster C
- n_C: the number of data points within the cluster C
- y_C: a probabilistic value that x^{new} belongs to the cluster C
- $flag_C$: a flag for the position of x^{new} in respect of the cluster C's boundaries
- j: the cluster j among C = 1..k which yields the highest y_C
- **DS**: a set of data streams with M data sources, N time points
- **Label(DS,C)**: a set of mapping from every data point within DS to C
- $CountDense_C$: a variable keeping the number of data points within the central region of the cluster C
- **CountMerge**: a variable keeping the number of data points with strong memberships to more than 1 cluster
- **S-threshold**: a threshold derived from the normal distribution for cluster splitting
- **M-threshold**: a threshold derived from the normal distribution for cluster merging
- $Bound_C$: a boundary set to 2σ or 3σ from the mean of the cluster C; the default value is 3σ
- λ: a fading factor with a default value of 0.1

Like clustering without cluster evolution, the POD-Clus algorithm starts by receiving a new data point, x^{new}, in line 2. Then, it determines if x^{new} is an outlier by using the *CheckBoundary* algorithm in line 3. Unless x^{new} is an outlier, POD-Clus assigns x^{new} to the closest existing cluster j, and updates the cluster synopsis (lines 7-9). The rest of the POD-Clus algorithm and other algorithms deal with cluster evolution (Figure 4, Figure 5, Figure 6, and Figure 7).

We now present the pseudo-code of the Split, Merge, and CheckBoundary algorithms, respectively. The Split and Merge algorithms are later

Figure 3. A 2-dimensional illustration of various cases of cluster evolution

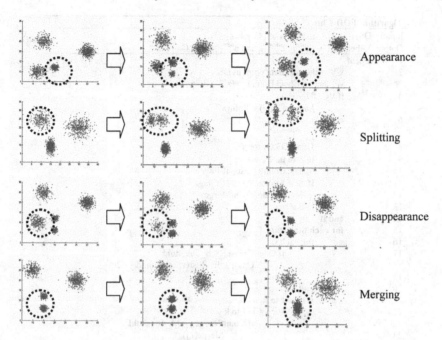

described in the section "Handling Cluster Evolution" and the CheckBoundary algorithm is described in the section "Determining Boundaries Using Probabilities" (Figure 5 and Figure 6).

An additional set of variables are introduced here for the Split algorithm:

- **kO**: the total number of outlier groups
- **(mO, SO)**: a synopsis of the outlier group O
- **nO**: the number of data points within the outlier group O
- **O-thresh**: a parameter indicating the minimum number of members required for an outlier group to become a cluster, the default value of which is 30
- **Label(x^{new},O)**: a set of mapping from every outlier to O.

Handling Cluster Evolution

The cluster synopses can also be utilized not only for cluster assignments to data points, but also for determining when data points are outside cluster boundaries. Since a cluster is a group of data points where data points are dense around the cluster centroid and sparse near the cluster's edge, data points beyond a cluster's boundary are identified as outliers of that cluster. Using the same principle, clusters for a potential merger are recognized by identifying overlapping clusters whose points are close to the centroid of both clusters.

The detection of appearance, splitting, disappearance, and merging is done by modeling each cluster by a Gaussian (normal) distribution. In Gaussian distribution about 68% of the data occur within ± 1σ from the mean, 27% occur between ± 1σ and ±2σ from the mean, and 4% occur between ± 2σ and ± 3σ from the mean; data points beyond ± 3σ from the mean are considered outliers.

The *CheckBoundary* algorithm handles the test of determining data points' positions with

Figure 4. Algorithm POD-Clus

Algorithm POD-Clus
Input: DS, (μ_C, Σ_C), and n_C, when C = 1..k
Output: Label(DS,C), $(\mu^{new}_C, \Sigma^{new}_C)$, and n^{new}_C, when C = 1..k

1	**repeat**
2	x^{new} = the next data point in DS
3	y_C, $flag_C$ = CheckBoundary(x^{new}, $Bound_C$)
4	**if** $\forall C$: $flag_C = 0$
5	Label(x^{new},O) = Split(x^{new})
6	**else**
7	$j = {}^{argmax(y_C)}_C$
8	Label(DS,C) for x^{new} = j
9	update μ_j, Σ_j, n_j
10	update $CountDense_C$ if $flag_C = 1$
11	**if** $|S| > 1$ when S = $\{\forall C|\ flag_C = 2\}$
12	update CountMerge
13	**end if**
14	**end if**
15	**for each** time point T
16	**for each** C
17	**if** $CountDense_C < S\_threshold$
18	C is a split cluster; set $Bound_C = 2\sigma_C$
19	**end**
20	**end**
21	**for** i = 1 to k
22	**for** j = i+1 to k
23	**if** $CountMerge_{ij} > M\_threshold$
24	Merge(i,j)
25	**end**
26	**end**
27	**end**
28	fade: $n_C = 2^{(-\lambda)}$ x n_C
29	**end**
30	**until** end-of-file
31	wait for new data

respect to cluster boundaries. It receives a single data point from the main POD-Clus algorithm and determines its degree of membership to every cluster C. Flag values for each C are then given to

the data point. More detailed explanation of the *CheckBoundary* algorithm can be found in the section called "Determining Boundaries Using Probabilities".

Figure 5. Algorithm split

Algorithm Split
Input: x^{new}, O-thresh = 30, (μ_O, Σ_O), and n_O
Output: Label(x^{new},O), $(\mu^{new}_O, \Sigma^{new}_O)$, and n^{new}_O, when O = 1.. k_O

1	**if** $\forall O$: x^{new} is beyond $\mu_O \pm 3\sigma_O$
2	create a new outlier group O
3	**else**
4	assign x^{new} to the nearest O
5	**if** $n^{new}_O > O\text{-thresh}$
6	convert O into a new cluster C_{k+1}
7	**end**
8	**end**

Figure 6. Algorithm merge

Algorithm Merge
Input: (μ, Σ), and n for i, j $\in$ C
Output: $(\mu^{merge}, \Sigma^{merge})$, and n^{merge}
1   Merge μ_i, Σ_i, and n_i with μ_j, Σ_j, and n_j

- For detecting *cluster appearance*, outliers may form a group if they are close to each other. When a new data point is considered an outlier, it is compared to existing outlier groups to determine if it should be added to any group. If the point does not fall within the $\pm 3\sigma$ from the centroid of any group (line 1 of the *Split* algorithm), it starts a new group (line 2); otherwise, we assign the point to the group whose centroid is the closest (line 4). Since we model clusters by the Gaussian distribution, we set the minimum number of points to be 30 for an outlier group to become a cluster (lines 5 to 7).

- Next we describe the heuristic for *cluster splitting*. When data points start to shift apart from an existing cluster, it starts to become sparse around the centroid. In our method the cluster density is monitored

(line 10 of the *POD-Clus* algorithm) and compared with a normal distribution (line 17). If the cluster distribution changes significantly from its expected distribution, we detect a split. Specifically, POD-Clus keeps count of the number of data points within the $\pm 1\sigma$ region of the cluster C in the variable CountDense$_C$ (line 10). We then use the chi-square test to calculate the splitting threshold (S-threshold) from the expected percentage of data points within $\pm 1\sigma$ from m region (68.2%). At the confidence level of 99.9%, the variable S-threshold is set to 48.68% in the POD-Clus algorithm (the derivation of the S-threshold is explained in detail in the section "Determining Thresholds in POD-Clus"). Therefore, if CountDense$_C$ falls below 48.68%, the cluster is ready to be split.

Figure 7. Algorithm CheckBoundary

Algorithm CheckBoundary
Input: x^{new}, Bound$_C$
Output: y_C, flag$_C$, C = 1..k
1   **for each** C
2         $y_C = p(x^{new}|(\mu_C, \Sigma_C))$
3   set imaginary points (e_1, e_2, e_3) at 1σ, 2σ, and 3σ edges
4         $\{p1, p2, p3\} = p(\{e_1, e_2, e_3\}|(\mu_C, \Sigma_C))$
5   **if** Bound$_C$ = 2
6   p3 = p2
7   **end**
8   **if** y_C < p3, flag$_C$ = 0, **end**
9   **if** y_C > p1, flag$_C$ = 1, **end**
10   **if** p1 > y_C > p2, flag$_C$ = 2, **end**
11   **end**

When a cluster C is detected for splitting, the splitting cluster's boundary, whose default value is 3σ and which is stored in the variable Bound$_C$, is reduced by one sigma (line 18). Future incoming data points of this cluster will become outliers when they are outside of the reduced boundary.

- *Cluster disappearance* is a form of cluster evolution that POD-Clus can handle automatically. As data points are assigned to different clusters based on their corresponding probabilities, a cluster will start to fade (line 28 of the *POD-Clus* algorithm) and disappear once no new data points are assigned into it. We explain fading later in this section.

- *Cluster merging* is done by observing the number of data points distributed within the clusters. When two clusters start to overlap with each other, data points within those clusters start to become members of both clusters. We use the probabilities of data points for each cluster (from the *CheckBoundary* algorithm) to determine if those points are members of more than one cluster, i.e. if their probabilities fall in the m ± 2σ region of both clusters. POD-Clus keeps track of the number of data points within a cluster in the region between ± 1σ to ± 2σ from the mean in the variable CountMerge (lines 11 to 13 of the *POD-Clus* algorithm). We employ a chi-square test to determine the merging threshold (M-threshold) from the expected percentage of points between ± 1σ and ± 2σ from m (27.2%). At a confidence level of 99.9%, the variable M-threshold is set to 15.06% (the derivation of the M-threshold is explained in detail in the section "Determining Thresholds in POD-Clus"). Therefore, the CountMerge variable needs to exceed 15.06% (line 23) for more than one cluster, in which case these clusters are merged and the cluster synopses are updated (line 1 of the *Merge* algorithm).

We use fading to assign more weights to recent data points as compared to the older data points. For each time T, the number of data points (n) in each cluster is weighted by a function of fading factor. Similar to other works in the field (Aggarwal et al., 2004; Udommanetanakit et al., 2007), we set our fading factor to 0.1. As a result, when m and σ (S) are updated with new data points, current data is given a higher weight than older data (line 28 of the *POD-Clus* algorithm). Further explanations of fading can be found in (Aggarwal et al., 2004).

Determining Boundaries Using Probabilities

For one dimensional data, a data point x is within range if $m_C - 3\sigma_C < x < m_C + 3\sigma_C$, and out-of-range otherwise, where $m_C \pm 3\sigma_C$ is defined as the cluster boundary. Applying the same principle for multi-dimensional data, we first identify cluster boundaries using a hypothetical point that is known to lie within the cluster boundary (line 3 of the *CheckBoundary* algorithm). A data point on the cluster boundary will have a value of $m_{Cd} + 3\sigma_{Cd}$ for every d, when d represents a dimension. Such a point is called a *3-sigma edge point*. However, when the cluster C is a split cluster (detected in line 17 of the *POD-Clus* algorithm) the cluster boundary becomes $m_{Cd} + 2\sigma_{Cd}$ for every d. Other types of edge point are also defined in line 3. These are points which lie on the $m_{Cd} + 1\sigma_{Cd}$ and $m_{Cd} + 2\sigma_{Cd}$, which are *1-sigma* and *2-sigma edge points*, respectively.

A new data point's probability is calculated (line 2) along with the probabilities of all edge points (line 4). If a new data point's probability is more than that of the *3-sigma edge point*, we will assign the new data point to the cluster; otherwise the new data point is detected as an outlier (line 8). The 1- and 2- sigma edge points are further used to determine split cluster (line 9), and clusters to merge (line 10), correspondingly.

Determining Thresholds in POD-Clus

POD-Clus is an algorithm which exploits the knowledge of data distribution. A cluster should be a group of data with dense area in the center and sparse area around its edge. In our attempt to theoretically establish the threshold selection, we count the number of data points in different regions as the observed frequency and compare it with the expected frequency of the normal distribution.

The expected frequencies for the region within $m\pm1\sigma$ and the region beyond $m\pm1\sigma$ but within $m\pm2\sigma$ are 68.2% and 27.2%, respectively. The standard chi-square test is carried out. In our implementation, we use a 99.9% confidence level. The critical value of chi-square is 10.83 ($\chi^2_{0.001,1}$ = 10.83). According to the standard chi-square test (Milenova & Campos, 2003), we derive two ranges of observed frequency for both regions as 48.98%-87.42% and 15.05%-39.34%, respectively. These ranges specify eligible percentages of data distribution for a cluster to still be normal.

For a cluster to split, the density of the center area decreases, hence we apply the lower bound of 48.98% as the S-threshold in order to detect splitting. For clusters to merge, data points increasingly belong to more than one cluster. These data points that belong to regions beyond $m\pm1\sigma$ but within $m\pm2\sigma$ of more than one cluster are called merge points. The count of merge points is stored in the variable CountMerge. We detect the merging by setting the M-threshold of the percentage of merge points to be the lower bound of the range, which is 15.05%, as the threshold needs to be crossed for more than one cluster.

Complexity Analysis

We now analyze the time and space complexities of the POD-Clus algorithm with cluster evolution. From the POD-Clus algorithm, the steps from lines 2 to 14 repeat n times, when n is the total number of data points. The steps from lines 15 to 29 repeat T times, when T is the number of time units in which data arrives. From the above two

components, the main POD-Clus algorithm has the time complexity of $O(n)$, which is the maximum of $O(n)$ and $O(T)$. The space required to store all cluster synopses is $O(k)$. We then analyze the various sub-processes involved as follows.

- **CheckBoundary:** The CheckBoundary algorithm is called from the main POD-Clus algorithm n times. For each time, it computes k probabilistic values of x^{new} and of three more edge points, when k is the number of clusters. Therefore, it incurs the time complexity of $O(k)$. From the space perspective, these edge points are designated and their probabilistic values are computed for each cluster. Hence, the CheckBoundary algorithm keeps extra $3*k$ edge points and $4*k$ probabilistic values (one for x^{new}, and three for edge points). Hence, the space requirement has the complexity of $O(k)$. Therefore, CheckBoundary has both the time and space complexities of $O(k)$.

- **Split:** The Split algorithm is called only when all flags ($\forall flag_C$) are zero. After the Split algorithm is triggered, it checks with l outlier groups whether the data point belong to any of the existing group; otherwise a new outlier group is formed. Thus, the Split algorithm has the complexity of $O(l)$, when l is the number of outlier groups. Moreover, the Split algorithm stores synopses of l outlier groups, which takes the space of $O(l)$. Accordingly, the Split algorithm has the time and space complexities of $O(l)$.

- **Merge:** The Merge algorithm is executed only when the percentages of merge points within clusters exceed the *M-threshold*. The process is very small and runs at a constant time ($O(1)$). It does not incur any additional space requirement.

- **Checking for clusters to split (lines 16 to 20 of the POD-Clus algorithm):** This part of the algorithm is processed T times, each time with a time complexity of O(k). The variables CountDense$_c$, S-threshold, and Bound$_c$ take a small space in memory with the complexity of O(k).

- **Checking for clusters to merge (lines 21 to 27 of the POD-Clus algorithm):** This part of the algorithm is processed T times, each time with a time complexity of O(k^2). The variables CountMerge and M-threshold take a small space in memory with the complexity of O(k^2).

EXPERIMENTS

This section reports an evaluation of the POD-Clus algorithm with one of the latest algorithms: E-Stream. As various clustering algorithms have been proposed, E-Stream and D-Stream are the most recent algorithms. However, E-Stream has a longer chain of comparisons with existing algorithms. E-Stream outperformed HPStream in terms of cluster quality (Udommanetanakit et al., 2007) and HPStream's clustering results surpassed CluStream's results when high-dimensional data are involved (Aggarwal et al., 2004). Prior to that, CluStream outperformed STREAM (Aggarwal et al., 2003). Therefore, we chose E-Stream for its comparison with a more recent algorithm (HPStream) rather than D-Stream, which was evaluated with CluStream. We show that our method improves on E-Stream in two phases: without cluster evolution and with cluster evolution.

Implementation Notes

We implemented E-Stream in MATLAB™ as described by Udommanetanakit et al. (2007). However, for clustering without cluster evolution, we allow a more direct comparison between the two algorithms by implementing the E-Stream algorithm without the part which handles cluster evolution. POD-Clus was implemented using

MATLAB™ as described in the Methodology section.

All tests assumed the same initial cluster formations for both E-Stream and POD-Clus to give an equal starting point for data streams clustering.

Evaluation Criteria

We evaluated the clustering techniques using two main aspects: cluster quality and efficiency of the algorithms. The former aspect of evaluation devised several evaluation criteria. The latter was obtained from measuring the elapsed execution time of the algorithms.

For cluster quality, we evaluated the algorithms using external validity criteria, which measure the cluster quality with pre-defined correct cluster assignment, and internal validity criteria, which measure the cluster quality based on the cluster formations themselves (Brun et al., 2007; Halkidi, Batistakis, & Vazirgiannis, 2002a, 2002b). External criteria validation is possible when information of pre-defined correct clusters is available; otherwise internal criteria validation is the only option.

For our experiments, we measured external criteria when possible. External criteria in the literature included Hubert Γ statistics, Rand statistics, Jaccard coefficient, and Folkes and Mallows index. We also borrowed Precision, Recall, and the F-measure from the information retrieval field to complement the assessment as some clustering validity criteria are expensive to compute for large datasets.

We also measured internal criteria, especially when there was the lack of ground truth. Sum SQuare Error (SSQ) and Silhouette were selected for our evaluation. SSQ is the sum squared distance of data points to their respective cluster centers. Lower SSQ values suggest a better cluster formation. Silhouette function is the ratio of the difference between the average inter-cluster and the average intra-cluster distances, to the maximum of the inter-cluster and intra-cluster distances

(Kaufman & Rousseeuw, 1990). The positive Silhouette values approaching 1 indicate good cluster quality, and negative Silhouette values approaching -1 indicate incorrect cluster assignment. The Silhouette function measures the compactness and separation of the produced clusters.

Experimental Results without Cluster Evolution

In principle, our method differs from E-Stream in that we use the Gaussian distribution as our model for the cluster synopses as opposed to the histogram-based approach used by E-Stream. The histogram is a data summarization technique which roughly approximates data. The number of bins needs to be specified and can affect the performance of the algorithm. The Gaussian distribution offers a smoother summarization without many input parameters. POD-Clus and E-Stream are similar in many ways. First, both algorithms incrementally maintain a set of statistics which is a summarization of data points within each cluster. Thus, the experiments in this section can be regarded as an evaluation of how different cluster statistics affect the effectiveness and efficiency of clustering.

Datasets

Data were randomly generated from stationary processes with various controlled parameters to simulate the no-evolution condition. As biomedical signals such as ECG streams have repeated patterns, the regularity of these simulated data can represent that of biomedical streams. We also generated data using a non-normal distribution to illustrate that the POD-Clus algorithm is valid even when data is not normally distributed.

Experimental Results

Experimental results are arranged by datasets. The controlled parameters on these datasets were

used in naming the datasets. The parameters D, C, M, and N with adjacent numbers represent the number of dimensions, the number of clusters, the number of streams, and the number of time points, respectively. As an example, $M20kN100kD50C10$ denotes a dataset that consists of 20,000 streams. Each stream contains recorded values of 50 dimensions along 100,000 time points. All streams belong to 10 different clusters.

Experiment 1: Skew-Normally Distributed Data (1D4C400M1000N)

A dataset called *1D4C400M1000N* was a 1-dimensional dataset with 4 distinct clusters. The dataset was generated using the skew-normal distribution (Azzalini & Valle, 1996) using the following parameters: $SN(5, 0.2, 5)$, $SN(6, 0.2, -5)$, $SN(3, 0.2, 1)$, and $SN(1, 0.2, -3)$, for clusters 1 to 4 respectively. The first two parameters represented location and scale, while the third parameter was a shape parameter indicating the level of skewness. The further from zero the shape parameter value, the more skewed the cluster. The positive-valued shape parameter suggested a right-skewed distribution plot with a stretched tail on the right of the plot, while the negative-valued shape parameter suggested a left-skewed distribution plot with a stretched tail on the left of the plot. There were 400 streams, each with 1000 time points.

By evaluating clustering results, cluster qualities were very close in SSQ and Silhouette values for both algorithms. On average, both algorithms produced very small errors in relationship to data points' values (0.48%). They also produced compact and well-separated clusters (Silhouette values always > 0.95) (Figure 8).

Results for Rand statistics, Jaccard coefficient, and Folkes and Mallows indices all indicate similar cluster qualities from both algorithms and suggest a very strong agreement between the true and the obtained cluster assignments (Figure 9).

As it was never reported in (Udommanetanakit et al., 2007) how to select an appropriate number

Figure 8. Dataset 1D4C400M1000N's internal validity criteria on (left) SSQ, and (right) Silhouette value

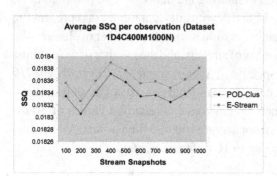 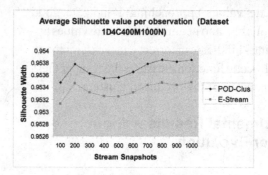

of histogram bins, we always used 10 (the default value in MATLAB) as the number of bins. In terms of efficiency, POD-Clus finished the clustering process much faster than E-Stream did, resulting in POD-Clus' total elapsed runtime at T_{1000} of 56.4% less than that of E-Stream A (Figure 10).

The above results demonstrate that although POD-Clus did not make a radical improvement in cluster quality over E-Stream, it did improve in clustering efficiency. Note that POD-Clus achieved the same result even though a stationary process other than normal distribution was used in data generation.

Experiment 2: 2-Dimensional Normally Distributed Data (2D3C300M100N)

Next we experimented on multi-dimensional data. A 2-dimensional dataset was created for twofold

benefits: to visualize clusters in a 2-dimensional space and to experiment with clusters of non-spherical shapes. With such aims in mind, some clusters were highly correlated between the two dimensions.

In Figure 11 (left), the 2-dimensional data streams for the time snapshot T_2 are viewable using scatter plots. The parameters used in data synthesis were: $N([5.5, 5.5], [1^2, 1^2])$, $N([4.5, 5.5], [1^2, 1^2])$, and $N([5, 3.5], [0.2^2, 0.2^2])$ for clusters 1 to 3, when values within the first square brackets represent means of the first and second dimensions and values within the second square brackets represent variances of the first and second dimensions. Clusters 1 and 2 (denoted by c1 and c2) were the clusters with very high correlations between dimensions, while cluster 3 (denoted by c3) was the cluster with a low correlation between dimensions. Three clusters were quite distinct from the plot.

Figure 9. Dataset 1D4C400M1000N's external validity criteria on (left) Rand statistics, (middle) Jaccard coefficient, and (right) Folkes-Mallows index

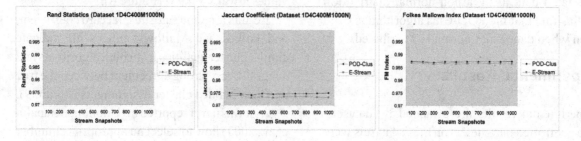

Figure 10. Dataset 1D4C400M1000N's evaluation on execution time

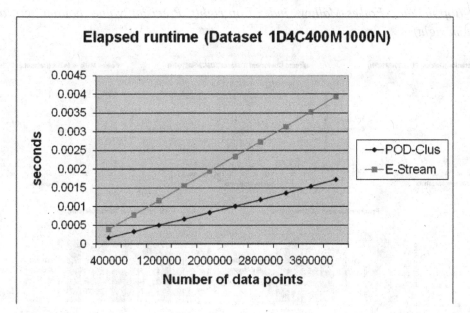

Testing POD-Clus and E-Stream algorithms on this dataset yielded interesting results. While POD-Clus was able to cluster the data points from T_2 to T_{100} most correctly, E-Stream clustered the streaming data points based on its distance function which favored spherical clusters. As a result, E-Stream detected clusters at T_2 in disagreement with the true cluster formation, despite the same correct initial assignment given to both algorithms. It clearly shows from visualization that POD-Clus produced clusters more correctly than E-Stream (Figure 11 and Figure 12).

The values of the external validity criteria computed from the clustering results validate the above claim. POD-Clus achieved almost the maximum values of 1 on all criteria (Rand statistics, Jaccard coefficient, and Folkes-Mallows index), while E-Stream attained values of approximately 0.75, 0.47, and 0.64, respectively. Precision and Recall values show results in the same direction with the above criteria. POD-Clus did extremely well in detecting the correct clusters, while E-Stream was very much confused between clusters 1 and 2 (Figure 13).

Figure 11. Dataset 2D3C300M100N's plots of true clusters at T_2 (left), clusters obtained from E-Stream at T_2 (middle), and clusters obtained from POD-Clus at T_2 (right)

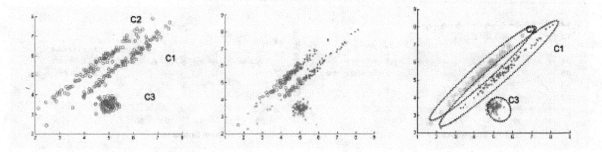

Figure 12. Dataset 2D3C300M100N's external validity criteria on Rand statistics (top left), Jaccard coefficient (top middle), Folkes-Mallows index (top right), Precision value (bottom left), and Recall value (bottom right)

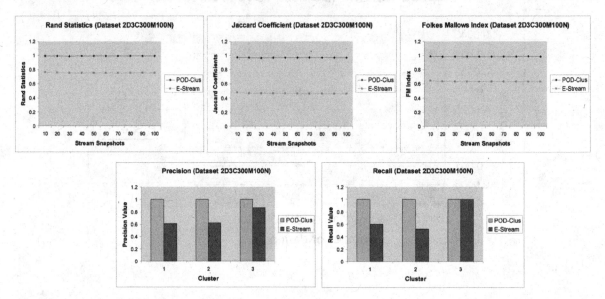

The results on the internal validity criteria demonstrate that POD-Clus produced about 14% of an average SSQ to a data point's value (9.83), whereas E-Stream produced about 7%. For Silhouette values, neither algorithms performed extremely well but E-Stream (0.6) still outperformed POD-Clus (0.3) on this aspect. This phenomenon of E-Stream's production of better SSQ values can be explained by E-Stream's ten-

dency to minimize distances of data points to cluster centers, leading to the lower SSQ values. To explain the Silhouette results, let us consider data points at the lower end of cluster 1 from Figure 11 (left). These data points were clustered by E-Stream as belonging to cluster 3. As Silhouette values are computed from intra-cluster and inter-cluster distances, their intra-cluster distances (when computed with data points at the

Figure 13. Dataset 2D3C300M100N's internal validity criteria on (left) SSQ, and (right) Silhouette value

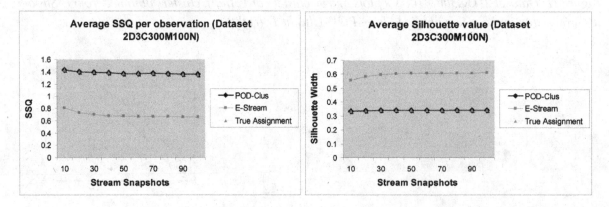

higher end of cluster 1) would be much larger than inter-cluster distances (when computed with data points at the lower end of cluster 2). Overall, this results in a low average Silhouette value of any algorithm which correctly clusters the data points. We verified this intuition by also plotting SSQ and Silhouette values of the true cluster assignment in Figure 13. The plots supported our hypothesis that the true cluster assignment of dataset 2D3C300M100N produced higher SSQ and lower Silhouette values, even as much as POD-Clus did.

For this dataset, POD-Clus produced the clustering results more efficiently than E-Stream did. Figure 14 illustrates a slightly faster execution time from POD-Clus. POD-Clus' runtime increased from the time when testing the one-dimensional data. However, POD-Clus presented a trade-off in clustering accuracy, especially when data are highly correlated between dimensions.

Experiment 3: 2-Dimensional Normally Distributed Data with Low Correlations between Dimensions and Oval-Shaped Clusters (2D4C400M100N)

We introduced a bias of highly-correlated data in the previous experiment, which worked in favor of POD-Clus. In this experiment, we constructed a 2-dimensional dataset with very low correlations among dimensions but with clusters of non-spherical shapes. The data's characteristics are summarized in Table 1.

The scatter plot of this dataset is illustrated in Figure 15 (left) with their corresponding cluster assignments in Figure 15 (middle and right). While all clusters had low correlations among dimensions, POD-Clus clustered data with non-spherical shapes better than E-Stream. This conclusion is confirmed by the internal cluster validity and external cluster validity of the dataset. However, the execution times of POD-Clus were slightly slower than those of E-Stream in this case (Figure 16, Figure 17, and Figure 18).

Table 1. Characteristics of datasets 2D6C-600M100N and 2D4C400M100N

Dataset	**2D4C400M100N**
Number of clusters (C)	4
Parameters	Cluster 1 = $N([5, 3.5], [0.2^2, 0.2^2])$, corr(X,Y) = -0.0261 Cluster 2 = $N([5, 2], [0.4^2, 0.02^2])$, corr(X,Y) = -0.0584 Cluster 3 = $N([5, 2.5], [0.75^2, 0.1^2])$, corr(X,Y) = 0.0940 Cluster 4 = $N([3.5, 3], [1^2, 0.2^2])$, corr(X,Y) = -0.0752
Number of time series (M)	400
Number of time points (N)	100

Experiment 4: Scalability Test (18D40C800M100N)

From the previous experiments, we have shown that POD-Clus is a feasible algorithm for clustering data streams as it always produced superior clustering results compared with E-Stream in external validity criteria. When tested with one-dimensional data, POD-Clus performed much faster than E-Stream. When tested with two-dimensional data, POD-Clus ensured better accuracies than E-Stream did. However, we need to establish that POD-Clus is linearly scalable in order to be applicable for large datasets.

For this scalability experiment, a set of 18-dimensional normally distributed data streams was generated. There were a total of 800 streams belonging to 40 clusters (20 streams per cluster). The number of time points per stream was 100. Then, the dataset was varied by the variables C and D. When the number of data dimensions (D) was varied, the number of clusters (C) was always set to 40. Therefore, all 800 streams were clustered. Figure 19 (left) illustrates the average runtime per data point when varying the number of data dimensions. The values are plotted along different time snapshots. From Figure 19, the POD-Clus algorithm spent from approximately 0.009 to

Figure 14. Dataset 2D3C300M100N's evaluation on execution time

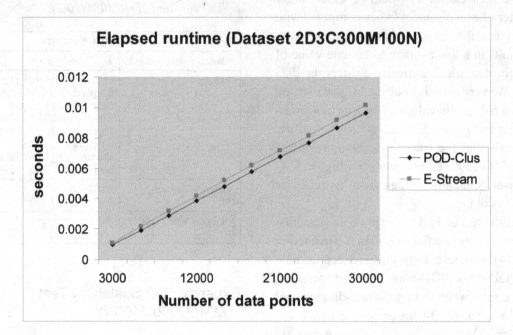

0.016 seconds per data point when D was varied from 2 to 18. The execution time increased only twice when the number of dimensions increased 9 times. This indicates a sub-linear scalability of POD-Clus to the number of dimensions. Figure 19 illustrates the elapsed execution time of the same experiment.

When the number of clusters (C) was varied, the number of dimensions (D) was set to 2. Note that varying C also impacted the number of streams (M) being clustered by POD-Clus. Figure 20 (left) illustrates the average runtime per data point

(0.0009 to 0.0092 seconds) when C varied from 3 to 40, and also implying that the number of streams varied from 60 to 800. The increase in execution time was linear to the increase in C, as shown in Figure 20.

In conclusion, POD-Clus was extensively tested against E-Stream. From the Experiment 1, POD-Clus executed the clustering on data streams more efficiently than E-Stream. From the Experiments 2 and 3, POD-Clus clustered particularly non-spherical clusters better than E-Stream. From the Experiment 5, POD-Clus

Figure 15. Dataset 2D4C400M100N's plots of true clusters at T_1- T_{100} (left), clusters obtained from E-Stream at T_2 (middle), and clusters obtained from POD-Clus at T_{100} (right)

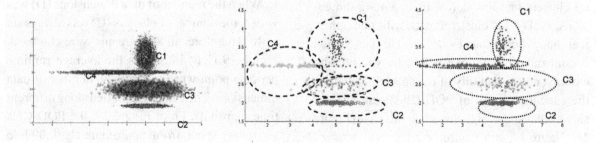

Figure 16. Dataset 2D4C400M100N's internal validity criteria on SSQs (left), and Silhouette values (right)

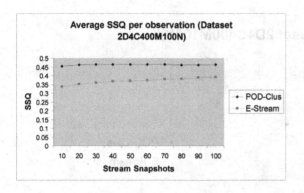 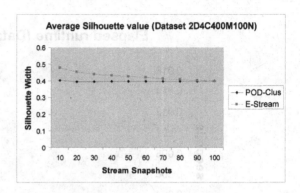

showed linear scalabilities on both the number of clusters and the number of data dimensions, in addition to the number of data points reported in the other previous experiments. We conclude that POD-Clus is an effective and efficient clustering algorithm in the case of clustering data streams without cluster evolution.

Experimental Results with Cluster Evolution

This section contains experimental results of both algorithms when cluster evolution is involved. Both POD-Clus and E-Stream have heuristics that help with the detection and handling of cluster evolution of many kinds, but they differ in how they handle the evolution of clusters.

We experimented with one synthetic dataset and one real-life dataset. A synthetic dataset

(named 2D-Evolution) was generated so that all types of cluster evolution were present. A real-life dataset (named 954Subotnick) was included so that the algorithms were tested against data with previously unknown characteristics.

Datasets

To assure that we tested our algorithms using a dataset which contained various forms of cluster evolution, we adapted the dataset from (Udom-manetanakit et al., 2007) as our 2D-Evolution dataset. This dataset contained two-dimensional 1500 data streams, each with 1000 time points and contained 3 to 5 normally-distributed clusters. Four types of cluster evolution were studied: cluster appearance, cluster disappearance, cluster merging, and cluster splitting. In order to describe the 2D-Evolution dataset, Figure 21 provides

Figure 17. Dataset 2D4C400M100N's external validity criteria on Rand statistics (left), Jaccard coefficient (middle), and Folkes-Mallows index (right)

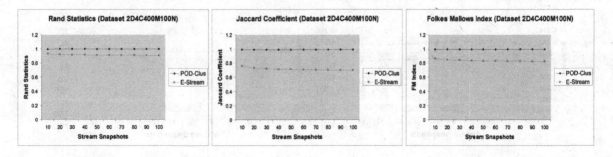

Figure 18. Dataset 2D4C400M100N's evaluation on execution time

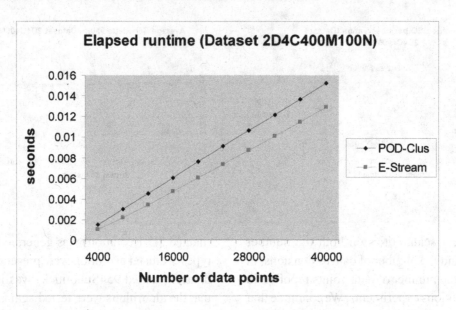

the dataset's 2-D visualization at different time snapshots. Each snapshot is denoted by T with a subscript number.

The cluster evolution simulated in this dataset is related to the patterns of biomedical signals. For example, in the case of ECG signals, the well-known sequence pattern of cardiac electrical activity (the P-R interval, the QRS complex, the ST segment, and the T wave) shows distinctly different groups of voltage values, with the QRS complex showing the highest peak of voltage values. Normal cardiac electrical signals comprise of all these components. However, ventricular fibrillation, a case of abnormal cardiac electrical activities, appears as chaotic waves and lacks the presence of the QRS complex found in the normal signals. Therefore, the appearance and disappearance of clusters are matched with the presence and absence of the QRS complex peaks. The irregular absence of the QRS complex can be

Figure 19. POD-Clus' scalability test on the number of dimensions

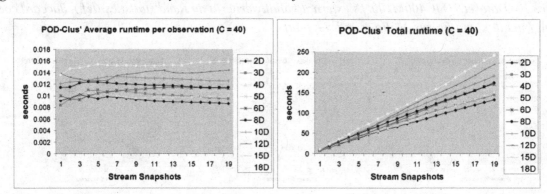

brought to attention with the help of a streams clustering algorithm which detects cluster evolution.

The second dataset was a real-life dataset obtained from the Baruch Data Warehouse at the Subotnick Financial Services Center[1]. The center collects stock market data with interesting features such as price, simple return, volume, and exchange. A total of 954 firms' stock trades from the Dow Jones Industrial Average, which was monitored during the month of January 2007, was extracted in 5-minute intervals. Since this stock market data was available only during trading hours (9:30am to 4:30pm), for each business day, the whole month's worth of trades constituted to a total of 1,700 time points. For 954 firms, it summed up to approximately 1.6 million data points. Missing data were discarded and only time slots with complete values were entered into the algorithms.

Many events may be revealed from clustering stock trade data. For example, one may find large market-moving events for an entire industry if a clustering is done around the simple returns feature. Clustering trade size may reveal when large trades tend to happen, e.g. at the beginning or the ending of the day.

As we had no prior knowledge of the true cluster formation, we executed an offline clustering algorithm, COMITS (Chaovalit & Gangopadhyay, 2007), on these data streams to obtain an initial clustering formation.

When evaluating cluster assignments from the POD-Clus algorithm for the case of clustering with cluster evolution, it was possible that some data points were assigned to outlier groups and therefore would not be associated to any cluster. If those data points belonged to some outlier groups which were not eventually converted to new clusters, they were evaluated as not belonging to any clusters. However, if some of those outlier groups eventually converted to new clusters, we evaluated the data points as if they belonged to the new clusters.

Experiment Results

We now present the experimental results, which are divided into results of the 2D-Evolution dataset and results of the 954Subotnick dataset. The former is divided into cluster appearance, cluster disappearance, cluster merging, and cluster splitting, according to the nature of data.

Experiment: The 2D-Evolution Dataset

The 2D-Evolution dataset contained 4 types of cluster evolution. Prior to the experiments, we pre-processed data into small subsets, each of which containing one type of cluster evolution. Data points were extracted during the time interval between $T_1 - T_{200}$, $T_{201} - T_{325}$, $T_{426} - T_{625}$, and $T_{626} - T_{1000}$ for cluster appearance, cluster disappearance, cluster merging, and cluster splitting, respectively. These subsets of data were then entered individually into two clustering algorithms (Figure 22).

For the data subset containing cluster appearance, the data points outside cluster boundaries were detected by POD-Clus' heuristics and enough outliers subsequently formed a new cluster, causing the F-measure values to be near 1. E-Stream was able to detect new cluster appearance. However, the split was overdone, causing the number of clusters at T_{200} to be 7. The scatter plot of E-Stream's cluster assignment with dotted ovals as a visual aid in cluster identification shows that there were 2 extra clusters (not within ovals) under cluster 2 which were split from the rest of the clusters. The results on F-measure and Silhouette values were plotted in Figure 23 under the column "Appearance". The plots showed lower F-measure and Silhouette width values of E-Stream than those of POD-Clus.

When testing with the data subset containing cluster disappearance, both algorithms handled the cluster disappearance well. The cluster assignments of both algorithms were close to the true cluster formations. The results on F-measure and Silhouette values were plotted in Figure 23 under

Figure 20. POD-Clus' scalability test on the number of clusters

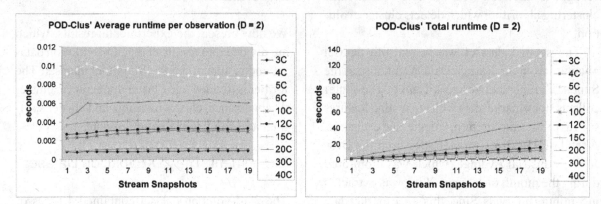

the column "Disappearance". Note that E-Stream's Silhouette values temporarily dropped around T_{110}, because E-Stream over-split clusters but corrected itself by the end of this time period.

For the data subset containing cluster merging, POD-Clus merged clusters 2 and 5 at T_{540}. Surprisingly, E-Stream was not yet able to merge these two clusters. This led to lower F-measure values of E-Stream than those of POD-Clus. As 1500 data points belonged to 3 or 4 clusters within this time period, the Precision and Recall values

of E-Stream were high for some clusters, resulting in quite high F-measure values of E-Stream. E-Stream not only failed to merge clusters, but also split and merged stable clusters. Silhouette widths reflected this over-splitting behavior of E-Stream. Whenever the Silhouette values dropped, it indicated that the over-splitting was taking place. The results on F-measure and Silhouette values were plotted in Figure 23 under the column "Merge".

When testing with the data subset containing cluster splitting, POD-Clus started to detect that the

Figure 21. Dataset 2-D Evolution's scatter plots at time snapshots T_{100}, T_{130}, T_{200}, T_{300}, T_{400}, T_{500}, T_{600}, T_{665}, and T_{800} (from left to right, top to bottom)

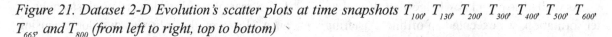

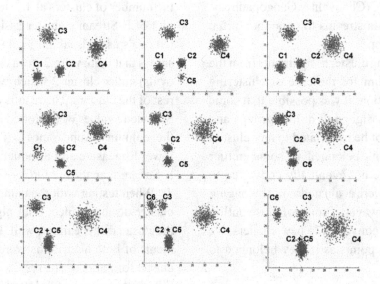

Figure 22. A scatter plot of E-Stream's cluster assignment at T_{200}

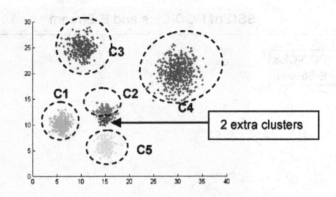

Figure 23. Cluster quality evaluation on F-measure (top) and average silhouette width (bottom) for four types of cluster evolution

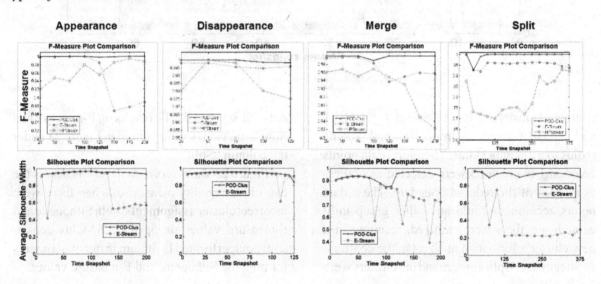

Figure 24. Execution time of the 2D-Evolution Dataset when testing with four types of cluster evolution

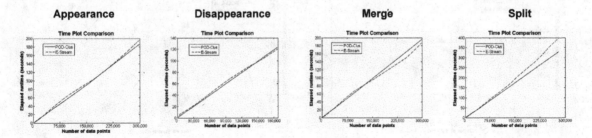

Figure 25. Cluster quality evaluation on SSQ of the 954Subotnick Dataset

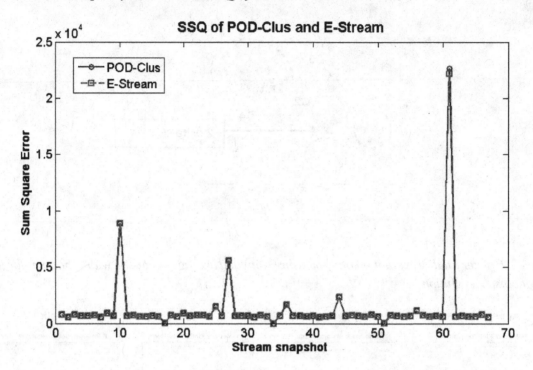

content of cluster 3 was not dense at T_{676}. Cluster 3's boundary was reduced from the normal 3-sigma radius to a 2-sigma radius. Therefore, data points belonging to cluster 3 were detected as outliers as a result of the reduced boundary. These data points accumulated into an outlier group until enough members were gathered, resulting in a new cluster's formation at T_{683}. On the contrary, E-Stream over-split clusters and the clusters were not well-separated. The results on F-measure and Silhouette values were plotted in Figure 23 under the column "Split".

Figure 23 shows consistent results across the two cluster quality measures. When there were incorrect cluster assignments, both Silhouette and F-measure values dropped. POD-Clus consistently outperformed E-Stream in our experiments for both the Silhouette and F-measure values.

Figure 26. Execution time of the 954Subotnick Dataset

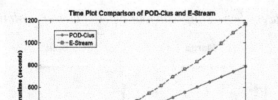

We set E-Stream's parameters as reported in (Udommanetanakit et al., 2007), and the F-measure values of E-Stream reported here are relatively consistent with those reported in (Udommanetanakit et al., 2007). We therefore plotted F-measure values of HPStream in Figure 23 as reported in (Udommanetanakit et al., 2007) for transitive comparison. POD-Clus certainly outperformed HPStream for detecting cluster evolution by transitivity.

Figure 24 illustrates efficiency results of POD-Clus and E-Stream algorithms in elapsed runtime against the number of data points. POD-Clus took slightly shorter time for the cases of appearance and split and slightly longer time for the cases of disappearance and merge. Even though the execution time were close between both algorithms, POD-Clus' overall runtime scaled more linearly to the number of data points due to E-Stream's constant splitting and merging.

Experiment: The 954Subotnick Dataset

The 954Subotnick dataset was a real-life dataset containing 954 firms' stock trade data. As clustering trading volume and exchange may reveal some exchanges which tend to report high-volume stock trades. We decided to cluster these 2 features "trading volume" and "exchange". The pre-processing of data was performed as follows.

The feature "exchange" was categorical and therefore data was converted into numerical values of 1-10. Since data values of both features "exchange" and "trading volume" had different scales, these features were normalized using a z-score normalization.

Executing the offline clustering algorithm offline revealed 2 groups of data: one with values in the normal range and another with outliers. For this reason, we decided to initially assign all pre-processed data to one cluster. POD-Clus detected outliers and formed 2 outlier groups at T_1. Then, a new cluster was founded from those outliers at T_{47} and became cluster 2. POD-Clus continued to find outliers and assigned them to either cluster

2 or outlier groups. The clustering process ended with 2 clusters and 5 outlier groups (Figure 25).

POD-Clus and E-Stream produced 2 clusters which were close in quality, as can be seen from the SSQ plot. However, POD-Clus executed linearly to the number of data points, while E-Stream did not. By looking at Figure 26 (right), POD-Clus' execution time per snapshot was more stable than E-Stream's execution time. The experiment log showed that E-Stream was constantly detecting cluster evolution. However, E-Stream's final number of clusters was 2, like that of POD-Clus and the cluster evolution detection by E-Stream did not contribute to better cluster qualities in terms of SSQ.

The experimental results of POD-Clus and E-Stream when cluster evolution was present suggest that POD-Clus was able to detect and handle the different types of cluster evolution with a better effectiveness. Moreover, they suggest that POD-Clus' runtime performance was more linear than that of E-Stream, which tended to reflect the over-splitting behavior of E-Stream.

DISCUSSION

This paper provides a theoretical framework for data streams clustering and proposes POD-Clus as a new approach for this framework. POD-Clus requires only one pass of data and processes data streams using a small constant time. POD-Clus' runtime per data point ranged from 0.0002 seconds in the case of 1-dimensional data to 0.009 seconds in the case of 2-dimensional data, and to 0.016 seconds in the case of 18-dimensional data. As an ECG signal may arrive at the rate of 0.001 – 0.01 seconds per sample, POD-Clus fits as a potential application in healthcare industry for real-time clustering of biomedical signals. POD-Clus effectively captured clusters with evolving nature, therefore making it an excellent candidate for systems which constantly monitor fast evolving events such as health monitoring systems.

The research presented in this paper can be further extended in many ways. The fading factor in the Methodology section introduces a fading effect on data observations at a uniform rate. Even though the appropriate lambda parameters fall in the range of 0.1-0.2 by the empirical results shown in this paper, an appropriate parameter in general is dependent on the test datasets. Also, the currently proposed fading factor approach lets POD-Clus store only the latest cluster information and hence cannot analyze clusters at past time snapshots with different lambdas. To overcome this limitation, a variant of the current approach can be proposed by storing various snapshots of information with an increase in storage cost. The issues of selecting and fine-tuning an appropriate fading factor warrant further research. Finally, developing this promising approach into practical healthcare applications remains an interesting open research area.

REFERENCES

Aggarwal, C. C., Han, J., Wang, J., & Yu, P. S. (2003). *A framework for clustering evolving data streams.* Paper presented at the 29th International Conference on Very Large Data Bases (VLDB'03), Berlin.

Aggarwal, C. C., Han, J., Wang, J., & Yu, P. S. (2004, August 31 - September 3, 2004). *A framework for projected clustering of high dimensional data streams.* Paper presented at the 30th International Conference on Very Large Data Bases (VLDB'04), Toronto, Canada.

Azzalini, A., & Valle, A. D. (1996). The multivariate skew-normal distribution. *Biometrika, 83*(4), 715–726. doi:doi:10.1093/biomet/83.4.715

Babcock, B., Babu, S., Datar, M., Motwani, R., & Widom, J. (2002, June 3-6, 2002). *Models and issues in data stream systems.* Paper presented at the 21st ACM SIGMOD-SIGACT-SIGART Symposium on Principles of Database Systems (ACM PODS'02), Madison, WI.

Barbará, D. (2002). Requirements for clustering data streams. *ACM SIGKDD Explorations Newsletter, 3*(2), 23–27. doi:doi:10.1145/507515.507519

Bragge, T., Tarvainen, M. P., & Karjalainen, P. A. (2004). *High-resolution QRS detection algorithm for sparsely sampled ECG recordings* (Tech. Rep. No. 1/2004). Kuopio, Finland: University of Kuopio, Department of Applied Physics.

Brun, M., Sima, C., Hua, J., Lowey, J., Carroll, B., & Suh, E. (2007). Model-based evaluation of clustering validation measures. *Pattern Recognition, 40*(3), 807–824. doi:doi:10.1016/j.patcog.2006.06.026

Chaovalit, P., & Gangopadhyay, A. (2007). *A method for clustering time series using connected components.* Paper presented at the 17th Annual Workshop on Information Technologies and Systems (WITS'07), Montreal, Canada.

Chen, Y., & Tu, L. (2007, August 12-15, 2007). *Density-based clustering for real-time stream data.* Paper presented at the 13th International Conference on Knowledge Discovery and Data Mining (SIGKDD'07), San Jose, CA.

Cowley, M. (2006, January 8). *Electrodes, leads & wires: A practical guide to ecg monitoring and recording.* Retrieved August 15, 2010, from www.mikecowley.co.uk/leads.htm

Domingos, P., & Hulten, G. (2000). *Mining high-speed data streams.* Paper presented at the 6th International Conference on Knowledge Discovery and Data Mining (SIGKDD'00).

Domingos, P., & Hulten, G. (2001, May 20). *Catching up with the data: research issues in mining data streams.* Paper presented at Workshop on Research Issues in Data Mining and Knowledge Discovery (DMKD 2001), Santa Barbara, CA.

Gama, J., Rodrigues, P., & Aguilar-Ruiz, J. (2007). An overview on learning from data streams. *New Generation Computing, 25,* 1–4. doi:doi:10.1007/s00354-006-0001-5

Golab, L., & Özsu, M. T. (2003). Issues in data stream management. *SIGMOD Record, 32*(2), 5–14. doi:doi:10.1145/776985.776986

Guha, S., Meyerson, A., Mishra, N., Motwani, R., & O'Callaghan, L. (2003). Clustering data streams: Theory and practice. *IEEE Transactions on Knowledge and Data Engineering, 15*(3), 515–528. doi:doi:10.1109/TKDE.2003.1198387

Halkidi, M., Batistakis, Y., & Vazirgiannis, M. (2002a). Cluster Validity Methods: Part I. *SIGMOD Record, 31,* 40–45. doi:doi:10.1145/565117.565124

Halkidi, M., Batistakis, Y., & Vazirgiannis, M. (2002b). Clustering Validity Checking Methods: Part II. *SIGMOD Record, 31,* 19–27. doi:doi:10.1145/601858.601862

Kaufman, L., & Rousseeuw, P. J. (1990). *Finding Groups in Data: An Introduction to Cluster Analysis.* New York: Wiley.

Liao, T. W. (2005). Clustering of time series data - a survey. *Pattern Recognition, 38*(11), 1857–1874. doi:doi:10.1016/j.patcog.2005.01.025

Lu, Y.-H., & Huang, Y. (2005, August 18-21). *Mining data streams using clustering.* Paper presented at the 4th International Conference on Machine Learning and Cybernatics, Guangzhou, China.

Milenova, B. L., & Campos, M. M. (2003). *Clustering large databases with numeric and nominal values using orthogonal projections.* Paper presented at the 29th VLDB Conference.

Sun, M., & Sclabassi, R. J. (1999, October 13-16). *Optimal selection of the sampling rate for efficient EEG data acquisition.* Paper presented at Proceedings of the First Joint BMES/EMBS Conference on Serving Humanity, Advancing Technology, Atlanta, GA.

Thompson, J. R., & Tapia, R. A. (1990). *Nonparametric Function Estimation, Modeling, and Simulation.* Philadelphia: Society for Industrial and Applied Mathematics (SIAM).

Udommanetanakit, K., Rakthanmanon, T., & Waiyamai, K. (2007, August 6-8). *E-Stream: evolution-based technique for stream clustering.* Paper presented at the 3rd International Conference on Advanced Data Mining and Applications (ADMA'07), Harbin, China.

Yang, J. (2003). *Dynamic clustering of evolving streams with a single pass.* Paper presented at the 19th International Conference on Data Engineering (ICDE'03).

ENDNOTE

[1] http://zicklin.baruch.cuny.edu/about/campus/subotnick.html

This work was previously published in International Journal of Computational Models and Algorithms in Medicine, Volume 1, Issue 3, edited by Aryya Gangopadhyay, pp. 1-30, copyright 2010 by IGI Publishing (an imprint of IGI Global).

Chapter 11
Privacy Preserving Clustering for Distributed Homogeneous Gene Expression Data Sets

Xin Li

Georgetown University, USA

ABSTRACT

In this paper, the authors present a new approach to perform principal component analysis (PCA)-based gene clustering on genomic data distributed in multiple sites (horizontal partitions) with privacy protection. This approach allows data providers to collaborate together to identify gene profiles from a global viewpoint, and at the same time, protect the sensitive genomic data from possible privacy leaks. The authors developed a framework for privacy preserving PCA-based gene clustering, which includes two types of participants such as data providers and a trusted central site. Within this mechanism, distributed horizontal partitions of genomic data can be globally clustered with privacy preservation. Compared to results from centralized scenarios, the result generated from distributed partitions achieves 100% accuracy by using this approach. An experiment on a real genomic data set is conducted, and result shows that the proposed framework produces exactly the same cluster formation as that from the centralized data set.

INTRODUCTION

In recent years, new bioinformatics technologies, such as gene expression microarrays, have been widely used to simultaneously identify a huge number of human genomic biomarkers, generate a tremendously large amount of data, dramatically increase the knowledge on human genomic information, and thereafter, significantly improve biomedical research.

A DNA microarray (Wikipedia, 2010), which is the practical realized technology of the Gene Expression (BioChemWeb.org, 2010), is a multiplex technology used in molecular biology. It consists of an arrayed series of thousands of microscopic spots of DNA oligonucleotides, called features, each containing picomoles (10^{-12} moles) of a specific DNA sequence, known as probes (or reporters). This can be a short section of a gene or other DNA element that is used to hybridize a

DOI: 10.4018/978-1-4666-0282-3.ch011

cDNA or cRNA sample (called target) under high-stringency conditions. Probe-target hybridization is usually detected and quantified by detection of fluorophore-, silver-, or chemiluminescence-labeled targets to determine relative abundance of nucleic acid sequences in the target. Since an array can contain tens of thousands of probes, a microarray experiment can accomplish many genetic tests in parallel. Therefore arrays have dramatically accelerated many types of investigation. The microarray data processing pipeline (Hackl, Sanchez Cabo et al., 2004) includes a variety of statistical steps: pre-processing (including background correction, normalization, and sum-

marization), differential analysis which contains raw p-value computation and false discovery rate (FDR) correction, and gene clustering / profiling analysis. Figure 1 shows that microarray experiment process in the lab and Figure 2 illustrates its gene clustering result.

However, these exciting advances do come with an inevitable issue, that is, the richer and richer human genomic data contains privacy sensitive information, such as, genetic markers, diseases, *etc.*, which may further lead to an individual's race, family, or even identity. Unfortunately, because genomic data does not directly carry individual identity information and it used

Figure 1. DNA microarray experiment

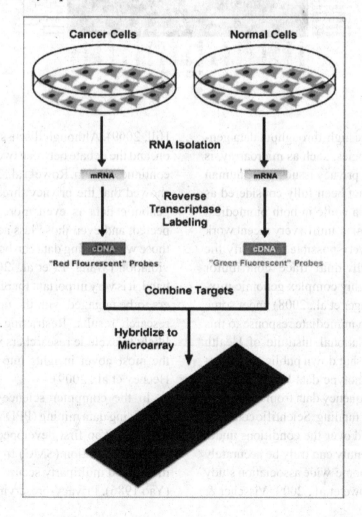

Figure 2. The gene clustering result (heatmap) of a microarray experiment

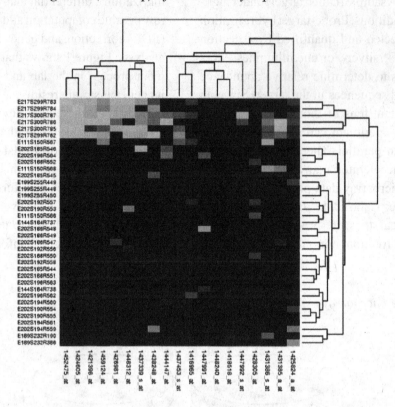

to be believed that the high-throughput data generated from technologies, such as microarray, is not accurate enough, privacy issues in the human genomic data have not been fully considered as a big issue for quite a while in both biomedical and informatics domains, until a very recent work showed that it was very possible to identify the presence of an individual trace contributor within a series of highly complex genomic mixtures (Homer, Szelinger et al., 2008) under some circumstances. As an immediate response to this new finding, The National Institute of Health (NIH) has agreed to shut down public access not just to individual genotype data but even to aggregate genotype frequency data from each study published using their funding. Scientific concerns have also been raised over the conditions under which individual identity can truly be accurately determined from genome-wide association study (GWAS) (Braun, Rowe et al., 2009; Visscher &

Hill, 2009). Although discussions are still going on, and the debate between two opposite opinions continues (Braun, Rowe et al., 2009), further study showed that the privacy threat on using human genomic data is even more realistic than expected, and even those less accurate data sets or those with missing data can be victims of privacy violation (Wang, Li et al., 2009). On the other hand, it is very important for biomedical researchers to be engaged with the up-to-date genomics research results. Restricting data accesses are likely to exclude researchers who might provide the most novel insights into the data (Church, Heeney et al., 2009).

In the computer science domain, privacy-preserving data mining (PPDM) has been studied for years. Yao first developed the secure multi-party computation (SMC) to theoretically solve distributed multiparty secure evaluation process (Yao 1986). Privacy-preserving data mining was introduced by Agarwal and Srikant (Agrawal & Srikant, 2000) and Lindell and Pinkas (Lindell & Pinkas, 2002), although using completely different methods, both work attempted to securely construct decision trees. The former paper utilized perturbation to randomize the original data, and correspondingly alter the mining algorithm. While the other paper applied secure multiparty computation (SMC)-like cryptography techniques (Goldreich, 1997) to preserve privacy during collaborative computation. Privacy preserving data clustering has been studied by a variety of research work. (Vaidya & Clifton, 2003; Jagannathan & Wright, 2005; Bunn & Ostrovsky, 2007; Natarajan, Rajalaxmi et al., 2007; Hong & Mohaisen, 2010; Jagannathan, Pillaipakkamnatt et al., 2010) Among these studies, Natarajan (Natarajan, Rajalaxmi et al., 2007) and Hong (Hong & Mohaisen 2010) utilized data transformation in conjunction with partition based hierarchical clustering algorithm, while others applied secure multiparty computation (SMC) techniques to make the *k*-means algorithm privacy-preserved. As observed, nearly all attempts can be categorized into two groups: data transformation and cryptographic (SMC) techniques.

Principal component analysis (PCA) was first introduced by Pearson (Pearson, 1901). It involves a mathematical procedure that transforms a number of possibly correlated variables into a smaller number of uncorrelated variables called principal components. The first principal component accounts for most of the variability in the data, and each succeeding component accounts for the next highest variability and so on. Now PCA is mostly used as a tool in exploratory data analysis and for making predictive models. PCA involves the calculation of the eigenvalue decomposition of a data covariance matrix or singular value decomposition of a data matrix, usually after mean centering of the data for each attribute. The

results of a PCA are usually discussed in terms of component scores and loadings (Shaw, 2003).

This paper concentrates on providing a specific methodology for the privacy preserving principal component analysis (PCA)-based gene clustering among distributed horizontal partitions. It applies the data transformation technology, and together with some restricted constraints, it can preserve the data privacy, and at the same time ensure 100% accuracy compared to the situation of centralized data set.

PRIVACY PRESERVED GENE CLUSTERING – METHODOLOGY

Scenario

Horizontal Partition

In this research, we only consider the scenario of horizontal partitioning, where the data is distributed among various parties but all parties have the same set of attributes. Equation (1) describes this horizontal partitioning scenario. Vertical partitioning and more complex generic scenarios will not be discussed in this paper, although they are very important and more common in the reality, and not just a mere extension of the horizontal partition.

$$x = \begin{pmatrix} S^1 \\ S^2 \\ . \\ . \\ S^k \end{pmatrix}$$

$$S^1 = \begin{pmatrix} S_1^1 & . & . & . & S_n^1 \end{pmatrix} = \begin{pmatrix} S_1^1 & S_2^1 & . & . & S_n^1 \end{pmatrix} = \begin{pmatrix} s_{11}^1 & s_{12}^1 & . & . & s_{1n}^1 \\ . & . & & & \\ . & & . & & \\ . & & & . & \\ s_{m_11}^1 & s_{m_12}^1 & . & . & s_{m_1n}^1 \end{pmatrix}$$

$$(1)$$

Overview of the Workflow

Figure 3 illustrates the detailed workflow of the proposed privacy preserving gene clustering architecture and methodology: every site calculates its local mean vector, from which the overall mean vector can be found; with the overall mean vector, every site computes its local contribution to the global covariance matrix, with which the global covariance matrix can be calculated by taking a weighted average; from the global covariance matrix, eigenvalues and eigenvectors are derived, and based on a pre-defined threshold, a set of eigenvectors are chosen; based on the chosen eigenvectors and the overall mean vector, every site projects its local data on this new basis which is identical for all parties; after the trusted central site (TCS) receives all pc-projected data, it combines all partitions, performs gene clustering, and sends back the result to all sites.

In Figure 3, each site has a clear boundary, which protects its local data privacy from their peers and the TCS. The overall mean vector and overall covariance matrix are only available to all participating data sources but is NOT accessible to the TCS. The merged PC-projected data from all participating sites only belongs to the TCS, and none of participating sites can access to it.

Figure 3. The workflow of proposed methodology on privacy preserving gene clustering

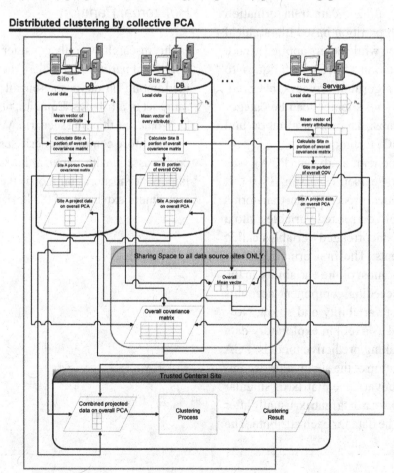

Mean Vectors Calculation

Reason to Have the Overall Mean

Each participating site needs to calculate the mean of each attribute in its local gene expression data (one horizontal partition), which results in local mean vectors of all attributes owned by every participating site. SMC can be used for participating sites to apply weighted average to calculate the overall mean of each attribute in the overall data (all horizontal partitions together).

In our proposed methodology, the overall mean vector of all attributes is critical to compute the overall covariance matrix in a distributed manner. When computing the local covariance matrix from a local horizontal partition, the local mean vector is used, which only covers the local variability of that partition. However, what we want to do is to compute the contribution to the overall covariance matrix from this local partition, which should cover the overall variability of the whole data set rather the partitioned one only. Therefore, we need to use the overall mean vector of attributes to substitute the local ones in the calculation, and the result is no longer the local covariance matrix but the local contribution to the overall covariance matrix, which can be computed from combined original gene expression data if there were no privacy issues in the data.

Methods and Algorithm

As described in Equation (1), the overall data set X with n attributes has k horizontal partitions which correspond to the k local participating sites. Therefore, site (i) has n horizontal partitioned column vectors: $S_1^i \; S_2^i \; ... \; ... \; S_n^i$ ($i \in \{1 \; 2 \; ... \; ... \; k\}$). The mean of the jth column in the ith partition $\overline{S_j^i}$ can be calculated by Equation (2), where m_i is the number of observations (rows) in this partition, and therefore, the mean vector $\overline{S^i}$ can be computed by Equation (3).

$$\overline{S_j^i} = \frac{\sum_{q=1}^{m_i} s_{qj}^i}{m_i}, \qquad \begin{pmatrix} i \in \{1 \; 2 \; ... \; ... \; k\} \\ j \in \{1 \; 2 \; ... \; ... \; n\} \end{pmatrix}$$

(2)

$$\overline{S^i} = \begin{pmatrix} \overline{S_1^i} & ... & \overline{S_n^i} \end{pmatrix} = \begin{pmatrix} \dfrac{\sum_{q=1}^{m_i} s_{q1}^i}{m_i} & ... & \dfrac{\sum_{q=1}^{m_i} s_{qn}^i}{m_i} \end{pmatrix}, \qquad \begin{pmatrix} i \in \{1 \; 2 \; ... \; ... \; k\} \\ j \in \{1 \; 2 \; ... \; ... \; n\} \end{pmatrix}.$$

(3)

When all sites get their local mean $\overline{S_j^i}$, the overall mean $\overline{S_j}$ can be calculated by weighted average as described in Equation (6). And the overall mean vector of attributes $\overline{X}$ can be found by Equation (5).

$$\overline{S_j} = \frac{\sum_{i=1}^{k} m_i s_j^i}{\sum_{i=1}^{k} m_i}, \qquad \left(j \in \{1 \; 2 \; ... \; ... \; n\} \right)$$

(4)

$$\overline{X} = \begin{pmatrix} \overline{S_1} & \overline{S_2} & \overline{S_n} \end{pmatrix} = \begin{pmatrix} \dfrac{\sum_{i=1}^{k} m_i s_1^i}{\sum_{i=1}^{k} m_1} & ... & \dfrac{\sum_{i=1}^{k} m_i s_n^i}{\sum_{i=1}^{k} m_k} \end{pmatrix}.$$

(5)

Figure 4 gives the algorithm by which the overall mean vector of attributes are calculated from distributed sites without revealing the original gene expression data.

Secure Local Mean Vector by SMC

In the above distributed overall mean vector calculation, each site (i) $i \in \{1 \; 2 \; ... \; ... \; k\}$ only needs to provide its local mean vector $\overline{S^i}$ and the number of local observations m_i. Although both $\overline{S^i}$ and m_i are not original data, it is good to utilize the secure multi-party computation (SMC) to double protect privacy of participating sites.

Figure 4. Algorithm of distributed overall mean vector calculation

```
1:      for i =1 to k do
2:            for j = 1 to n do
3:                  for q = 1 to m[i,j] do
4:                        sum[i,j] = sum[i,j] + s^i_{qj}
5:                  end for
6:                  average[i,j] = sum[i,j] /m[i,j]
7:            end for
7:            vector[i] = all elements of average[,j]
8:      end for
9:      vector = weight average of all elements in vector[]
```

To calculate the weighted average of mean vectors, two parts need to be computed: the sum of all products of the number of observations and mean vector for every site $\sum_{i=1}^{k}\left(m_i \times \overline{S^i}\right)$, and the total number of observations $\sum_{i=1}^{k} m_i$. With these two parts the global can be computed by Equation (5).

Therefore if we can run two SMCs to get these two parts correspondingly, the overall mean vector can be got without sharing any information of local mean or the number of observations of each site.

To use the SMC compute $\sum_{i=1}^{k} m_i$, it can be initiated by the first site S^1, which generates a random number N_1 and sends the N_1+m_1 to the next site S^2. Because only S^1 know the number N_1, there is no way for any other parties to extract m_1 information from N_1+m_1. S^2 adds N_2+m_2 into the number it gets, and now the number it sends out to the next party is $N_1+m_1+N_2+m_2$. After this process circulates over all parties and returns to S^1, the number is $N_1+m_1+N_2+m_2+...+N_i+m_i+...+N_k+m_k$, and now S^1 can subtract N_1 that is he added to the number, and then sends the number which is $m_1+N_2+m_2+...+N_i+m_i+...+N_k+m_k$ to the next site. After the second circulation ends, all sites subtracted the noises they added to their original data, and what left is $\sum_{i=1}^{k} m_i$. As described above, for each site (i), since only it know the added number N_i, and what it sends out is N_i+m_i, the original data m_i cannot be available to any other parties.

Similarly to computing the global mean vector by SMC, it is not difficult to apply SMC on computing the $\sum_{i=1}^{k}\left(m_i \times \overline{S^i}\right)$. The only difference is that each site will send out the row vector $m_i \times \overline{S^i}$ with its added noise M which is a random generated vector with the same number of elements with $\overline{S^i}$ and known only by the site (i).

Once we get both $\sum_{i=1}^{k}\left(m_i \times \overline{S^i}\right)$ and $\sum_{i=1}^{k} m_i$ by SMC, we can easily get the global mean vector without letting any party lose its data of either individual mean and the number of observations.

Computing the Overall Covariance Matrix

Each horizontal partition site computes its local contribution to the covariance matrix on the overall data. To do so, each site computes the covariance matrix on its local partition as usual, but uses the overall mean vector of attributes to substitute the local mean in the computation. After all sites get their local contributions, they can utilize either global sharing (avoiding SMC to reduce the communication cost) or SMC, and weighted average to get the overall covariance matrix.

Interactively Computing the Covariance Matrix

The target of the proposed methodology is to get the overall gene clustering result without sharing the original gene expression data, and therefore, the privacy of each site is preserved. Hence, we have to make sure that the data transformation does not lose or distort too much information, compared to the original data. Serving as the transformation algorithm, the PCA is utilized in our methodology, and the idea is to let local sites transform their original gene expression data into PC-projected data locally, which will be provided to the trusted central site (TCS) for combination and clustering processing, so that the TCS cannot have access to the original data, and the privacy is preserved. However, the problem is that, if each site conducts PCA solely and projects its local data to the new basis, the combination of all locally PC-projected data cannot remain consistent with the original or PC-projected whole data set. This is because when one site conducts PCA individually, the covariance matrix it gets is solely based on its local data, and therefore, this covariance matrix covers only the variability of its local data. In this way, the covariance matrices resulting from all sites should be different, which derive different eigenvalues and eigenvectors, and therefore let every site have a distinguished new basis when it conducts PC-projection for it local data. Thus, to ensure all participating sites project their local data on an identical new basis, it is necessary to get the overall covariance matrix, which covers the variability of there overall data set. With this overall covariance matrix, all sites derive identical eigenvalues and eigenvectors, which provide the same new basis to them.

Method and Algorithm

Each participating site applies Equation (6) to compute the contribution to the overall covariance matrix from its partition. It varies from the regu-

lar covariance matrix computation Equation (x) by using the overall mean vector $\overline{X}$ to substitute the local mean vector $\overline{S^i}$. Therefore, the result $\mathrm{cov}_{overall}(S^i)$ is no longer the local covariance matrix for the partition (i), but the contribution to the overall covariance matrix on the whole data set, which contains the local contribution of the variability from the view of the whole data set.

$$\mathrm{cov}_{overall}(S^i) = E\left[\left(S^i - \overline{X}\right)\left(S^i - \overline{X}\right)^T\right]$$

$$= \begin{bmatrix} E\left[\left(s_1^i - \overline{X_1}\right)\left(s_1^i - \overline{X_1}\right)^T\right] & E\left[\left(s_1^i - \overline{X_1}\right)\left(s_2^i - \overline{X_2}\right)^T\right] & \cdots \cdots & E\left[\left(s_1^i - \overline{X_1}\right)\left(s_n^i - \overline{X_n}\right)^T\right] \\ \vdots & \vdots & \cdots \cdots & \vdots \\ E\left[\left(s_n^i - \overline{X_n}\right)\times\left(s_1^i - \overline{X_1}\right)^T\right] & E\left[\left(s_n^i - \overline{X_n}\right)\left(s_2^i - \overline{X_2}\right)^T\right] & \cdots \cdots & E\left[\left(s_n^i - \overline{X_n}\right)\left(s_n^i - \overline{X_n}\right)^T\right] \end{bmatrix}$$

$$\left(i \in \left\{1 \quad 2 \quad \ldots \quad \ldots \quad k\right\}\right), \tag{6}$$

After all participating sites get their local contribution to the overall covariance matrix, they share them with each other, and therefore, weighted average can be used to calculate the overall covariance matrix, as shown in Equation (7).

$$\mathrm{cov}(X) = \frac{\sum_{i=1}^{k}\left(m_i \times \mathrm{cov}_{overall}(S^i)\right)}{\sum_{i=1}^{k} m_i}. \tag{7}$$

Figure 5 gives the algorithm to compute the global covariance matrix from every local data set $S^i\left(i \in \left\{1 \quad 2 \quad \ldots \quad \ldots \quad k\right\}\right)$, the number of observations in each local site m_i, and the overall mean vector $\overline{X}$.

Secured Multi-Party Computation (SMC)

During the distributed global covariance matrix computation, we did not apply the SMC but let each local party directly share its contribution to the global covariance matrix (CGC) $\text{cov}_{overall}(S^i)$ to its peers, mostly because of the high communication cost it occurs. However, the privacy is still preserved without utilizing SMC in this computation.

As shown in Equation (7), for each partition site (i), one of its CGC elements, the covariance contribution between the pth and q^{th} columns, $Cov_{overall}(S_p^i, S_q^i)$, can be determined by Equation (8), where S_p^i is its pth column vector, S_q^i is its qth column vector, $\overline{S_p}$ is the overall mean of pth column, $\overline{S_q}$ is the overall mean of the qth column of the whole data set X. Here, the $\overline{S_p}\,\overline{S_q}$ is known by other participating sites, and if SMC is applied in the local mean calculation the $\overline{S_q}S_p^i - \overline{S_p}S_q^i$ is unknown, so that the accessibility to $Cov_{overall}(S_p^i, S_q^i)$ cannot by uniquely determined by the $E(S_p^i S_q^i)$. Furthermore, even if SMC is not utilized to calculate the overall mean, and $\overline{S_q}S_p^i - \overline{S_p}S_q^i$ is known to other participating parties, one party may find $E(S_p^i S_q^i)$ but cannot get S_p^i and S_q^i which are the original data need to be protected.

Thus, we can conclude that even if SMC is not used in the global covariance matrix computation, and no matter if SMC is used in the overall mean calculation, by having access to the covariance contribution of site (i) $Cov_{overall}(S_p^i, S_q^i)$, it is still impossible for another party to invert PCA to get its original data S_p^i and S_q^i.

$$Cov_{overall}(S_p^i, S_q^i) = E\left(\left(S_p^i - \overline{S_p}\right)\left(S_q^i - \overline{S_q}\right)\right) = E\left(S_p^i S_q^i\right) - \overline{S_q}\,\overline{S_p^i} - \overline{S_p}\,\overline{S_q^i} + \overline{S_p}\,\overline{S_q}$$
$$i \in \{1 \quad 2 \quad ... \quad ... \quad k\}$$
$$p, q \in \{1 \quad 2 \quad ... \quad ... \quad n\} \tag{8}$$

Also, it is impossible for one party to perform an inverse PCA to get back the original data S_p^i and S_q^i that belong to another party by having

access to the covariance contribution of site (i) $Cov_{overall}(S_p^i, S_q^i)$.

Accuracy

After collecting all k local contributions to the global covariance matrix, we can simply take weighted average on both sides in Equation (8), and the right side becomes $E(S_p S_q) - \overline{S_p}\,\overline{S_q}$. It can be transformed to

$$E(S_p S_q) - \overline{S_q}E(S_p) - \overline{S_p}E(S_q) + \overline{S_p}\,\overline{S_q},$$

and further be changed to $E\left(\left(S_p - \overline{S_p}\right)\left(S_q - \overline{S_q}\right)\right)$, which is the global covariance between S_p and S_q by the definition of covariance. Therefore, it is proved that the global covariance matrix computed from multiple data sources by our distributed methodology is the same as the one directly calculated from the whole original data X.

PCA Computation

Based on the overall covariance matrix, each site computes its eigenvalues and eigenvectors. Every local site rearranges the eigenvalues in the descending order, and using a pre-defined percentage of variance of the overall data, all local sites pick up the first few eigenvalues and corresponding eigenvectors to fulfill the requirement.

Eigen Analysis

From Equation (9) and (10) it is not difficult to compute the eigenvalues λ and eigenvectors Evc.

$$Cov(X) \times Evc_i = \lambda_i \times Evc_i \tag{9}$$

$$| Cov(X) - \lambda \times I | = 0. \tag{10}$$

Figure 5. The algorithm to compute the global covariance matrix

```
1:     for i=1 to k do
2:            for j = 1 to n do
3:                   for q = 1 to n do
4:                          cov[q,j,i] = average((s_q^i - X̄_q)×(s_j^i - X̄_j)^Y)
5:                   end for
6:            end for
7:     end for
7:     cov_matrix[1:n , 1:n]=weight average of all elements in cov[,,i]
8:
```

There are multiple ways to calculate λ and Evc, and if all local parties agree to use a pre-selected one, they can all get the identical λ and Evc by computing locally from the global covariance matrix $Cov(X)$.

PC Selection

Once a single local site (i) gets the eigenvalues λ and eigenvectors Evc, it needs to pick up a set of PCs to be a new basis. To ensure that all local sites choose the same basis, it is necessary to have a pre-defined threshold, which is a percentage that determines how much variance the chosen PCs should cover. To do so, each local site rearranges the eigenvalues λ in descending order, and also rearranges the eigenvectors to make each eigenvector Evc_j to be in the same position as its corresponding eigenvalue λ_j. The site picks up the first several eigenvalues whose sum accounts for more or equal to the threshold over the sum of all eigenvalues.

$$\lambda = \{\lambda_1 \quad \lambda_2 \quad \cdots \quad \cdots \quad \lambda_i \quad \cdots \quad \lambda_n\} \tag{11}$$

$$t \leq \frac{\sum_{j=1}^{l} \lambda_j}{\sum_{j=1}^{n} \lambda_j}. \tag{12}$$

As shown in Equation (11) and (12), after arrangement, site (i) has chosen the first l eigenvalues λ_P, and the sum of the chosen l eigenvalues over the sum of all n eigenvalues is larger or equal to the threshold t.

Corresponding the chosen eigenvalues λ_P, the first l eigenvectors are picked up to be the chosen eigenvectors E, which together with λ_P represents the selected principal components (PCs).

Accuracy

Although the eigenvalues and eigenvectors are computed and selected by each site individually, the PCs selected by all sites should be identical. Because 1) they are all computed from an identical covariance, which is the sole source for both eigenvalues and eigenvectors; 2) all sites utilize the same method to compute eigenvalues and eigenvector, which is pre-determined; 3) when choosing the eigenvalues and vectors, all sites follow the same pre-defined threshold, which makes the chosen eigenvalues and corresponding eigenvectors identical. Therefore, although the PC-selection is done by multiple sites individually, the result by every site remains identical.

PC Projection

Based on the picked eigenvectors, each site projects it horizontal partition of the overall gene expression data on the new basis. Since each site uses the overall mean and the same set of selected eigenvectors, which are derived from the overall covariance matrix on the whole data set, the projected data is on the global new basis, and it is identical for every site.

$$S_{PC}^i = (S^i - \overline{X}) \times E = \left(\begin{pmatrix} S_1^i & S_2^i & ... & ... & S_n^i \end{pmatrix} - \begin{pmatrix} \overline{X_1} & \overline{X_2} & ... & ... & \overline{X_n} \end{pmatrix} \right) \times E$$

$$\left(i \in \left\{ 1 \quad 2 \quad ... \quad ... \quad k \right\} \right). \tag{13}$$

According to Equation (13), the global projection of local data S_{PC}^i is the product of the different between the local data (horizontal partition) S^i and the overall mean vector $\overline{X}$.

Because all horizontal partitions use the same new basis, E and $\overline{X}$, which are the same of the new basis of the global PCA, each projection S_{PC}^i is part of the global PC-projected data, that is, the combination of those locally projected data is identical to the PC-projected data directly computed from the overall data set X.

After the TCS receives all PC-projected local gene expression data sets from every site (all horizontal partitions), it can apply a variety of algorithms, *e.g.*, hierarchical, *k*-means, *etc.*, to cluster the combined overall data set, and sends part of the clustering result (clusters of genes) back to every local site.

Trusted Central Site (TCS)

Merging Projected Data

Because all horizontal partitions use the same new basis, E and $\overline{X}$, which are the same as the new basis of the global PCA, each projection S_{PC}^i is part of the global PC-projected data, that is, the combination of those local projected data is identical to the PC-projected data directly computed from the overall data set X.

$$X_{PC} = \begin{pmatrix} S_{PC}^1 \\ S_{PC}^2 \\ . \\ . \\ . \\ S_{PC}^k \end{pmatrix}. \tag{14}$$

Therefore, according to Equation (14) the combined PC-projected data X_{PC} is composed by vertically put all PC-projected horizontal partitions. Figure 6 below gives the algorithm to compose all PC-projected partitions into the overall PC projection data.

Although in the Equation (14) and Figure 6, the PC-projected partitions are ordered by numbers from 1 to k during processing, the TCS has no idea as to which partition is on which original position, therefore, the orders of partitions in the combination of PC projections is irrelevant to the order of partitions in the original data. However, although the order of the partitions might not be the same as in the original data, each PC partition composed from multiple distributed sites is identical to the corresponding partition of the overall PC-projected data directly calculated from the original data X.

Cluster Merged PC Projected Data

After composing all of the PC-projected partitions S_{PC}^i, $i \in \left\{ 1 \quad 2 \quad ... \quad ... \quad k \right\}$ into a whole projected data set X_{PC}, the TCS can use a variety methods, *e.g.*, hierarchical, k-means, and *etc.*, to perform the gene clustering. Here in this paper, we use the hierarchical clustering as an example to illustrate how it works on the combination of PC-projected partitions.

In hierarchical clustering (Ward, 1963; Wikipedia, 2010), each cluster is subdivided into smaller clusters, forming a tree-shaped data structure or dendrogram. Agglomerative hierarchical clustering starts with the single-gene clusters and successively joins the closest clusters until all genes have been joined into the super-cluster. In fact, there is

Figure 6. Algorithm of combining all PC-projected partitions

```
1:      row=0
2:      for i=1 to k do
3:              for  q = 1 to m[i] do
4:                      row=row+i
5:                      for j =1 to n do
6:                              X_PC[row, q] = S_PC^i[q , j]
7:                      end for
8:              end for
9:      end for
10:     X_PC[1:∑_{i=1}^{k} m_i ,1:n] is the combination of all PC-projected partitions.
```

a whole family of clustering methods, differing only in the way inter-cluster distance is defined (the 'linkage function'). Some of the more common ones are single linkage (the distance between clusters is the shortest distance between any two members of the cluster), complete linkage (largest distance between any two members), average linkage/UPGMA (un-weighted pair-group method using arithmetic averages; average distance between any two members) and centroid linkage/ UPGMC (un-weighted pair-group method using centroids; distance between the cluster centroids).

Figure 7 shows the procedure of building the hierarchy from the individual elements by progressively merging clusters (Wikipedia 2010). To do so, one can construct a distance matrix, where the number in the ith row, j^{th} column is the distance between the ith and j^{th} elements. Then, as clustering progresses, rows and columns are merged as the clusters are merged and the distances updated. This is a common way to implement this type of clustering, and has the benefit of caching distances between clusters.

$$\min \left\{ d\left(x , y\right) : \quad x \in A \quad y \in B \right\}. \tag{15}$$

In this paper we use single linkage (or "nearest neighbor"), a simple agglomerative clustering algorithm, which is a method of calculating distances between clusters in hierarchical clustering. As shown in Equation (15), in single linkage, the distance between two clusters is computed as the distance between the two closest elements in the two clusters.

Figure 8 shows a hierarchical gene clustering result (Mathworks 2007), rows represent genes (observations), and columns represent treatments (attributes). As described above, from the beginning of the gene clustering process, each gene is a single cluster, and then nearest gene clusters merged together to be an aggregative gene cluster which continues to merge into another bigger one, and finally, all clusters merged together to be a super-cluster. Therefore, a tree structure is generated as shown on the left of Figure 8.

In our proposed methodology, the TCS performs a nearest neighbor clustering to obtain the gene clustering using the combined PC-projected partitions. Because the PCA projection retains most of the variability of the original data, the projected data behaves similar to the original during the gene clustering processing, therefore, the gene clusters resulting from the PC-projected data is similar to those from the original data.

TCS Sends Result to All Parties

Once the TCS completes the gene clustering, it will send the gene clustering information back to local sites. Because all local sites have access to the overall mean vector and select eigenvectors, with which one might conduct inverse PCA to get the original gene expression, therefore the PC-projected values are not included in the gene clustering result sent to local sites. The local sites get the gene clusters and the list of genes from the TCS.

Local Parties Compose Gene Profile

After receiving the gene clustering result, each local site calculates the mean vector of all attributes for every cluster. SMC can be used again for all local sites to get the overall mean vectors of every cluster by weighted average, and therefore, the overall gene profile is computed.

A gene profile is a measurement on the gene(s) activities, which shows how one or in most cases a group of gene is (are) expressed in response to a series of treatments (attributes). When multiple genes are clustered together, it indicates that they behave similarly and therefore form a gene profile. In most of cases, the gene profile is calculated by averaging all genes in the cluster for each attribute, which thereafter results in a mean vector, which is the gene profile.

Gene profiles are important for biologists to study the behaviors and interactions among gene(s), and to generate new or enhanced new pathways (gene networks). However, from the gene clustering result obtained at the TCS, one cannot get the gene profiles, because 1) the data the TCS uses is not original data, and has no complete attributes; 2) although, it is possible to use PC-projected values to substitute original data, due to the privacy issue addressed in Step 5, the PC-projected data is not shared among all local sites. Thus, it is necessary to design an alternative way to compose gene profile.

Figure 7. Hierarchical clustering

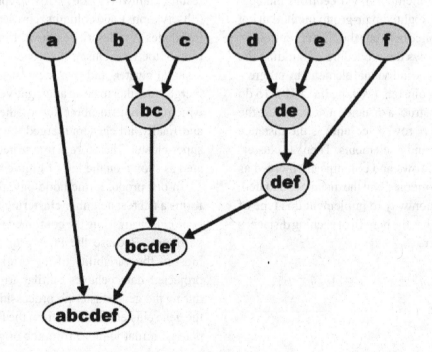

Figure 8. Hierarchical gene clustering result

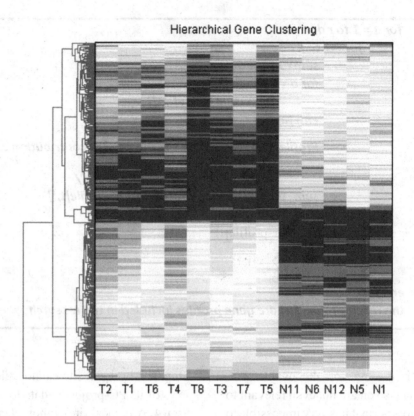

Gene Profiles

As described in the step 5, each local site will receive the names of the gene clustered in multiple gene clusters. Each site (i) scans every cluster, and picks up the genes that belong to its local partition in each gene clusters. Suppose we are considering r clusters in total, with gene cluster t ($t \in (1 \quad . \quad . \quad . \quad r)$), site (i) has genes involved, and it calculates the mean of all gene expression values for every attribute, and thus, resulting in a mean vector, which is the local contribution of gene profile (t). Once all local sites get their local contribution to the gene profile (t), a weighted average can be applied to calculate the overall mean vector for this gene cluster which is the gene profile (t). We can repeat this process r times to get all r gene profiles we are interested in.

Figure 9 above provides the algorithm for local sites to calculate gene profiles corresponding to those gene clusters resulted from the TCS by distributed PCA processing.

SMC and Privacy

Similar to the step 2, which also uses weighted average to calculate the global mean from local means provided by distributed sites, SMC can be applied to doubly ensure the privacy of the original expression data. However, this is not necessary, because, what each site shares out are the mean vectors of those genes involved in corresponding gene clusters. Since the site-wise allocation of genes in each gene clusters is unknown to any local site, which means, other sites do not even know the source of each mean vector that any site provides, therefore other information like

Figure 9. Algorithm to compose gene profiles

```
1:    for t = 1 to r do
2:        for i=1 to k do
3:            sum=0
4:            for o =1 to v[i, t] do
5:                sum=sum+C[i, v[i, t]]
6:            end for
7:            Profile[t,i]= sum/v[i,t]  /*this is the site(i)'s contribution to gene
                                          profile (t)*/
8:            sum_profile[t]=sum_profile+v[i] X Profile[t,i]
9:        end for
10:       profile[t]= sum_profile[t] / ∑(i=1 to k) v[i, t]
11:   end for
12:   the result profile[1:r] are gene profiles included in the research
```

covariance matrix, eigenvectors, eigenvalues, PC-projected data, and so on are not even relevant to those mean vectors, so that it is very impossible to use those local mean and number of genes in the cluster to trace back to the original data. Therefore, we can conclude that it is safe for site (i) to share its mean of gene expression values in every gene clusters, and SMC is not necessary for protecting the privacy of original gene expression data.

Steps to Preserve Privacy

The proposed methodology is based on a semi-trusted architecture, and to preserve privacy during the distributed gene clustering procedure, certain disciplines must be enforced by both TCS and every local site.

Step 1: The TCS cannot release either partitioned or overall PC-projected data to any local site.
Step 2: Any local site cannot release either overall mean vector or global covariance matrix to the TCS.

Step 3: Any local site cannot release part or all of its PC-projected data to any of its peers.
Step 4: Any local site cannot release part or all of its original data to the TCS pr any of its peers.

Proof of Privacy in the Proposed Methodology

Individual Local PC-Projected Data

Figure 10 shows the privacy sensitive information allocated to each party during projecting local data to the selected global PCs. As shown in Figure 10, the original local data S^i is owned by site (i), and no any other party can access it. Each site (i) also owns its PC-projected data S^i_{PC}, which is only provided to the TCS, any other data source site cannot access it. The overall mean vector $\overline{X}$ and the selected set of eigenvectors E are available to all data source sites but not to the TCS.

Also from the Figure 10, if some one other than site (i) want to access the original data S^i, it has to have both the PC-projected data S^i_{PC} and

Figure 10. The privacy allocation during local PC-projection

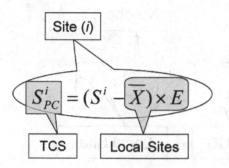

the selected set of eigenvectors E with overall mean vector $\overline{X}$, which are not accessible simultaneously to any party other than the site (i), therefore, the privacy of S^i is preserved.

Overall PC Projected Data

After the PC-projected data are sent to the TCS, the accessibility allocation of each part of data is shown in Figure 11. In the left part of Figure 11, every site (i) owns it PC-projected local data S^i_{PC}, and sends it to the TCS. The TCS then composes them into the overall PC-projected data X_{PC}. The TSC cannot do an inverse PCA to get S^i from S^i_{PC} as described above and shown in Figure 11. The left part of Figure 11 shows an alternative way to get X_{PC} from the combined original data set X, which does not exist in our scenario. From the Equation, we can see if someone wants to compute X, it has to have simultaneous access to X_{PC}, E, and $\overline{X}$, which are actually separately accessible to TCS and all local sites, thus no one can compute the overall original data X, and therefore the privacy is preserved.

Privacy Violation Scenarios

As described and illustrated above, it is impossible to hack part or overall of the original data if both the TCS and all local sites enforce the disciplines mentioned before. However, even if some of the parties are not completely honest, the privacy may still be preserved.

Figure 12 enumerates all scenarios that the proposed methodology faces. Rows represent the privacy violence situation of each participating site, and columns represent the situation of how the TCS violates the protocols.

Accuracy

The accuracy of the PC-projected data computed from distributed data sources is compared with the PC-projected data directly calculated from the overall data set X which does not happen in the proposed methodology and the scenario described in the paper. Using the definition of the covariance matrix and the method we use to compute global covariance matrix from distributed sites, it can be theoretically proven that our distributed covariance matrix computation result is exactly the same as the one calculated directly from X. Because the eigenvalues and eigenvectors are solely derived from the covariance matrix, and the new PCA basis is dependent on the selected eigenvalues and the overall mean vector $\overline{X}$ of X, which can also be calculated from distributed sites in our methodology, we can safe draw the conclusion that our distributed PC projection method can gain exactly the same result as that from overall original data X.

EXPERIMENTS AND RESULTS

Experiment Overview

In our experiments, a real gene expression data set is chosen to test the proposed privacy preserving gene clustering methodology. This data set is generated by using customized cDNA microarray chips.

Figure 11. The privacy allocation in with the TCS

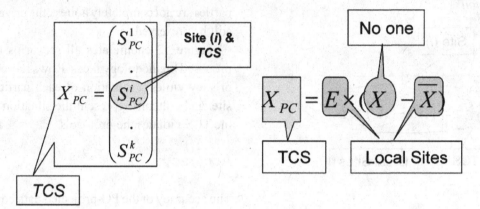

During the experiments, for each data set, two process pipelines are conducted: 1) centralized scenario – which assumes that the data set is completely accessible and analyzed directly; and 2) distributed scenario where each data set is randomly split into multiple horizontal partitions multiple times (usually greater than 30), where that no single party can directly access all partitions, and therefore the proposed privacy preserving gene clustering methodology is utilized to analyze the data. For each data set, comparisons are made between the centralized scenario and every split of the distributed scenario. The results show that using the proposed methodology in the distributed scenario can gain exactly the same result as that of the centralized scenario.

The steps followed in the experiment consisted of, first, processing PCA on the whole data set, and getting the clustering results for the centralized result, and second, simulating the distributed scenario by splitting the data set, and then utilizing the proposed scenario to calculate the PCA over the distributed partitions of the data set. But before this procedure is conducted, some standard processing, including data filtering and pre-processing, need to be done.

Filtering Data

The microarray data set is usually quite large and a lot of the information corresponds to genes that do not show any interesting changes during the experiment. To make it easier to find the interesting genes, it is necessary to reduce the size of the data set by removing genes with expression profiles that do not show anything of interest.

The sample microarray data set is cNDA dual color array, and it has same empty spots, so it is necessary to remove them from the data, since for the purpose of the experiment, these empty spots can be considered as noise. There are also some missing data where the expression level is marked as "NaN". One approach to dealing with these missing values would be to impute them using the mean or median of data for the particular gene over time. Our experiments used a less rigorous approach of simply throwing away the data for any genes where one or more expression levels were not measured. Since there also some values inside the data set are extremely small, it is very be useful to either filter out those genes with extreme values or raise them into a minimum value which would not affect the later differential test much. In our experiments, we choose to simply remove those genes with extremely small values.

Figure 12. Privacy preserving analysis

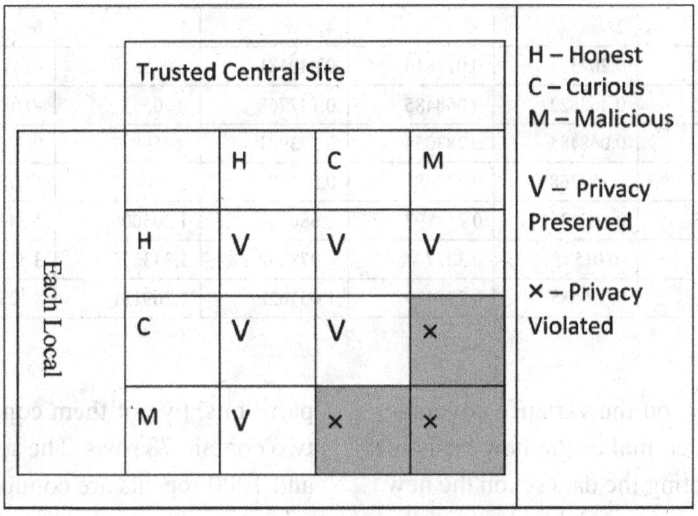

Pre-Processing Data

In the remaining data, it is found that most profiles are flat which means that there are no significant differences among them. This flat data is obviously of use as it indicates that the genes associated with these profiles are not significantly affected by the diauxic shift. However, in this example, researchers are interested in the genes with large changes in expression accompanying the diauxic shift. Therefore, we need to use some statistical filtering functions to remove genes with various types of profiles that do not provide useful information about genes affected by the metabolic change. Before doing so, it is necessary to normalize all conditions (columns) to be a same level to reduce the array chip and other noise effects, and Loess is employed to conduct it in this experiment, other methods like quantile may also work well if one needs fast result. After normalization, we use variance greater than the 10th percentile and zeros corresponding to those below as the threshold which returns a logical array of the same size as the variable genes with ones corresponding to rows of yeast gene expression values. One can also utilize other statistical methods like Local-Pooled-Error (LPE) test or

Linear Model for Microarray Analysis (Limma) to extract significantly expressed genes accompanying the diauxic shift.

Data Set

The data set is yeast gene expression data to study temporal gene expression of almost all genes in Saccharomyces cerevisiae during the metabolic shift from fermentation to respiration. Expression levels were measured at seven time points during the diauxic shift (DeRisi, Iyer et al., 1997). There are 7 columns which represents sample collected at 7 different time spots. After the data filtering and pre-processing, there leaves 310 out of 4540 genes in the data set, which is corresponded to 310 rows.

PCA Gene Clustering on the Centralized Scenario

With the filtered and pre-processed data, which has 310 rows and 7 columns, the PCA computation is conducted by: 1) calculating the covariance matrix of the data set, where the results are shown in Table 1 ; 2) performing eigen analysis, which results in eigen vectors and eigen values; 3) se-

Table 1. The covariance matrix of the centralized scenario

Columns	1	2	3	4	5	6	7
1	0.193249	0.207552	0.017816	0.040581	0.098516	-0.17915	-0.16453
2	0.207552	0.463822	0.068485	0.147768	0.30533	-0.01535	0.030585
3	0.017816	0.068485	0.283058	0.223981	0.259897	0.3277	0.272479
4	0.040581	0.147768	0.223981	0.574186	0.680369	1.078833	1.004622
5	0.098516	0.30533	0.259897	0.680369	1.204006	1.343275	1.269131
6	-0.17915	-0.01535	0.3277	1.078833	1.343275	3.511943	3.120871
7	-0.16453	0.030585	0.272479	1.004622	1.269131	3.120871	3.45888

lecting the PCS based on the variance coverage of 90% or more, which makes the new basis of the data set; 4) projecting the data set on the new basis to get the PC transformed data; and finally, 5) hierarchically clustering the projected data.

The result is shown on Figure 13, the number of clusters, which is 6 in this case, is pre-defined.

Splitting the Data Set

As stated before, in this paper only the horizontal partition is handled, and therefore, in this experiment, 310 rows o f the data set is split into 4 partitions, two of them contain 77 and the other two contain 78 rows. The split is randomly done, and 1000 repeats are conducted.

Using Privacy Preserving Gene Clustering on the Distributed Scenario

During this process, the proposed privacy preserving gene clustering methodology is applied in every split situation: 1) calculating the mean vector in each partition; 2) merging all local partitions into the overall covariance matrix by weighted

Figure 13. The PCA gene clustering result of the centralized scenario

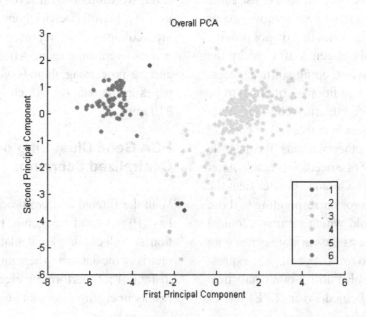

average; 3) having every partition compute its local portion of the overall covariance matrix by using the overall mean vector, (Table 2 shows the result of all these 4 portions); 4) merging the portions into the overall covariance matrix (shown in Table 3); 5) calculating (in each partition) the eigenvectors and eigenvalues from the overall covariance matrix; 6) selecting PCs by assuring that more than 90% of variance is covered, and therefore, the new basis is constructed; 7) projecting at each partition its local data on the new basis; 8) merging the local PC projected data into the overall one; 9) and performing the hierarchical clustering on the overall projected data.

Figure 14 shows one final gene clustering result of the 1000 splitting repeats, which is calculated by the proposed Privacy Preserving Gene Clustering methodology under the distributed scenario.

Comparison

After checking results of 1000 splitting situations, we found that all global covariance matrices are identical, and they are also identical to the one under the centralized scenario. Table 1 demonstrates the covariance matrix calculated from the centralized data set. Table 2 shows 4 portions of the global covariance matrix which are calculated from 4 participating sites under the distributed scenario. Table 3 shows the global covariance matrix under the distributed scenario, which is

Table 2. 4 local portions of the overall covariance matrix under one of the 1000 split situation

Local portions of the overall covariance matrix								
		Covariance Matrix						
Partition	Columns	1	2	3	4	5	6	7
S1	1	0.0490	0.0926	0.0022	0.0196	0.0581	-0.0410	-0.0279
	2	0.0926	0.2813	-0.0056	0.0518	0.1485	0.0024	0.0415
	3	0.0022	-0.0056	0.0522	0.0309	0.0338	0.0528	0.0156
	4	0.0196	0.0518	0.0309	0.1160	0.1547	0.2162	0.1964
	5	0.0581	0.1485	0.0338	0.1547	0.3314	0.2792	0.2705
	6	0.0410	0.0024	0.0528	0.2162	0.2792	0.7875	0.6985
	7	0.0279	0.0415	0.0156	0.1964	0.2705	0.6985	0.8212
S2	1	0.0368	0.0425	0.0113	0.0078	0.0210	-0.0307	-0.0378
	2	0.0425	0.0940	0.0394	0.0461	0.0763	-0.0000	-0.0038
	3	0.0113	0.0394	0.0844	0.0853	0.0939	0.0877	0.0705
	4	0.0078	0.0461	0.0853	0.1718	0.1986	0.3046	0.2739
	5	0.0210	0.0763	0.0939	0.1986	0.3580	0.3519	0.3182
	6	0.0307	0.0000	0.0877	0.3046	0.3519	0.9367	0.8415
	7	0.0378	0.0038	0.0705	0.2739	0.3182	0.8415	0.8854
S3	1	0.0916	0.0604	0.0069	0.0247	0.0291	-0.0493	-0.0420
	2	0.0604	0.0639	0.0229	0.0430	0.0578	0.0085	0.0128
	3	0.0069	0.0229	0.0682	0.0523	0.0633	0.1052	0.1077
	4	0.0247	0.0430	0.0523	0.1572	0.1787	0.2761	0.2847
	5	0.0291	0.0578	0.0633	0.1787	0.2773	0.3626	0.3556
	6	0.0493	0.0085	0.1052	0.2761	0.3626	0.8577	0.7731
	7	0.0420	0.0128	0.1077	0.2847	0.3556	0.7731	0.8986
S4	1	0.0159	0.0121	-0.0027	-0.0116	-0.0097	-0.0581	-0.0568
	2	0.0121	0.0247	0.0118	0.0069	0.0226	-0.0263	-0.0199
	3	0.0027	0.0118	0.0783	0.0555	0.0690	0.0819	0.0787
	4	0.0116	0.0069	0.0555	0.1292	0.1484	0.2819	0.2496
	5	0.0097	0.0226	0.0690	0.1484	0.2373	0.3496	0.3249
	6	0.0581	0.0263	0.0819	0.2819	0.3496	0.9301	0.8078
	7	0.0568	0.0199	0.0787	0.2496	0.3249	0.8078	0.8536

Table 3. The overall covariance matrix calculated by merging 4 local portions shown above in Table2 under one of the 1000 split situations in the distributed scenario

Columns	1	2	3	4	5	6	7
1	0.193249	0.207552	0.017816	0.040581	0.098516	-0.17915	-0.16453
2	0.207552	0.463822	0.068485	0.147768	0.30533	-0.01535	0.030585
3	0.017816	0.068485	0.283058	0.223981	0.259897	0.3277	0.272479
4	0.040581	0.147768	0.223981	0.574186	0.680369	1.078833	1.004622
5	0.098516	0.30533	0.259897	0.680369	1.204006	1.343275	1.269131
6	-0.17915	-0.01535	0.3277	1.078833	1.343275	3.511943	3.120871
7	-0.16453	0.030585	0.272479	1.004622	1.269131	3.120871	3.45888

the merged result of 4 portions shown in Table 2. As one can easily find out, Table 1 and 3 give exactly the same covariance matrix. Furthermore, all 1000 gene clustering results are identical to each other, and they are also identical to the one under the centralized scenario. As shown in Figure 13 and 14, they are exactly the same two-dimensional clustering result. Therefore, it has 100% accuracy as compared with the results under the centralized scenario.

CONCLUSION

This paper presents a novel methodology to handle distributed Principal Component Analysis (PCA)-based cluster analysis on gene expression (microarray) data, and at the same time to preserve the data privacy of every site in a horizontally partitioned data. Each data provider does not need to reveal its data directly to others in order to gain a comprehensive analysis from a global point of view. Towards this goal, the proposed

Figure 14. The PCA result of by the proposed Privacy Preserving Gene Clustering methodology under one of 1000 split situations calculated in the distributed scenario

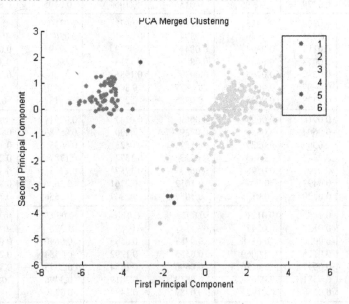

methodology provides a framework to allow all horizontal partitions to interactively conduct the PCA computation. Data providers covertly and interactively calculate the overall covariance matrix, and project their data on an identical global new basis. All participating sites send their projected data to the trusted central site (TCS). Finally the TSC combines all projected data and performs the global gene clustering analysis.

During the process, only participating sites can access the covariance matrix, and only the TCS can access to the global projected data. Thus, no one can successfully hack into the system to get original data that belongs to others by inverse PCA, and therefore, the data privacy is preserved.

In proposed methodology, the global covariance matrix is calculated interactively by all individual sites, which results in exactly the same outcome as when calculated from merging all data, so that the new basis in the distributed scenario is identical to that of the centralized scenario.

Compared to current popular perturbation based approaches, the proposed methodology does not need to refine the clustering algorithms and provides more accurate results; and compared to pure secure multi-party computation (SMC) approaches, it significantly saves communication cost and also improves accuracy.

LIMITATION AND FUTURE WORK

Although the proposed Privacy Preserving Gene Clustering methodology preserves original data privacy, simplifies the distributed clustering by avoiding changing algorithms, and achieves 100% accuracy, it does have limitations. First, it requires a trusted central site (TCS) is needed to perform the final clustering analysis on the global projected data. Although the TCS is not assumed to have access to the global covariance matrix so that it cannot get the projected data by an inverse PCA computation, there could be situations where one

or more partitions are malicious and might leaks the covariance matrix to the TCS. If the TCS is also malicious, it is possible that it can get the original data by inverse PCA, although it may not be able to identify the sources of data portions. Thus, strict policies, which are described in this paper, must be enforced to doubly ensure privacy. The second limitation is that in this paper only the situation of horizontal partition, which accounts for only homogenous data sets, is considered, but in the reality, heterogeneous data sets (vertical partition) and more complex mixed partition / generic situation is also very popular. Extending the proposed methodology from the horizontal partition to the vertical and mixed partitions is not simple or straightforward. Significant efforts need to be made to extend the method to address such scenarios.

Future work to improve the current methodology includes: trying to find a solution to block the way that TCS reaches the original data by inverting PCA; extending this current methodology to vertical partition and even more complex mixed partition (heterogeneous data sets).

REFERENCES

Agrawal, R., & Srikant, R. (2000). Privacy-preserving data mining. *SIGMOD Record, 29*(2), 439–450. doi:10.1145/335191.335438

BioChemWeb.org. (2010). Genes & Gene Expression. *The Virtual Library of Biochemistry and Cell Biology*. BioChemWeb.org.

Braun, R., & Rowe, W. (2009). Needles in the haystack: identifying individuals present in pooled genomic data. *PLOS Genetics, 5*(10), e1000668. doi:10.1371/journal.pgen.1000668

Bunn, P., & Ostrovsky, R. (2007). Secure Two-Party k-Means Clustering. In *Proceedings of the 14th Acm Conference on Computer and Communications Security* (pp. 486-497, 612).

Church, G., & Heeney, C. (2009). Public access to genome-wide data: five views on balancing research with privacy and protection. *PLOS Genetics*, *5*(10), e1000665. doi:10.1371/journal.pgen.1000665

DeRisi, J. L., & Iyer, V. R. (1997). Exploring the metabolic and genetic control of gene expression on a genomic scale. *Science*, *278*(5338), 680–686. doi:10.1126/science.278.5338.680

Goldreich, O. (1997). On the foundations of modern cryptography. In *Proceedings of the Advances in Cryptology (Crypto '97)* (Vol. 1294, pp. 46-74).

Hackl, H., & Sanchez Cabo, F. (2004). Analysis of DNA microarray data. *Current Topics in Medicinal Chemistry*, *4*(13), 1357–1370. doi:10.2174/1568026043387773

Homer, N., & Szelinger, S. (2008). Resolving individuals contributing trace amounts of DNA to highly complex mixtures using high-density SNP genotyping microarrays. *PLOS Genetics*, *4*(8), e1000167. doi:10.1371/journal.pgen.1000167

Hong, D., & Mohaisen, A. (2010). Augmented Rotation-Based Transformation for Privacy-Preserving Data Clustering. *Etri Journal*, *32*(3), 351–361. doi:10.4218/etrij.10.0109.0333

Jagannathan, G., & Pillaipakkamnatt, K. (2010). Communication-Efficient Privacy-Preserving Clustering. *Trans. Data Privacy*, *3*(1), 1–25.

Jagannathan, G., & Wright, R. N. (2005). Privacy-preserving distributed k-means clustering over arbitrarily partitioned data. In *Proceedings of the eleventh ACM SIGKDD international conference on Knowledge discovery in data mining*, Chicago (pp. 593-599). New York: ACM.

Lindell, Y., & Pinkas, B. (2002). Privacy preserving data mining. *Journal of Cryptology*, *15*(3), 177–206. doi:10.1007/s00145-001-0019-2

Mathworks. (2007). *Analyzing Illumina Bead Summary Gene Expression Data*. Retrieved from http://www.mathworks.com/matlabcentral/fx_files/16171/1/content/illuminageneexpdemo.html

Natarajan, A. M., Rajalaxmi, R. R., et al. (2007). A hybrid data transformation approach for privacy preserving clustering of categorical data. *Innovations and Advanced Techniques in Computer and Information Sciences and Engineering*, 403-408, 562.

Pearson, K. (1901). On lines and planes of closest fit to systems of points in space. *Philosophical Magazine*, *2*, 559–572.

Shaw, P. (2003). *Multivariate statistics for the Environmental Sciences*. London: Hodder-Arnold.

Vaidya, J., & Clifton, C. (2003). Privacy-preserving k-means clustering over vertically partitioned data. In *Proceedings of the ninth ACM SIGKDD international conference on Knowledge discovery and data mining*, Washington, DC (pp. 206-215). New York: ACM.

Visscher, P. M., & Hill, W. G. (2009). The limits of individual identification from sample allele frequencies: theory and statistical analysis. *PLOS Genetics*, *5*(10), e1000628. doi:10.1371/journal.pgen.1000628

Wang, R., Li, Y. F., et al. (2009). Learning your identity and disease from research papers: information leaks in genome wide association study. In Proceedings of the 16th ACM conference on Computer and communications security, Chicago (pp. 534-544). New, York: ACM.

Ward, J. H. (1963). Hierarchical Grouping to Optimize an Objective Function. *Journal of the American Statistical Association*, *58*(301), 236. doi:10.2307/2282967

Wikipedia. (2010). *Cluster Analysis*. Retrieved from en.wikipedia.org/wiki/Cluster_analysis

Wikipedia. (2010). *DNA Microarray*. Retrieved from en.wikipedia.org/wiki/DNA_microarray

Yao, A. C.-C. (1986). How to generate and exchange secrets. In *Proceedings of the 27th Annual Symposium on Foundations of Computer Science* (pp. 162-167). Washington, DC: IEEE Computer Society.

This work was previously published in International Journal of Computational Models and Algorithms in Medicine, Volume 1, Issue 3, edited by Aryya Gangopadhyay, pp. 31-54, copyright 2010 by IGI Publishing (an imprint of IGI Global).

Chapter 12
Upper GI Bleed, Etiology, Role of Endoscopy in Rural Population of Punjab

Ravinder Singh Malhotra
Sri Guru Ram Das Institute of Medical Sciences & Research and Center for Public Health Informatics, India

Arun Gupta
Sri Guru Ram Das Institute of Medical Sciences & Research and Center for Public Health Informatics, India

K. S. Ded
Sri Guru Ram Das Institute of Medical Sciences & Research and Center for Public Health Informatics, India

Darpan Bansal
Sri Guru Ram Das Institute of Medical Sciences & Research and Center for Public Health Informatics, India

Harneet Singh
Sri Guru Ram Das Institute of Medical Sciences & Research and Center for Public Health Informatics, India

ABSTRACT

Haematemesis and malena are the two most important symptoms of upper gastrointestinal bleeding. The most common cause of upper gastrointestinal bleeding is due to a peptic ulcer. In this paper, the authors research the cause of bleeding. Contrary to previous studies, results favor esophageal varices, e.g., alcoholism or cirrhosis liver post necrotic, as the most common cause of bleeding rather than a peptic ulcer. The authors' study is based on an observational retrospective protocol with records of 50 consecutive patients with GI bleeding, attending the emergency room from February 2007 until September 2009. Results show that the treatment of UGI bleeding has made important progress since the introduction of emergency endoscopy and endoscopic techniques for haemostasis. The application of specific protocols significantly decreases rebleeding and the need for surgery, whereas mortality is still high. The data highlight the decreasing trend of peptic ulcer as the sole cause of bleeding, as shown in previous literature, ascertaining that varices are now the most common variable.

DOI: 10.4018/978-1-4666-0282-3.ch012

BACKGROUND

Gastrointestinal bleeding is one of the few frightening things that the patient experiences, which can indicate simple, benign, complex or malignant disorders and result in disaster if proper steps are not taken to identify the source of bleeding and treat it. Bleeding proximal to ligament of Treitz, i.e., from esophagus, stomach and duodenum is called upper gastrointestinal bleeding while bleeding from jejunum, ileum, colon, rectum are grouped under lower gastrointestinal bleeding. Various causes of upper GI bleed being esophageal, gastric, duodenal ulcers (40%), followed by erosions (20%), varices (10%), Mallory Weiss tear, tumors, vascular lesions and others constituting the rest. Haematemesis and malena are the two important symptoms of upper gastrointestinal bleeding.

Endoscopy remains the gold standard in the diagnosis and management of acute upper gastrointestinal bleeding. (Russell, 2004) Major advantage of endoscopy is that it gives direct visualization, and ability to perform therapeutic interventions. For most upper gastrointestinal lesions the sensitivity (about 90%) and specificity (about 100%) of endoscopy are far higher than those of barium radiography (about 50 and 90% respectively). Endoscopic therapy controls bleeding in greater than 90% of patients and reduces rebleeding (up to 50%), thus decreasing morbidity and improving survival. Endoscopic sclerotherapy/banding has been the most successful and safest procedure in the management of first bleed of oesophageal varices. It can stop bleeding in 80-90% of patients. (D'Amico, 1995)

With the advent of newer modalities of endoscopic treatment and latest facilities, this life threatening sequence can be arrested. So looking at all the various facts, we undertook this study to see the applicability of endoscopy in diagnosis and management of UGI bleed, with its demographic profile in our setup.

Causes of Upper Gastrointestinal Bleeding

Accurate estimation of true frequency with which various diseases cause bleeding is less difficult now than in previous years. Identification of the source often depends on how soon after the onset of bleeding diagnostic measures are employed. However approximately 10% of cases still remain in which no cause is demonstrated or proved despite vigorous use of various diagnostic measures currently available. Overall mortality for all sources of upper gastrointestinal bleeding is approximately 10%. (Gupta, 1993) Leonardo et al conducted a study to see for various causes of UGI bleeding, published in 2008. As per this study, endoscopic findings and stigmata of recent hemorrhage (SRH) were detected in study population (Dagradi, 1979) According to another study by Caestecker J, Endoscopic findings and the incidence rate in patients with upper Gastro Intestinal Bleeding were [5] Duodenal ulcer - 24.3%, gastric erosion - 23.4%, gastric ulcer - 21.3%, esophageal varices - 10.3%, Mallory-Weiss tear - 7.2%, esophagitis - 6.3%, duodenitis - 5.8%, neoplasm - 2.9%, stomal (marginal) ulcer - 1.8% esophageal ulcer - 1.7% and other/miscellaneous-6.8%.

Endoscopic Findings in Case of Bleeding

Varices

In most cases, the diagnosis of varices can be made endoscopically without difficulty as they have characteristic endoscopic appearance. The veins appear irregular, serpiginous, often bluish structures running longitudinally in the sub mucosa of the esophageal wall. Dagradi classified esophageal varices as their appearance on endoscopy: [6]

Grade-1: Blue red varices <2mm in diameter.
Grade-2: Blue varices 2-3mm in diameter.

Grade-3: Elevated blue veins 3-4mm in diameter.

Grade-4: Tortuous blue varices >4mm in diameter almost meeting in midline.

Grade-5: Grape like varices occluding the lumen and showing presence of small cherry-red varices overlying blue grey varices.

In some instances, a portion of the surface of veins appears red known as red color sign. It is associated with risk of hemorrhage (Ali, 2007).

Overall, any red color sign increases the risk of bleeding from 12-52%.

Ulcer

Most patients with a bleeding upper gastrointestinal lesion undergo an endoscopic examination of stomach & the first and second portion of the duodenum. Forrest endoscopically categorized bleeding peptic ulcers into 3 categories (Cales, 1990):- In those who have recurrent bleeding, it has been shown that a second endoscopic attempt at control of bleeding will fail in 25% of patients, who will then require emergency surgery (Lebrec, 1980)

Sources of Bleeding

*   **Oesophagogastric varices**: Normal portal pressure is about 7 mm Hg. If this portal pressure rises then varices develop and the portal blood is carried to systemic veins. Normally 100% of portal blood can be recovered from hepatic veins but in cirrhosis only 13% is obtained.
*   **Predicting rupture:** Cales et al told that in sixty three percent of cirrhotic patients will not bleed within 2 yrs of diagnosis but 50% will die of first hemorrhage. There is a strong correlation between variceal size, assessed endoscopically and the probability of bleeding (Levine, 1987). Lebrec D, Defleury and Rueff B were of the view that intravariceal pressure is less important al-

though a portal pressure above 12 mmHg appears necessary for varices to form & subsequently bleed (Longstreth, 1995)

Why Do Varices Bleed?

Two main theories have been put forward- erosive and eruptive. Erosive theory states that gastroesophageal mucosal damage is frequently accompanied with varices in cirrhotic due to alcoholism especially. Eruptive theory states that rupture of varices can be pictured secondary to: (a) increased pressure in vein, (b) large diameter of the vein, (c) an abnormality or structural weakness of the vein and (d) a combination of any of these three features.

Portal hypertension is a necessary pre-requisite for the development of varices and portal pressure of 12 mm of Hg is required to produce bleeding from the esophageal varices. Variceal bleeding presents greater problem because one third will rebleed during same hospitalization and patients are at high risk for complications due to underlying liver disease. Associated abnormality in renal, cardiovascular and immune system contributes to their mortality of 20 to 65% (Longstreth, 1995). Other causes of esophageal bleeding are: - esophagitis, Mallory-Weiss Syndrome, tumor including surface of polypoidal lesion and Telengiectasia of either familial or sporadic type.

Stomach and Duodenum

*   **Peptic ulcers:** The leading cause of severe UGI bleed and accounts for 50% of bleeds from UGI tract. Bleeding ensues from erosion of an ulcer base through the wall of a blood vessel. The likelihood of bleeding depends on size and depth of ulcer. Severity depends on size of vessel eroded. Erosion of vessel occurs from side of vessel not terminal end. Most common cause of peptic ulcer bleed is erosion of gastro duodenal artery and is seen in posterior

Table 1.

Site	Portal component	Systemic component	Consequence
Umbilicus	Left branch of portal vein	Anterior abdominal wall veins (paraumbilical veins)	Caput medusae
Cardia of stomach	Oesophageal branches of left gastric vein, posterior gastric, short gastric veins	Oesophageal tributaries of accessory hemiazygous vein	Varices
Bare area of liver	Hepatic venules	Phrenic and intercostals veins	Dilated veins
Anal canal	Superior rectal vein	Middle and inferior rectal	Rectal varices (Haemorrhoids)
Posterior abdominal wall	Veins of duodenum, ascending colon, descending colon	Retroperitoneal veins of abdominal wall and of renal capsule	Prominent veins
Liver	Patent ductus venosus connects left branch of portal vein	Inferior vena cava	Prominent veins

placed ulcers. Bleeding from peptic ulcer occurs about 5 times more often after age of 50 than before. Moreover, an ulcer that first appears late in life is more likely to bleed than an ulcer that begins earlier. The frequent use of H2 blockers and proton pump inhibitors resulted in decrease of incidence of peptic ulcer disease and its complication.

- **Acute stress ulcers**: They account for 5% of all cases of bleeding ulcers. Stress ulcers are more often multiple than single and may occur in both the stomach and duodenum

- (Levine, 1987) Many patients have no pain, bleeding is only manifestation. They are mostly seen in patients of severe burns (curling ulcers) and head injury (Cushing ulcers).

- **Gastro duodenal Erosions**: Small, often minute, typically numerous, circumscribed, mucosal defects, in contrast to frank ulcers do not penetrate the muscularis mucosa. They are associated usually with gastritis.

- **Portal gastropathy**: The mucosa is affected by the increased portal pressure and may exude blood, even in the absence of well developed visible varices.

- **Gastric varices**: Very challenging to control bleeding from these varices. One may go for sclerotherapy or banding, but both these procedures are very difficult in gastric varices.

- **Hiatus Hernia**: The less frequently encountered paraesophageal hiatus hernia is notorious as a source of bleeding due to strangulation. Bleeding is usually slow and presents as iron deficiency anemia rather than melaena and seldom is haematemesis. Bleeding sometimes massive is a frequent feature of this bizarre configuration.

- **Tumors**: Although anemia caused by steady seepage of blood from eroded or ulcerated tumors of stomach and duodenum is common, gross bleeding is seldom a feature. Adenomas of stomach or duodenum, especially when large and pedunculated may bleed, sometimes massively.

- **Diseases of Blood and Blood Vessels**: Polycythemia rubra Vera GI bleeding may be an initial manifestation of this disorder. A duodenal or gastric ulcer is found in 20% of patients. Bleeding may also arise from gastric erosion. Leukemia and the lymphomas may cause blood loss due to leukemic ulceration of mouth, stomach or upper intestinal tract abetted by thrombocytopenia related to the disease or induced by intensive chemotherapy. However gastro duodenal mucosal ulceration or erosions are frequent sources of haematemesis and melaena in leukemic patients. Platelet disorders like ITP where platelet count falls below 30000/mm³, may present as UGI bleed. Hemophilic in about 20% of cases present as gastrointestinal hemorrhage with duodenal ulcer being main cause. Various blood vessel diseases like Diafouley's disease, hereditary haemorrhagic telangiectasia (Rendu Osler Weber disease), cavernous haemangiomatosis malformation, Pseudoxanthoma elasticum, present as UGI bleed. In most cases it is from stomach or proximal small bowel.

- **Non variceal bleeding**: Peptic ulcer bleeding in 70% of patients stop spontaneously. Endoscopic appearance of the ulcer predicts chances of rebleeding and chooses treatment option.

OBJECTIVE

The objectives of the present study are:

1. To assess the important etiological factors for Upper Gastrointestinal bleeding.
2. To evaluate the age and sex incidence in relation to etiological factors for Upper Gastrointestinal Bleeding
3. To study the role of oesophagogastroduodenoscopy in Diagnosis, Management and Prognosis of Upper Gastrointestinal Bleeding

MATERIAL AND METHODS

The present study was conducted on 50 patients from time period of February 2007 till September 2009, presenting with haematemesis and melaena or history of same, at Sri Guru Ram Das Institute of Medical Sciences and Research Vallah, Sri Amritsar after attaining approval from hospital ethics committee. Before subjecting the patient to endoscopic studies, detailed history was taken from the patient and also from patient's attendants to elaborate the cause of bleeding.

Following variables were collected: hemoglobin, bleeding and clotting time, and blood urea and serum creatinine, serum Calcium, Glucose levels, liver function tests, prothrombin index, platelet count, Blood grouping and cross matching and viral Markers- HB_sAg, Hepatitis C Virus and HIV. Endoscopy was done using FUJINON 200 VIDEOENDOSCOPE [that consist of a end viewing Oesophagogastrodudonoscope, video processor and monitor] Other material kept available will be Bite guard, Xylocaine local spray, Surgical gloves, 6 shooter ligation bands with handle, Sclerosant injection, ligation clips, Sclerotherapy needle No.23G and No. 21G, Cyanoacrylate Glue, Epinephrine 1:10000.

Statistical Analysis: Descriptive analysis was performed to determine the overall frequency distribution of the etiology of bleeding followed by an age and gender stratified analysis. All results have been reported as percentage distribution.

PROCEDURE

Patient presenting with acute upper gastrointestinal bleeding were resuscitated first with intravenous fluid therapy. Blood transfusions were given as per need. Gastric lavage with tap water/ cold normal saline was done after placing nasogastric tube. Intravenous vasopressin/octreotide infusion, proton pump inhibitors were started. Then patients underwent diagnostic and therapeutic oesophagogastroduodenoscopy using FUJINON 200 VIDEOENDOSCOPE, after taking informed consent and stabilizing the patient. Patients were in left lateral position. After explaining whole procedure to conscious and cooperative patient, local xylocaine spray 15% was done in the posterior pharyngeal wall and patient was asked to swallow it. After that a bite guard was put in between teeth of patient. Then the video endoscope was introduced into mouth of patient and negotiated through cricopharynx to enter esophagus and then stomach. Direct viewing technique was used for the procedure. Whole of esophagus, stomach and duodenum was visualized for any ooze or bleeding and therapeutic procedures were undertaken accordingly. Data was collected. Data was being age incidence of bleeding in males and females, number of cases according to the various causes; various symptoms according to which the patient presents smokers and alcoholics having the symptoms of gastrointestinal bleed, results of various methods during follow up period after completing full course of therapy. The exclusion criteria included patient with severe cardiopulmonary instability where risk to patient outweighs potential benefit of patient were excluded and any patient with known/ suspected perforated viscous was excluded.

RESULTS

This detailed study of upper gastrointestinal bleeding was conducted on 50 patients and endoscopic diagnosis and subsequent management was undertaken and following observations were made.

Out of 50 cases 41 were males and 9 were female patients. All patients belonged to age group between 10-80 years and majority of patients 19(38%) were in age group of 41-50years. In this 15(30%) were males and 4(8%) were females. Alcohol intake was the cause in majority 32 (64%) patients and all the patients were males. Hepatitis C Virus (HCV) was the causative factor in 10(20%) males and 6(12%) female patients. Out of 10 males with HCV positivity, 8 were alcoholics as well. One male (2%) and one female (2%) were hepatitis B positive. The same female was positive for HCV also. In 2 (4%) patients there was portal vein thrombosis. Two (4%) males and

1(2%) females were taking NSAIDS. Five (10%) patients were taking NSAIDS and were alcoholics as well. The majority of patients complained of retro sternal pain 20(40%). 21(42%) presented with haematemesis alone and 22% presented with both haematemesis and melaena. 24% patients presented with melaena alone. Pain was aggravated by food in 12% of patients and reduced in 10% patients.

Other Medical History

In this study, only some patients with chronic duodenal ulcer gave a history of abdominal pain and 40(80%) gave history suggestive of portal hypertension. About 10 of them gave history of taking treatment with H2 antagonists and antacids (Table 2).

On physical examination, 35(70%) of them had pallor, tachycardia and 14 (28%) patients with acute bleeding were in a state of shock. Patients with Portal hypertension (68%) had either splenomegaly or ascites.

Hemoglobin estimated in majority of patients' revealed anemia. 27(54%) of patients had hemoglobin levels less than 8gm% at the time of admission. Renal function test (blood urea, serum Creatinine) was deranged in 6(12%) patients. Prothrombin index (PTI) was deranged in 36(72%) of patients. 16(32%) of patients were Hepatitis C positive. 1(2%) was Hepatitis B positive. 1(2%)

Table 2. Etiology of bleeding

Etiology	Male		Female	
	No	%	No	%
Alcohol	32	64	-	-
HCV	10	20	6	60
HbsAg	1	2	1	10
NSAIDS	2	4	1	10
Portal vein Thrombosis	-	-	2	20
Alcohol & NSAIDS	5	10	-	-

was positive for both of them. Abdominal ultrasound was done in all the patients. 37(74%) of patients had features of portal hypertension with cirrhosis. About 11 (22%) patients had incidental finding in form of cholelithiasis & renal stones. One patient positive for hepatitis C had hepatocellular carcinoma as well. Endoscopy was done in all the patients.

Table 3 shows endoscopic diagnosis of the study group resulted in upper gastrointestinal bleeding. The study reveals that esophageal varices remain the most common cause of bleeding. Esophageal varices and esophageal gastric varices were found in 45(90%) of patients. Ulcers were seen in 3(6%) patients. The remaining rare causes were esophagitis, gastritis, and duodenitis. Only 3(6%) patients had varices with peptic ulcers (Figure 1).

Of all patients with bleeding, 8(16%) cases underwent endoscopic sclerotherapy. We used 1% Sodium tetradecyl sulphate as the sclerosant and about 1-2 cc was injected to every column, usually intravariceally. 35 (70%) patients underwent banding alone. There were only 2(4%) patients who underwent both banding & sclerotherapy for varices and ulcers respectively. In 2(4%) patients with mucosal erosions (gastritis/ Duodenitis/ esophagitis) only medical management was done. Recurrent bleeding was seen in 7 out of 45 patients of variceal bleed.

Table 3. Endoscopic diagnosis

Diagnosis	No of cases	Percentage
Ulcer	3	6
Esophageal varices	38	76
Gastric varices	2	4
Esophageal varices with peptic ulcer	3	6
Esophagitis	1	2
Erosive gastritis/ duodenitis	1	2
Varices with gastritis/duodenitis	2	4

DISCUSSION

Upper gastrointestinal bleeding is the frequent presentation in emergency ward. This study was conducted to analyze the commonest etiology and age/ sex incidence of upper gastrointestinal bleeding in patients attending emergency. Assessment of the role of endoscopy in diagnosis & management of upper gastrointestinal bleeding was also done.

Age Incidence and Sex Incidence

In the present study (Table 4) male and female ratio was 4.5:1. In the study conducted by George F.Longstreth on Epidemiology of Hospitalization for Acute Upper GI hemorrhage, among 258 hospitalizations, the male to female ratio was 2:1 (Cuellar RE, 1990)

The present series established male preponderance for upper gastrointestinal bleeding, which may be due to the fact that nearly 70% of the patients encountered were alcoholics and had alcoholic liver disease (Figure 3).

Etiology of Acute Upper Gastrointestinal Hemorrhage

Alcohol intake was most common causative agent of upper gastrointestinal bleeding in our series, this factor was seen in 32(64%) of patients. It was followed by Hepatitis C virus infection. HCV positivity is more in males 10(20%) patients than females 6(12%). Other causes were portal vein thrombosis and NSAIDS use. Among 7 (14%)of the patients with history of Non-steroidal anti-inflammatory drugs intake, there was bleeding due

Table 4. Age and sex comparison in research

Age and Sex Comparison	Present Series	George Longstreth et al
Male: Female ratio	4.5:1	2:1
Mean age	40 yrs	41 yrs

Figure 1. Showing endoscopic diagnosis

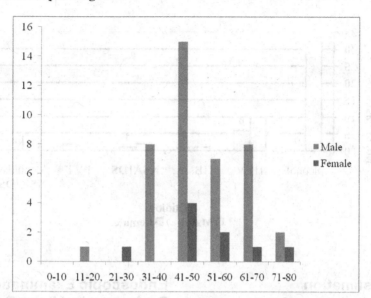

to gastric mucosal erosions in 3 patients, peptic ulcer 3 patients and esophagitis 1 patient. Alcohol intake is a common practice prevalent in male population of our area. A fraction of the population is also drug abusers. These males are addicted to oral or intravenous drugs. These addictions are the cause of alcoholic liver disease and Hepatitis B & C liver diseases in our patients. Hepatitis B & C is also spread by the local practitioners (quacks) who have poor knowledge of the spread of these diseases and sterilization of syringes.

A prospective endoscopic evaluation of the cause of upper gastrointestinal hemorrhage in alcoholics conducted by C. Mel Willcox et al. (1996) has been compared here with the present study (Table 5).

In our study about 79% of alcoholic patients had variceal bleeding, as compared to 16% in study by C. Mel Wilcox. There is significant association of consumption of alcohol with variceal bleeding both in the present study & in the comparable study. Both gastric and duodenal ulcers were seen in our study and by C. Mel Wilcox. In our study both types of ulcers were seen in 6.25% patients, while gastric ulcers were seen

in more (21%) patients by other study. Erosive gastritis also features commonly with alcoholics.

Clinical Features

In the present study 28% of the patients had hypotension & 70% had tachycardia (pulse rate more than 100/min) 54% had hemoglobin of less than 8g% & they all required blood transfusion of 2 to 4 units. Among 28% of the patients who presented in the state of shock 22% presented 6 to 12hrs after the initial episode & 6% had massive haematemesis & presented within the first 6 hrs of initial bleed.

Schiller et al in their study of upper gastro-intestinal hemorrhage have found hypotension in 23.04%, tachycardia in 27%, and hemoglobin less than 7g% in 20.19%.

In this study the percentage is higher than Schiller et al mostly because of delay in seeking medical attention and also the small number of patients studied.

Figure 2. Showing sex incidence with etiology

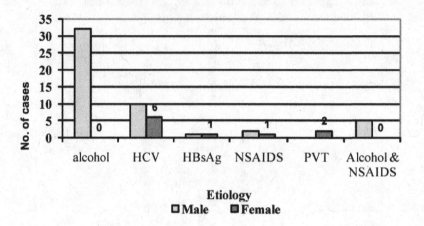

Hemoglobin Estimation

It was done in all patients in the present study at the time of admission. About 54% of patients had hemoglobin levels less than 8g% at the time of admission. At the maximum 4 units of blood was transfused within the first 24 hrs after admission. Serial estimation of haemoglobin levels was useful in identifying the amount of blood loss and for further management. Schiller et al in their study of upper gastrointestinal hemorrhage have found hemoglobin less than 7g% in 20.19%.

Endoscopic Examination Was Performed in All the Cases

In the present study, the site of bleeding was correctly, demonstrated by endoscopy in all the patients (100%). In ASGE survey, endoscopy was diagnostic in 87% of patients with upper gastrointestinal bleeding (Massimo, 1994). The accuracy of detecting lesions through endoscopy is probably due to the skill of an endoscopist and stabilization of patients by medical means before taking them up for Endoscopy.

Figure 3. Showing age and sex distribution

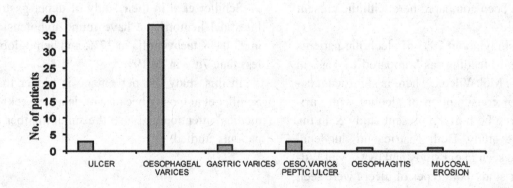

Table 5. Etiology of Upper Gastrointestinal Hemorrhage in relation to alcohol use

Cause	Present series (N= 32)	C. Mel Wilcox et al (n=212)
Gastric ulcer	2(6.25%)	45(21.2%)
Varices	25(78.12%)	34(16.0%)
Duodenal ulcer	2*(6.25%)	31(14.6%)
Mallory Weiss Tear	-	15(7.07%)
Esophagitis	1(3.13%)	10(4.7%)
Erosive Gastritis	2** (6.25%)	6(2.8%)
Others	-	11(5.1%)

*1 out of 2 patients was having Varices as well
** Both these patients were having Varices

Endoscopic Diagnosis

In our study the commonest cause of upper GI bleed was esophageal varices in about 90% of cases, whereas second common cause was peptic ulcer. In contrast to Longstreth and American society of Gastrointestinal survey (Massimo, 1994) where peptic ulcer remains the commonest source of upper gastrointestinal bleeding. In other study conducted by Leonardo et al on 436 patients (Leonardo et al, 2008), 50% of cases were of peptic ulcer, only 12% had varices as cause followed closely by esophagitis 10%. But study conducted by Caestecker J, 24% were having duodenal ulcer, 23% gastric erosions, varices were seen only in 10% of cases. The reason for this discrepancy between our study and the other studies is three folds

1. Among males alcohol consumption is very high in the rural population of Punjab.
2. There is a very large number of quacks and untrained medical practitioners who use unsterilized single syringe on multiple patients thus putting them to risk of blood borne infections
3. The incidence of iv drug abusers is on the increase

Table 6. Incidence as percent of total diagnosis

Diagnosis	Present series (n=50)	ASGE (n=2225 pts)	Longstreth et al (n=258)
Peptic ulcer	6	47.4	61.7
Gastritis/ Duodenitis	2	29.2	10.5
Esophagitis	2	6.3	3.9
Varices	90*	10.3	6.2
Mallory Weiss syndrome	-	7.2	3.5
Malignancy	-	2.9	1.6
others	-	6.5	1.9

*In two cases (4%) which were associated with gastritis/Duodenitis, 1 (2%) case had associated peptic ulcer disease also.

Survival after Endoscopic Intervention

Forty five cases of esophageal & oesophagogastric varices were detected by endoscopy. Among 45 patients, 14 cases had hypotension at the time of presentation & all the patients underwent emergency sclerotherapy/ banding within 12 to 24 hrs after admission, the remaining 31 cases underwent elective intervention. 1% sodium tetra decal sulphate was used as sclerosant for all patients in our study & six band ligator was used as banding agent. Among these 45 cases, 4 deaths were reported in the first week after the procedure. Of the remaining 41 cases, 12 cases are still in follow up undergoing repeated sclerotherapy/banding at the interval of 3 weeks for complete obliteration of varices. And no incidence of recurrence of bleeding has been reported in any of the remaining 30 cases. Of the 4 deaths reported, 1 patient died due to hepatic encephalopathy& the other 3 due to recurrent bleeding.

The result of the present study is compared with a study conducted by Massimo Graffeo et al from the University of Brescia, Brescia, Italy.

The present study indicates that endoscopic intervention is very useful in arresting the first episode of bleeding and in preventing rebleed. The study done by Massino Graffeo et al indicates that the only way of reducing the high incidence of recurrence of varices after initial obliteration appears to include complete obliteration.

In a recent study by Hashizume et al. (2005), esophageal varices were completely eradicated in 78% of patient. In our study this rate was of range of 91.11%.

In our study the percentage of death by hemorrhage within the first week was found to be 8.89%. In a recent study by Hashizume et al, 2.8 percent of deaths by hemorrhage were observed during follow up.

In a study done by Massimo Graffeo et al when true eradication was confirmed after endos-copy, no recurrences were noted. Eradication of varices certainly reduced the risk of further fatal hemorrhages in short term & also medium/ long term & therefore it was associated with survival. However variceal eradication is a long term process & Massimo Graffeo et al achieved it on the average 26 months after the initial sclerotherapy by repeating treatments. Therefore, only patients who did not die in the first months of follow up could have obtained the eradication.

In our study esophageal sclerotherapy as well as banding had no complications. Esophageal sclerotherapy and banding has shown fairly good results in the initial arrest of bleeding due to esophageal varices with a low incidence of major side effects and also helped in their long term management.

SUMMARY AND CONCLUSION

Fifty cases of acute upper gastrointestinal bleeding were studied in this series (January 2008 until September 2009). All the cases were subjected to upper gastrointestinal endoscopy. Each case history was recorded individually as per the pro forma and investigations were done as the cases demanded.

- Upper gastrointestinal bleeding was 4.5 times more common in males than in females and the mean age in this series was 40 years with the range falling from 10 to 80 years.
- Most common cause of upper gastrointestinal bleeding in the present study was found to be secondary to esophageal varices(About 90%) major cause being alcoholic cirrhosis (74%), peptic ulcers(6%) and 4% secondary to mucosal erosions.
- About 22% of patients had both haematemesis and malena. In all the patients studied about 28% had hypotension and 70% had tachycardia at the time of presen-

tation. 54% of them had hemoglobin value less than 8 gm% and they were given blood transfusion as per requirement

- In all cases in the series the site of bleeding was correctly demonstrated with the help of Endoscopy.
- Oesophago-gastroduodenoscopy was very useful in Locating the site of bleed in all cases, for banding/sclerotherapy in cases with variceal bleeding, for taking biopsy for histopathological study in suspicious cases of gastric ulcers.
- Endoscopic banding has been found to be most successful and safe procedure in the initial arrest of bleeding due to esophageal varices with least complications.
- All the cases of upper gastrointestinal hemorrhage secondary to esophageal varices were subjected to endoscopic banding and sclerotherapy with 1% sodium tetradecylsulphate. Gastric ulcers with bleeding were subjected to biopsy through endoscopy.
- Almost all the patients in the study group were treated conservatively until the condition of the patient was stable. Then they were subjected to definitive line of management like medical or surgical line which was suitable for them.
- Overall mortality in the present series was 8% which was due to rebleeding and hepatic failure. This mortality rate was correlating well with other studies.

In the end we conclude that another study is required in upper GI bleed etiology as in our study the main cause of upper GI bleed is esophageal varices which is in contrast to the study done by Longstreth and American society of Gastrointestinal survey where peptic ulcer remains the commonest source of upper gastrointestinal bleeding. Since 64% of the patient population had a positive history of alcohol consumption and another 20% of the male patients were HbsAg positive, similarly 70% of the female patient population were HbsAg (60%) and HCV (10%) and this is a big preventable risk factor in the etiology of upper GI bleed.

ACKNOWLEDGMENT

We would like to thank Dr. Ashish Joshi M.D., M.P.H. at Center for Public Health Informatics, India for help in the preparation and review of the manuscript.

REFERENCES

Ali, T., & Stanley, W. (2007). *Shackelford's Surgery of the alimentary tract* (6th ed., p. 802).

Caestecker, J., & Straus, J. (2007, December 23). *Upper Gastrointestinal Bleeding: Surgical Perspective.eMedicine*. Retrieved from http:/ www. emedicine.com/ MED/topic3566.htm

Cales, P., Zabotto, B., & Meskens, C. (1990). Gastroesophageal endoscopic features in cirrhosis. Observer variability, in there associations and relationship to hepatic dysfunction. *Gastroenterology*, *98*, 186.

Cuellar, R. E., Gavaler, J., & Alexander, A. (1990). Gastrointestinal Hemorrhage. *Archives of Internal Medicine*, *150*, 1381. doi:10.1001/ archinte.150.7.1381

D'Amico, G., Pagliaro, L., & Bosch, J. (1995). The treatment of portal hypertension: A metaanalytic review. *Hepatology (Baltimore, Md.)*, *22*, 332–354.

Dagradi, A. E., & Weingarten, A. J. F. (1979). Failure of endoscopy to establish a source of upper gastrointestinal bleeding. *The American Journal of Gastroenterology*, *72*, 395–402.

Gupta, P. K., & Fleisher, D. E. (1993). Nonvariceal upper gastrointestinal bleeding. *The Medical Clinics of North America*, *77*(5), 973–1012.

Hashizume, M., Kitano, S., Yamaga, H., Wada, H., & Sugimachi, K. (2005). Eradication of oesophageal varices recurring after portal non-decompressive surgery by injection sclerotherapy. *British Journal of Surgery, 7,* 940–943.

Lebrec, D., & Defleury, R. B. (1980). Portal hypertension, size of esophageal varices and risk of gastrointestinal bleeding in alcoholic cirrhosis. *Gastroenterology, 79,* 1139.

Leonardo, T., Maria, C. P., & Angelo, Z. (2008). Endoscopic finding in pts with UGI bleeding clinically classified in three risk groups prior to endoscopy. *World Journal of Gastroenterology, 14*(32), 5046–5050. doi:10.3748/wjg.14.5046

Levine, B. A. (1987). Stress ulcer. *Problems in General Surgery, 4,* 208–222.

Longstreth, G. F. (1995). Epidemiology of Hospitalization for acute upper gastrointestinal hemorrhage: A population based study. *The American Journal of Gastroenterology, 90*(2), 206–210.

Massimo, G., Federico, B., & Giovanna, L. (1994). Survival after endoscopic sclerotherapy for esophageal varices in cirrhotics. *The American Journal of Gastroenterology,* 1815–1822.

Planas, R., Quer, J. C., & Boix, J. (1994). A prospective randomized trial comparing somatostatin and sclerotherapy in the treatment of acute variceal bleeding. *Hepatology (Baltimore, Md.), 20,* 370. doi:10.1002/hep.1840200216

Russell, R. C., Williams, N. S., & Bulstrode, C. J. (Eds.). (2004). *Bailey and Love's Short Practice of Surgery* (24th ed., p. 1030). New York: Arnold.

Tyatgat, G. N. J., Classen, M., Waye, J., & Nakazawa, S. (2000). Practical Management of Non-Variceal Upper Gastrointestinal Bleed. In *Practice of Therapeutic Endoscopy* (2nd ed., p. 4).

Wilcox, C. M., Alexander, L. N., & Straub, R. F. (1996). A prospective endoscopic evaluation of the causes of upper gastrointestinal hemorrhage in alcoholics. A focus on alcoholic gastropathy. *The American Journal of Gastroenterology, 91*(7), 1343–1347.

APPENDIX OF ABBREVIATIONS

BUN: Blood urea nitrogen

DLC: Differential Leukocyte Count

GI: Gastro Intestinal

HB: Hemoglobin

HIV: Human Immunodeficiency Virus

HCV: Hepatitis C Virus

HBs: Ag Hepatitis B antigen

IVC: inferior vena cava

ICU: intensive care unit

NSAIDS: Non Steroidal Anti Inflammatory Drugs

PTI: Prothrombin Time Index

PHT: Portal Hypertension

SMV: Superior Mesenteric Vein

SGOT: Serum Glutamate Oxaloacetate Transaminase

SGPT: Serum Glutamate Pyruvate Transaminase

TIPS: Transjuglar Intrahepatic Porto Systemic Shunt

TLC: Total leukocyte count

UGI: Upper Gastro Intestinal

USG: Ultra Sonography

This work was previously published in International Journal of Computational Models and Algorithms in Medicine, Volume 1, Issue 3, edited by Aryya Gangopadhyay, pp. 55-68, copyright 2010 by IGI Publishing (an imprint of IGI Global).

Chapter 13
Evaluation of Clustering Patterns using Singular Value Decomposition (SVD):
A Case Study of Metabolic Syndrome

Josephine M. Namayanja
University of Maryland, Baltimore County (UMBC), USA

ABSTRACT

Computational techniques, such as Simple K, have been used for exploratory analysis in applications ranging from data mining research, machine learning, and computational biology. The medical domain has benefitted from these applications, and in this regard, the authors analyze patterns in individuals of selected age groups linked with the possibility of Metabolic Syndrome (MetS), a disorder affecting approximately 45% of the elderly. The study identifies groups of individuals behaving in two defined categories, that is, those diagnosed with MetS (MetS Positive) and those who are not (MetS Negative), comparing the pattern definition. The paper compares the cluster formation in patterns when using a data reduction technique referred to as Singular Value Decomposition (SVD) versus eliminating its application in clustering. Data reduction techniques like SVD have proved to be very useful in projecting only what is considered to be key relations in the data by suppressing the less important ones. With the existence of high dimensionality, the importance of SVD can be highly effective. By applying two internal measures to validate the cluster quality, findings in this study prove interesting in context to both approaches.

INTRODUCTION

In a realistic sense humans by nature are different, however it might seem that if individuals are affected by similar factors – either internal or external, they tend to exhibit similar characteristics. What if these characteristics vary from one individual to another or between groups of individuals? This study identifies groups of clusters in individuals that are diagnosed with MetS (MetS Positive) and is furthered with a comparison of those do not fit into the diagnosis (MetS Nega-

DOI: 10.4018/978-1-4666-0282-3.ch013

tive). In order to understand the patterns of the clusters formed, there are two techniques applied – 1) Simple K – Means clustering and 2) Singular Value Decomposition (SVD) as a pre-processing task performed prior to the former. Because the process of collecting medical data can be quite tasking on the part of health professionals due to the limitless number of features that surround its domain, it presents even more of a problem for those, such as researchers and analysts, who try to expand the use of this type of data. Such datasets are highly dimensional and thus contain just about too many attributes for a single record. This often makes it difficult for knowledge workers to not only make a viable selection but to also represent this information in a manner that supports both visualization and clarity. Therefore (Thomasian, Castelli, & Li, 1998) commend that computational research presents data reduction techniques such as SVD and Principle Component Analysis (PCA) that can be applied to manage this curse of dimensionality.

In the first approach (also referred to as Non-SVD) of this study, a Simple K-means clustering algorithm is used as an exploratory analysis technique to group individuals of selected age groups with similar characteristics into k clusters where k refers to the ideal number of clusters (Bunn & Ostrovsky, 2007) with an aim of maximizing intra cluster similarity and minimizing inter cluster similarity. While in the second approach SVD (also referred to as SVD- based clustering in this study) is initially applied to create a factorization of a given matrix X and hence reduce the dimensionality of its underlying data structure to produce a more appropriate subspace of the data based on some ranking system (Phillips, Watson, & Wynne, 2008). This ranking system describes the linear independence of a data matrix which is determined by the dependency of rows/columns on each other. Further still, this technique can be applied to any type of data set D represented

as any size of matrix but the linearity may differ depending on the distribution of the data. (Martin, 2005) adds that it also provides a method for mathematically discovering correlations within data and in this study the use of SVD is followed by clustering the reduced dataset into k clusters. The purpose of both approaches sums up into a comparison of clusters formed at both iterations to determine the performance of the clustering algorithm depending on the quality of clusters formed. As the technique of clustering has previously been applied to numerous applications such as information retrieval, machine learning, data mining research (Bunn & Ostrovsky, 2007) and computational biology (Frahling & Sohler, 2006), SVD has taken phase in face recognition, medical imaging as stated in (Hsu et al., 2007; Lee et al., 2004; Lui et al., 2009; Ma et al., 2009; Zanderigo et al., 2009) and is also used as a complimentary technique on Latent Semantic Indexing (LSI) and clustering which is the case in this study. More so, computational methods such as Markov Chains and SVD itself have been looked at previously in alliance with several aspects of the health domain from brain functionality (Brockwell, Kass, & Schwartz, 2007) and Alzheimer's disease (Li et al., 2005) to cardio (Brinegar et al., 2009) plus gene related studies (Alshalalfa, Alhaji, & Rokne, 2008). With the objective of this study in mind, the comparison of cluster quality is validated using two internal measures which include: 1) Sum of Square Error (SSE) which looks at the distance (Euclidean distance) of the data point x from the cluster centroid c and 2) Silhouette Coefficient (Sil) which considers the distances of individual data points to other points internally within a cluster and externally to other clusters formed (Frahling & Sohler, 2006). This foreword on the study is extended with a motivation that describes Metabolic Syndrome in depth and samples on real statistical based examples of its effects.

Motivation

With close to 72 million obese Americans (Ascribe Newswire: Health, 2008), the prevalence of Metabolic Syndrome (Met S) is alarming. An estimation of 45% of the population highlights that the older generation (Sherman, 2009; Howe, 2008; The Consumer's Medical Journal, 2009; Miner, 2010) within the age of 60 and 70 years plus, has a diagnosed rate of approximately 60% and 40% respectively (Sherman, 2009; Howe, 2008). Having no particular definition for MetS, previous studies define the latter also called Insulin resistance syndrome (Nutrition Action Health Letter, 2009) or Syndrome X, as a group of conditions when combined, put an individual at an increasing risk of having heart disease, and diabetes (Sherman, 2009; The Consumer's Medical Journal, 2009; Miner, 2010; Uemura et al., 2009; Brzycki, 2010; National Institutes of Health (NIH), 2009; Chan et al, 2008). According to the National Cholesterol Education Program – Adult Treatment Panel III and other health bodies, there are five risk factors associated with Met S (Ascribe Newswire: Health, 2008; Nutrition Action Health Letter, 2009) which include: blood pressure $>=130/85$ mmHg; fasting glucose $>= 110$ mm/dL; triglycerides $>= 150$ mm/dL; HDL cholesterol which varies for men and women with < 40 mm/dL and < 50 mm/dL respectively; abdominal obesity of > 40in for men and > 35in for women (Sherman, 2009).

It has been indicated that if an individual has any three or more of the five symptoms then one can be diagnosed as having Metabolic Syndrome (American Heart Association (AHA), 2010). More emphasis is placed on the fact that higher risks are linked to the existence of abdominal obesity and insulin resistance (Ascribe Newswire: Health, 2008; Howe, 2008; Roan, 2010). National health organizations, particularly AHA and National Heart, Lung and Blood Institute (NHLB1) confirm this criterion with slightly varying specifics (Sherman, 2009; AHA, 2010; Grundy et al., 2004).

A large percentage of the older group suffering from MetS face high mortality risks with elevated levels of blood sugar and high blood pressure, while the middle aged are stroked with Cardio Vascular Disease (CVD) (Sherman, 2009). Due to what seems like controllable but highly desirable factors, mainly poor diet and lack of exercise, MetS has managed to pave its way through. Infants (Howe, 2008) and 7% of those at age 20 (Miner, 2010) are no exception to becoming victims. After-birth effects in women (Kuznar, 2009) such as increased abdominal obesity, hypertension and more, have proved to create fertile ground for MetS and 13.7% of those in menopause are estimated to suffer from this disorder (The Consumer's Medical Journal, 2009).

Emerging evidence has shown that having MetS plays a critical role in one's health - one that escalates the risk of having cardiovascular disease and type 2 diabetes (Sherman, 2009; AHA, 2010). More downside on Met S includes an increase in erectile dysfunction in men at a rate of 26.7% (Miner, 2010) with an interesting upside of preventing prostate cancer especially in Diabetic patients (Kuznar, 2009). Since Met S is linked to such fatality, it is indeed necessary to watch out for signs that can predict chances of having this disorder, which undoubtedly can endanger one's life. Further still, restrictions on certain foods such as high carbohydrate intake and fatty foods like fish that are associated with Persistent Organic Pollutants (POPs) need to be enforced ((Uemura et al., 2009; Ruzzin, 2010; Palmer, 2009) with no disregard to physical exercise plus necessary medication to manage risk factors.

The later sections of the study follow up with an approach (methodology) used to obtain results and then experimental results are discussed to describe the findings. Finally, the study concludes by providing remarks on which approach is more appropriate in the cluster analysis of these individuals.

APPROACH

The course of approach followed during this study is summarized in Figure 1. It indicates the initial step where the data is extracted and stratified into bins and follows through two distinct steps, one that includes the direct application of k–means clustering (without SVD application) to the data bins represented by the selected age groups and the second approach takes on another pre-processing task – SVD that reduces each data bin into a rank k approximation of linearly independent columns, before applying k-means clustering. In both approaches, the clusters are validated using the two internal measures mentioned earlier – SSE and Sil, and the patterns formed by these clusters are evaluated. The sub-sections in this approach go on to discuss in detail the specifics of each technique used, how it works and how it relates to this study.

Given a rectangular matrix D_1 (m * n) where $D_1 = \{d_1...d_n\}$ in the form $\begin{pmatrix} x_{11} & \cdots & x_{1n} \\ x_{21} & \cdots & x_{2n} \\ x_{m1} & \cdots & x_{mn} \end{pmatrix}$ of a general sample population, each data item d_i has a set of corresponding attributes $A_{ij} = \{a_{i1}...a_{in}\}$.

Also matrices D_2 (o * n) as $\begin{pmatrix} y_{11} & \cdots & y_{1n} \\ y_{21} & \cdots & y_{2n} \\ y_{m1} & \cdots & y_{mn} \end{pmatrix}$ and D_3 (p * n) as $\begin{pmatrix} z_{11} & \cdots & z_{1n} \\ z_{21} & \cdots & z_{2n} \\ z_{m1} & \cdots & z_{mn} \end{pmatrix}$, are $\subset$ of D_1 representing a group of individuals classified as having Metabolic Syndrome (MetS Positive) and those without (MetS Negative), respectively (Figure 1).

Singular Value Decomposition

The purpose of SVD in this study is to create a more appropriate subspace of the data that highlights greater significance among the relations of the data.

Definition 1: Singular Value Decomposition (SVD)

For a data set D_i where $D_i = U \sum V^T$, $U = D_iD_i^T$, an m * n orthogonal left eigenvector matrix, $\sum = \sqrt{D}$, an n * n diagonal Eigen value matrix represented as $\begin{pmatrix} a_1 & & 0 \\ & \ddots & \\ 0 & & a_n \end{pmatrix}$ where all non-diagonal elements = 0 and $V^T = D_i^TD_i$, a transpose of a p * n orthogonal right eigenvector matrix.

This form represents a decomposition of D_i and reduces the dimensionality of its underlying data structure.

Figure 1. An illustration of the approach followed during the study

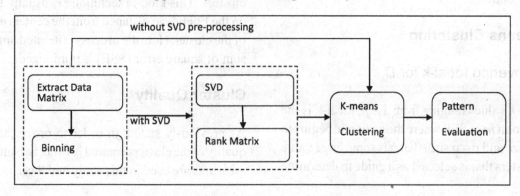

Figure 2. Determining Ideal k for clustering individuals

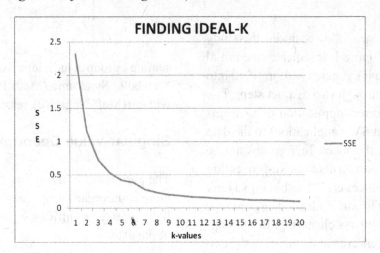

Rank Approximation

Based on a given number k of linearly independent columns, an approximation of a rank k matrix D_k for D_i states that $D_k = U_k * \sum_k$ denoted as

$$\begin{pmatrix} k_{11} & k_{12} & \cdots \\ \vdots & \vdots & \cdots \\ k_{m1} & k_{m2} & \cdots \end{pmatrix} * \begin{pmatrix} k_1 & & 0 \\ & \ddots & \\ 0 & & k_n \end{pmatrix}$$ respectively,

where U_k represents k left eigenvectors and $\sum_k$ represents the k most significant Eigen values.

$D_k \approx D_i$ represented as a low rank approximation which suppresses the insignificant relations in the data such that D_k is a linear representation of values $d_{k1} \ldots d_{kn}$. In that case if D_i is partitioned, clusters are represented along dimensions of D_k. In this study, rank $k = 2$ is the approximation used mainly because there are two significant Eigen values.

K-Means Clustering

Discovering Ideal-k for D_k

Given k values ranging from $1 \ldots p$, ideal-k is the mid-point m of SSE where the error rate begins to stabilize and $p \approx n$ such that n is some large value of clusters that is selected as a guide to determine

which ideal number of clusters should be used to group individuals. Therefore $m = k$ such that k is the ideal number of clusters to partition D_k. Figure 2 shows how ideal k is discovered.

It should be taken into account that D_k is stratified into bins $b_1 \ldots b_n$, where b_n is the maximum number of bins. In this study, the bins represent the age groups of individuals and these include Young (18-44), Middle (45-55) and Old (> 55). There is no specific binning technique applied in this case and hence the size of each bin b_i in terms of $|b_i|$ is determined by the total number of existing records per age group. It should also be considered that due to this, the bins are unequal.

For ideal $k = 4$, K-means clustering is an algorithm that allows for individuals with similar behavior in this study to be grouped into four clusters. This kind of technique is usually based on the Euclidean distance from the center (mean) of the cluster. Here the process is iterated until the sum of square error (SSE) is minimized.

Cluster Quality

As previously stated, in order to prove that the quality of the clusters created is valid, two internal measures are used in this study and these include

SSE and Sil. Their definitions are specified in the text that follows.

Definition 2: Sum of Square Error (SSE)

For $SSE = \sum_{i=1}^{K} \sum_{x \in C_i} dist^2(m_i, x)$ where ideal k ranges from 1 to k, the sum of the square distance of data point x (refer to d_{ki}) from the cluster center c is obtained for all data points per given cluster. The lower the SSE value, the more defined a cluster is. It further describes a higher intra-cluster similarity and lower inter-cluster similarity (Jain, Murty, & Flynn, 1999).

Definition 3: Silhouette Coefficient (Sil)

For Sil = $1 - a/b$ if $a < b$ where a = average distance of point d_{ki} to the points in its cluster and b = the average distance of d_{ki} to the points in another cluster (Frahling & Sohler, 2006). Sil values range from -1 to 1, where -1 describes a poor clustering and thus high cluster overlaps, whereas 1 describes a good clustering with less or no overlaps between clusters. Therefore the higher the value, the more defined the cluster.

Protocol of Analysis

The patterns defined by D_k which refers to the reduced data set, are evaluated focusing on the behavior of clusters per stratification – age group. More so, there is a comparison of the MetS Positive and MetS Negative group of individuals to determine the level of similarity in one group versus the other. Also the results from both internal measures, that is, SSE and Sil are validated for any similarities and contrasts in the error rate of patterns. And finally, the clusters formed with SVD and without SVD are evaluated in order to determine which approach defines clusters with a minimal error rate.

EXPERIMENTAL RESULTS

Following the approach taken above, the findings of the study presented in this section are of various forms; 1) Using SVD and Non-SVD for the cluster formation, 2) Using SSE and Sil for the internal measures to validate the clusters and 3) MetS Positive and MetS Negative patterns of analysis for the individuals diagnosed with MetS and those who are not respectively. Further still, all these forms are represented across the selected age groups defined as bins. In the next sub-section, the specifics pertaining to the original data set and it source are described.

Data Set Used

As mentioned in the motivation example, this study is based upon a combinatorial analysis of the attributes that relate to the possibility of Metabolic Syndrome in selected age groups. The data used to facilitate this study is in reference to the Third National Health and Nutrition Examination Survey (NHANES III), one of the various health statistical surveys performed by Center for Disease Control (CDC) (CDC, 1997). This data set contains data collected over a period of six years with over 2000 variables used to describe each instance. However, for purposes of this study, seven variables were selected and a total of 16848 instances fitted the age threshold which is > 18 years. These instances initially were referred to as a General population (D_1), but later divided and classified to form two other data sets, a MetS Positive (D_2) and MetS Negative (D_3) groups of individuals. A detailed analysis of the results follows in the next sub-section.

Results

Datasets $D_2 \wedge D_3$ represented as matrices with sizes o*n (MetS Positive) and p*n (MetS Negative) respectively, had all instances stratified into 3 age groups: Young (18-44); Middle (45-55) and Old

(> 55), and clusters were defined per age group given ideal $k = 4$. With two internal measures – SSE and Sil used to evaluate the quality of clusters formed by the application of SVD before clustering (SVD-Based) and without SVD (Non-SVD), a detailed comparison of the findings (Figure 3).

Measure 1: Sum of Square Error (SSE)

From the general point of view, the patterns defined by applying SVD and those without SVD for both the MetS Positive and MetS Negative individuals are the opposite of one another.

In SVD-based clustering, the patterns formed by the two groups of individuals – MetS Positive and MetS Negative as shown above is similar in that case where both have clusters more defined in the Young and Old age groups as indicated by the lower SSE values which shows that the error in the clusters is significantly < 1. This further explains that individuals in these two age groups possess similar behavior, with characteristics that are closely related for all variables linked to Metabolic Syndrome. On the contrary, the Middle age group shows less defined clusters based on the higher SSE values with cluster error > 2 for MetS Negative and > 4 for MetS Positive, an indication of more distinct behavior for both MetS Positive and MetS Negative individuals.

However, without the application of SVD, the patterns formed are similar for MetS Positive and MetS Negative, but the clusters are less defined in the Young and Old age groups as indicated by the higher SSE values where cluster error > 8 in both cases. Here the individuals behave more differently from one another. For the Middle age group, the clusters are more defined based on lower SSE values where cluster error < 8 for MetS Positive and < 4 for MetS Negative which shows that individuals have more similar behavior. Also individuals in the Old age group behave similar in both MetS Positive and Negative, though the behavior in the Young group strongly differs.

In general, the quality of the clusters formed using SVD in SSE is better because the error rate is significantly lower compared to that without SVD.

Measure 2: Silhouette Coefficient (Sil)

In using Sil to validate clusters without the application of SVD, the MetS Positive groups seem to strike out with less cluster overlaps for the Old and Middle age vs. the MetS Negative group for the Old and Young in SVD-based clustering. This is noted as a contradiction of results represented by both approaches (Figure 4).

In the general sense, SVD presents the clustering with less overlaps, hence more cohesiveness with 4/6 of the clustering having an average width > 0.6 whereas, non-SVD presents the clustering with more overlaps, hence less cohesiveness with 4/6 of the clustering having an average width < 0.6.

Figure 3. a) Pattern definition using SVD b) Pattern definition without SVD

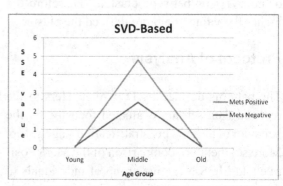

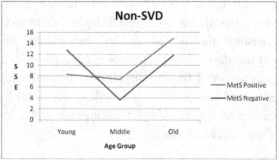

Figure 4. a) Pattern definition using SVD b) Pattern definition without SVD

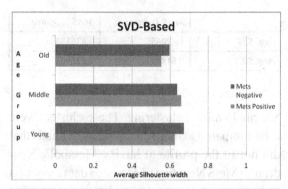

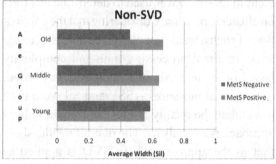

Without the application of SVD, it is also interesting to notice that the overlaps in the clusters decrease as the age decreases i.e. from Old to Young in the MetS Negative individuals while cluster overlaps decrease as age increases i.e. from Young to Old in the MetS Positive individuals. Using SVD, the same pattern follows for the MetS Negative individuals as those in Non-SVD and what is even more interesting is that the MetS Positive closely matches the Negative except that the Middle age group stands out more than the Young age group.

Also in SVD-based clustering, the best clustering is demonstrated in the Young MetS Negative and the worst goes to the Old MetS Positive groups. While in Non-SVD clustering, the best clustering is seen in Old Positive and worst is seen in Old Negative groups. All in all, the application of SVD still presents better clusters in Sil based on the less cluster overlaps defined above.

Observations

With the notion of trying to understand the findings in this study, some factors are mentioned below that could explain the outcome. This further explains the qualitative nature surrounding the analysis of the results. These factors are categorized according to cluster quality measures used – SSE and Sil, and the application of binning.

Measures

While both measures can be applied to validate clusters, their evaluation method is different. SSE considers a centroid-based approach to cluster objects (Jain et al., 1999), and Sil considers distances of individual data points to other points internally within a cluster and externally to other clusters formed (Frahling et al., 2006). It is not justifiable to determine which measure is better since both have similar results when applied to the use of SVD and without SVD as portrayed above. However it is has been noted that SSE has been noted to overlook outliers while Sil actually focuses on the outliers individually. However, this study is not evaluating the performance of internal measures but is inclined to analyzing cluster formation in individuals related to the possibility of MetS.

Application of Binning

The lack of a proper binning technique such as equal frequency binning can have an effect on the results obtained. But in this case the results show that SVD – based clustering forms better clusters than "straight forward" clustering. Tables 1 and 2 present a comparison of the average cluster error in all 3 age groups (bins) obtained using SVD and without.

Better clusters are formed in both SSE and Sil with SVD which is determined by calculating the average error rate of all age groups (bins). There is a thin margin in the cluster quality determined by Sil where Sil > 0.6 in both MetS Positive and

Table 1. Showing average error per clustering using SVD

	MetS Positive	MetS Negative
Avg. SSE	1.638867	0.881633
Avg. Sil.	0.6122	0.6357

Table 2. Showing average error per clustering without using SVD

	MetS Positive	MetS Negative
Avg. SSE	10.2065	9.436133
Avg. Sil.	0.6184	0.526933

MetS Negative with SVD and Sil < 0.6 in the Negative group without the application of SVD. Comparatively, the error margin is significantly larger in SSE where SSE < 2 for both MetS Positive and Negative groups with SVD and SSE > 9 with no SVD. From an interpretivist point of view, by using SSE it is possible that SVD looks at the underlying structure hence creating a suitable decomposition of the data altogether regardless of the existing number of records per bin, whereas Non-SVD simply focuses on the data at hand considering the data records available in each bin and hence basing its clustering technique on that. The latter can present biased results especially if the number of records is more in a given stratification (bin) compared to others and thus distorting the data somehow which increases the cluster error. But again this study is not examining binning techniques and their effect on clusters but to compare the clusters formed at both iterations (SVD–Based vs. Non–SVD) and determine which direction is more ideal especially when trying to analyze high dimensional datasets – a factor common in medical datasets. Future studies should take this observation into consideration to determine the effect of binning on the results particularly in this case.

CONCLUSION

At the beginning of this study, it was stated that the goal was to identify groups of clusters in individuals that are diagnosed with the possibility of Metabolic Syndrome (Mets Positive) using Simple K-means clustering. These clusters were then compared to those grouping individuals that did not fit the profile of having Metabolic Syndrome (MetS Negative). More so, a data reduction technique – SVD was used to determine its effect on cluster formation. Considering that the application of such a technique should be able to provide some minimal processing time and complexity based on an analysis of a smaller data portion, two internal measures – SSE and Sil were used to validate the quality of clusters formed in both approaches of analysis. The overall results show that in the approach where SVD is applied as pre-processing step, the clusters formed are more defined (with SSE) in both MetS Positive and Negative in the Young and Old age groups with almost no cluster error, and less cluster overlaps (with Sil) in both MetS Positive and Negative in the Young and Middle age groups, an indication of better cluster formation compared to the approach where SVD is not applied indicating less defined clusters (in SSE) in both MetS Positive and Negative especially in the Old age group and more cluster overlaps (in Sil) among the MetS Negative especially in the Old age group. It should be noted that in both approaches, all mechanisms followed were similar. These include; clustering technique (Simple K-means), number of clusters (four) and binning technique (age groups), thus there were no exceptions made in either approach that would have any post-effect on the results. Again, future research can explore outside the scope of this study, considering the effect of other factors such as proper binning techniques and the performance of measures used to validate cluster quality.

REFERENCES

Alshalalfa, M., Alhajj, R., & Rokne, J. (2008). Combining Singular Value Decomposition and t-test into Hybrid Approach for Significant Gene Extraction from Microarray Data. In *Proceedings of the 8th IEEE International Conference on BioInformatics and BioEngineering (BIBE)* (pp. 1-6). Washington, DC: IEEE.

American Heart Association. (2010). *Metabolic Syndrome*. Retrieved July 13, 2010, from http://www.americanheart.org/presenter. jhtml?identifier=4756

American Heart Association. (2010). *Statistical fact sheet risk factors 2010 update*. Retrieved July 13, 2010, from http://www.americanheart.org/downloadable/heart/1260809371480FS15META10. pdf

Brinegar, C., Zhang, H., Wu, Y. L., Foley, L. M., Hitchens, T. K., Ye, Q., et al. (2009). Real-Time Cardiac MRI using Prior Spatial-Spectral Information. In *Proceedings of the Annual International Conference of the IEEE Engineering in Medicine and Biology Society (EMBC)* (pp. 4383-4386). Washington, DC: IEEE.

Brockwell, A. E., Kass, R. E., & Schwartz, A. B. (2007). Statistical Signal Processing and the Motor Cortex. *Proceedings of the IEEE*, *95*, 881–898. doi:10.1109/JPROC.2007.894703

Brzycki, M. (2010). AF Q & A. *American Fitness*, *28*, 15–15.

Bunn, P., & Ostrovsky, R. (2007). Secure two-party k-means clustering. In P. Ning (Ed.), *Proceedings of the 14th ACM conference on Computer and communications security* (pp. 486-497). New York: ACM.

Center for Disease Control (CDC). *(1997)*. NHANES III: Series 11 Data Files. *Retrieved May 30, 2009, from* http://www.cdc.gov/nchs/nhanes/ nh3data.htm#1a

Chan, C.-L., Chen, C. W., & Liu, B. J. (2008). Discovery of association rules in metabolic syndrome related diseases. In *Proceedings of the IEEE International Joint Conference on Neural Networks (IJCNN 2008)* (pp. 856-862). Washington, DC: IEEE.

Frahling, G., & Sohler, C. (2006). A fast k-means implementation using corsets. In N. Amenta and O. Cheong, editors. In *Proceedings of the twenty-second annual symposium on Computational geometry* (pp. 135-143). New York: ACM.

Grundy, S., Brewer, H. B., Cleeman, J., Smith, S., & Lenfant, C. (2004). Definition of metabolic syndrome. In *Proceedings of the NHLBI/AHA Conference* (Vol. 24, pp. 13-18). Retrieved August 1, 2010, from http://circ.ahajournals.org/cgi/ content/full/109/3/433

Howe, D. K. (2008). Big Problems. *American Fitness*, *26*, 16–16.

Hsu, C. H., & Chen, C. C. (2007). Svd-based projection for face recognition. In *Proceedings of the IEEE International Conference on Electro/ Information Technology* (pp. 600-603). Washington, DC: IEEE.

Jain, A. K., Murty, M. N., & Flynn, P. J. (1999). Data Clustering: a review. *ACM Computing Surveys*, *31*, 264–323. doi:10.1145/331499.331504

Kuznar, W. (2009). Diabetes found to protect against prostate cancer. *Urology Times*, *37*, 8.

Lee, S., & Hayes, M. (2004). Properties of the singular value decomposition for efficient data clustering. *IEEE Signal Processing Letters*, *11*(11), 862–866. doi:10.1109/LSP.2004.833513

Li, J., Zhu, W., Wang, X., de Santi, S., & de Leon, M. J. (2005). Bayesian Applications to Longitudinal Analysis on Medical Data with Discrete Outcomes. In Proceedings of the *27th Annual International Conference of the Engineering in Medicine and Biology Society (IEEE-EMBS)* (pp. 1204-1207). Washington, DC: IEEE.

Liu, W., Yang, L., & Hanzo, L. (2009). Svd-assisted multiuser transmitter and multiuser detector design for MIMO systems. *IEEE Transactions on Vehicular Technology, 58*, 1016–1021. doi:10.1109/TVT.2008.927728

Ma, T., Yao, R., Shao, Y., & Zhou, R. (2009). A SVD-Based Method to Assess the Uniqueness and Accuracy of Spect Geometrical Calibration. *IEEE Transactions on Medical Imaging, 28*, 1929–1939. doi:10.1109/TMI.2009.2025696

Martin, J. G. (2005). Subproblem Optimization by Gene Correlation with Singular Value Decomposition. In H. Beyer (Ed.), *Proceedings of the 2005 conference on Genetic and evolutionary computation* (pp. 1507-1514). New York: ACM.

Miner, M. (2010). Metabolic Syndrome, Testosterone, and Lifestyle Modification: Impact on Erectile Dysfunction, Cardiovascular Disease and All-Cause Mortality. *Urology Times -. Sexual Health*, (Supplement), 16–21.

National Institutes of Health (NIH). (2009). *MetabolicSyndrome*. Retrieved July 13, 2010 from http://www.nlm.nih.gov/medlineplus/metabolic-syndrome.html

Ascribe Newswire: Health. (2008). *Study in 7,000 Men and Women Ties Obesity, Inflammatory Proteins to Heart Failure Risk; Obesity-Related Inflammation Also Pegged as Catalyst in Metabolic Syndrome* (p. 3). Health Source - Consumer Edition.

Nutrition, A. H. L. (2009)... *Inflammation & Beyond, 36*, 7–7.

Nutrition Health Review. (2009). Menopause and Metabolic Syndrome. *The Consumer's Medical Journal*, 15-15.

Palmer, S. (2009). Putting the Brakes on Inflammation Through Diet and Lifestyle Strategies. *Environmental Nutrition, 32*, 1–6.

Phillips, R. D., Watson, L. T., & Wynne, R. H. (2008). A Shared Memory Parallel Algorithm for Data Reduction Using the Singular Value Decomposition. In H. Rajaei (Ed.), *Proceedings of the 2008 Spring simulation multiconference* (pp. 459-466). New York: ACM.

Roan, S. (2010). A win-win for breastfeeding. *Fit Pregnancy, 17*, 22–22.

Ruzzin, J. (2010). Persistent Organic Pollutant Exposure Leads to Insulin Resistance Syndrome. *Environmental Health Perspectives, 118*, 465–471. doi:10.1289/ehp.0901321

Sherman, F. T. (2009). Baby Boomers court metabolic syndrome. *Geriatrics, 64*, 8–15.

Thomasian, A., Castelli, V., & Li, C. (1998). Clustering and Singular Value Decomposition for Approximate Indexing in High Dimensional Spaces. In N. Pissinou, C. Nicholas, J. French, & G. Gardarin (Eds.), *Proceedings of the seventh international conference on Information and knowledge management* (pp. 201-207). New York: ACM.

Uemura, H., Arisawa, K., Hiyoshi, M., Kitayama, A., Takami, H., & Sawachika, F. (2009). Prevalence of Metabolic Syndrome Associated with Body Burden Levels of Dioxin and Related Compounds among Japan's General Population. *Environmental Health Perspectives, 117*, 568–573.

Zanderigo, F., Bertoldo, A., Pillonetto, G., & Cobelli, C. (2009). Nonlinear Stochastic Regularization to Characterize Tissue Residue Function in Bolus-tracking MRI: Assessment and Comparison with SVD, Block-circulant SVD, and Tikhonov. *IEEE Transactions on Bio-Medical Engineering, 56*, 1287–1297. doi:10.1109/TBME.2009.2013820

This work was previously published in International Journal of Computational Models and Algorithms in Medicine, Volume 1, Issue 3, edited by Aryya Gangopadhyay, pp. 69-80, copyright 2010 by IGI Publishing (an imprint of IGI Global).

Chapter 14
Optimization Model and Algorithm Help to Screen and Treat Sexually Transmitted Diseases

Kun Zhao
Georgia State University, USA

Thomas Gift
Centers for Disease Control and Prevention, USA

Guantao Chen
Georgia State University, USA

Guoyu Tao
Centers for Disease Control and Prevention, USA

ABSTRACT

Chlamydia trachomatis (CT) and Neisseria gonorrhoeae (GC) are two common sexually transmitted diseases among women in the United States. Publicly funded programs usually do not have enough money to screen and treat all patients. Therefore, the authors propose a new resource allocation model to assist clinical managers to make decisions on identifying at-risk population groups, as well as selecting a screening and treatment strategy for CT and GC patients under a fixed budget. At the same time, the authors also develop a two-step branch-and-bound algorithm tailor-made for our model. Running on real-life data, the algorithm calculates the optimal solution within a very short time. The new algorithm also improves the accuracy of an approximate solution obtained by Excel Solver. This study has shown that a resource allocation model and algorithm might have a significant impact on real clinical issues.

INTRODUCTION

Background on Sexually Transmitted Diseases in the United States

Chlamydia trachomatis (CT) and *Neisseria gonorrhoeae* (GC) are the two most commonly reported sexually transmitted diseases (STDs)

in the United States. Most infections are asymptomatic and would not be detected without asymptomatic screening, especially for women. In 2008, 1,210,523 cases of chlamydia were reported to the Centers for Disease Control and Prevention (CDC) in the United States. This case count corresponds to a rate of 401.3 cases per 100,000 population, an increase of 9.2% com-

DOI: 10.4018/978-1-4666-0282-3.ch014

pared with the rate in 2007 (Centers for Disease Control and Prevention, 2010b). In 2008, 336,742 cases of gonorrhea were reported to CDC in the United States, corresponding to a rate of 111.6 per 100,000 population (Centers for Disease Control and Prevention, 2010b).

Many CT and GC infections are detected through screening and treatment in public clinics. In reality, these clinics may not have sufficient budgets to screen all eligible women with the most effective CT/GC tests and to offer patients more expensive, single-dose treatments that improve adherence. To use limited resources effectively, CT and GC control programs usually provide selective screening based on defined guidelines. For example, CDC and the U.S. Preventive Services Task Force (USPSTF) recommend annual screening for CT for all sexually active females 25 years and younger (Centers for Disease Control and Prevention, 2010a). In addition, USPSTF also recommends screening all sexually active women younger than 25 years, including those who are pregnant, for GC if they are at increased risk for infections (U.S. Preventive Services Task Force, 2005).

Identifying which subpopulations to screen for CT and GC is just one part of the real-life problem. The availability of several testing assays with various performance parameters and costs presents a challenge for screening strategies: newer diagnostic tests that are less invasive and more sensitive offer increased opportunities for screening, but at a greater cost. In other words, the problem is whether more infections can be diagnosed and treated using a more sensitive and expensive test to screen fewer patients, or to use a relatively cheaper and less sensitive test to screen a greater number of patients. To further complicate the issue, test manufacturers market combination tests or bundled tests at prices that are less expensive than the price of separate single-pathogen tests. This situation encourages the testing for GC even when its prevalence in the population is extremely low.

Overview of Creating Resource Allocation Models for STDs

There are not a lot of resource allocation (optimization) models regarding the control of CT and GC infections. But many efforts have been made to develop models to investigate and evaluate HIV prevention and control programs (Brandeau & Zaric, 2009; Kaplan & Pollack, 1998; Lasry, Zaric, & Carter, 2007; Sendi & Al, 2003). To correlate with the practical relevance to CT infections, researchers initially developed a resource allocation model to determine the optimal strategy for curing CT infections among asymptomatic women at clinics (Tao, Gift, Walsh, Irwin, & Kassler, 2002). Two years later, researchers proposed a mixed-integer program to model re-screening women who test positive for CT infections (Tao, Abban, Gift, Chen, & Irwin, 2004). These two optimization models are able to offer simple guidelines for clinics on the selection of test and treatment for certain populations. However, these models are not able to manage two or more infections (e.g. CT and GC) at the same time at given clinics.

Overview of Algorithms for Solving STDs Resource Allocation Models

Many health care researchers rely on existing resource allocation model software to solve their proposed models because some software applications are easy to use (Gift, Walsh, Haddix, & Irwin, 2002; Lasry, Carter, & Zaric, 2008; Tao et al., 2002, 2004). However, these applications sometimes may not provide the best outcomes due to the complexity of proposed models and the limitations of algorithms used in the software. For example, the resource allocation models used in the previous STD studies were nonlinear programming models and the optimal outcomes generated by the algorithm were never verified.

With respect to the nature of the resource allocation models that are typical nonlinear models, the algorithms for these models in general could be divided into two categories: exact algorithms (e.g. dynamic programming or branch-and-bound) (Kaplan & Pollack, 1998; Martello, Pisinger, & Toth, 2000; Martello & Toth, 1990) and approximation algorithm (e.g. generalized reduced gradient method) (Lasry et al., 2008; Microsoft, 2006; Rauner, Brailsford, & Flessa, 2005; Tao et al., 2004). The exact algorithms, which are exhaustive and are guaranteed to find an optimal solution with a small number of variables, may run in exponential time (Martello & Toth, 1990). In most cases, approximation algorithms, which may calculate near-optimal solutions, have to be used to speed up the computation time. This is the case for current commercial software applications, such as Excel Solver, MPL and Lingo (Hillier & Lieberman, 2001). When the resource allocation models become more complicated and various algorithms may lead to different outcomes, the knowledge of the limitations of various algorithms regarding computation accuracy and time is critical to the researchers. Unfortunately, comparing the computation accuracy and time of exact and approximation solutions to real-life STDs model has not yet been examined or published. In other words, we do not know how well an approximation algorithm could perform on real-life health care data. This may be due to the fact that the optimization modelers tend to focus on sophistication of the mathematical formulation rather than the practical relevance and algorithm accuracy and time (Lasry, Richter, & Lutscher, 2009; Tao et al., 2004).

Our Research Objectives

We have three main objectives in this study. First, to improve CT and GC control and prevention in the United States, we created a resource allocation model which is a cubic binary programming model to consider two STDs. The model is designed to recommend an optimal strategy for identifying at-risk groups with a certain screening assay and treating those with positive results under a fixed budget. Second, to solve this resource allocation

model, we developed a two-step branch-and-bound algorithm. Because our model had two diseases and limited number of constraints and our two-step branch-and-bound algorithm is an exact algorithm rather than approximation algorithm, our approach will always provide the optimal outcomes. Finally, we compared our computation results to those obtained by Excel Solver in terms of optimal outcome and computation time. The comparison can help us to better understand the characteristics of the resource allocation models and the advantages and disadvantages of the algorithms used to solve the model.

METHODS

Description of the Model

The object of the model is to *maximize the number of cured infections (cured cases) among women under a fixed budget*. One patient with both infections cured is counted as two cured cases. We assume that patients would be tested and treated according to one of the four options below using a nonrapid test that would require women with positive tests to be recalled for treatment. Option 1). Single screening test and single treatment for CT only. A CT screening test is given to women and then CT treatment is given to those who had positive tests. Option 2). Single screening test and single treatment for GC only. Similar to Option 1. Option 3). Sequence screening tests that tested for CT and then GC if a positive CT result. A CT screening test is performed and then a GC test is performed on those women who had positive CT tests; and CT treatment is given to those who had positive CT tests and GC treatment is given for those who had positive GC tests. Option 4). Combo screening test for both CT and GC. Women are screened for both CT and GC at the same time using a combo test. CT or GC or both are treated if patients had positive tests for CT or GC or both, respectively.

There are other options in theoretical situations, such as screening patients for GC first, then testing those with positive GC results for CT, or screening patients for CT and presumptively treat patients for GC if they have positive CT results. However, the options are not listed in this model because they are not realistic for use in the United States due to the much lower prevalence of GC than CT and concerns about GC drug resistance (Gift et al., 2002; Newman, Moran, & Workowski, 2007). We do not count uninfected women who test positive at screening ("false positive") and get treated as a cured case. But, we do include the additional costs for treatment and the treatment visit of false positive results.

Realistically, we assume that the same test and treatment are offered to all women in each group. The reason to make this assumption is that strategy involving more than one test or treatment may be more complicated to implement in routine clinic practice, although it may cure more women at a fixed budget level. For example, clinics will face the challenges related to specimen handling, storage, transport, and billing for each test, and providers may need additional training to explain test performance issues to women in each group (Tao et al., 2004; Tao et al., 2002). Two more simplifying assumptions are made in the model. First, we assume that all sexually active women who visit the clinic and are infected with CT or GC or both have no symptoms of infection. Second, no patients receive more than one test or treatment for the same infection at any one visit.

Data Used in the Model

As seen in Table 1, our model divides a theoretical cohort of 10,000 sexually active female patients into three age groups (younger than 20 years, 20-24 years, and 25-34 years) and four race/ethnicity groups (White, Black, Hispanic and Other). The age groups analyzed are similar

Table 1. Population distribution characteristics of theoretical cohort of 10,000 women

Age	Race/ethnicity			
	White	Black	Hispanics	Others
Number of patients				
<20 years 20-24 years 2680 640 480 200 25-34 years 2010 480 360 150	2010	480	360	150
20-24 years	2680	640	480	200
25-34 years	2010	480	360	150
CT prevalence[1]				
<20 years 20-24 years 2680 640 480 200 25-34 years 2010 480 360 150	3.8%	15.6%	9.2%	10.7%
20-24 years	2.5%	14.4%	6.3%	7.5%
25-34 years	1.2%	11.8%	2.5%	3.3%
GC prevalence[2]				
<20 years 20-24 years 2680 640 480 200 25-34 years 2010 480 360 150	0.1%	1.9%	0.1%	0.2%
20-24 years	0.2%	2.2%	0.1%	0.2%
25-34 years	0.2%	1.8%	0.1%	0.2%

[1,2] All prevalence rates are referenced from (Dicker, et al., 2000; Miller, et al., 2004).

to those classified in the CDC for screening and treating for CT infections (Tao et al., 2004). The prevalence rate of each group is referenced from (Dicker, Mosure, Levine, Black, & Berman, 2000; Miller et al., 2004).

Our model includes two CT tests (Pace 2 CT and BD ProbeTec CT), one GC test (culture), three combo tests (Pace 2C Combo, BD ProbeTec CT/GC, and APTIMA CT/GC), two CT treatments (doxycycline and azithromycin), and two GC treatments (ceftriaxone and cefixime). The test sensitivity and specificity are shown in Table 2. All costs and other parameters are shown in Table 3. Those parameters in Table 2 and Table 3 come from published literatures (Augenbraun et al., 1998; Black et al., 2002; Gaydos et al., 2003; Koumans, Johnson, Knapp, & St. Louis, 1998; Martin et al., 1992, 2000; Newman et al., 2007; Schachter, Chow, Howard, Bolan, & Moncada, 2006; Van Der Pol et al., 2001). When different values of a parameter were reported from multiple literatures, the baseline value was based on the investigators' assessment of the most strongly supported value given the evidence in the published literatures.

The Mathematical Model

Several mathematical notations in the model and the formulas are introduced here. More details are in the Appendices A and B.

- **Population notations.** The patient population is divided into m groups ($m = 12$ in real-life data). For each group i, let x_i be a binary variable such that $x_i = 1$ if all the patients in the group i is identified for screening and $x_i = 0$ otherwise. Let $P_t(i)$ and $P_g(i)$ be the prevalence of the group i with CT and GC, respectively. Pop_i is the number of patients in i th group.
- **Screening notations.** There are r available screening assays ($r = 6$ in real-life

data). Let y_j be a binary variable such that $y_j = 1$ if the screening assay j is used and $y_j = 0$ otherwise. For each assay j, let $Sn_t(j)$ and $Sp_t(j)$ be the sensitivity and specificity for CT; let $Sn_g(j)$ and $Sp_g(j)$ be the sensitivity and specificity for GC; let $Bc(j)$ and $Ac(j)$ be the unit-based costs and additional costs of the j th test. Let Vc be the costs per patient for the visit in which screening is done.
- **Treatment notations.** There are s available treatment regimens for CT and t available for GC ($s = 2$ and $t = 2$ in real-life data). Let $z_{(k,l)}$ be a binary variable such that $z_{(k,l)} = 1$ where $k > 0$ and $l > 0$ if the regimen k is used for treating CT together with regimen l used for treating GC. $z_{(0,l)} = 1$ is that only the GC treatment regimen l is selected and CT will not be treated, and $z_{(k,0)} = 1$ is that only CT is treated. For each CT treatment regimen k, let $E_t(k)$ be the effectiveness of the k th regimen. Similarly, let $E_g(l)$ be the effectiveness of the l th regimen for GC treatment. We also denote costs of drugs $Dc_t(k)$ for CT and $Dc_g(l)$ for GC, respectively. Let Tc be the costs per patient for the visit in which a treatment is done.
- **Number of cured cases and unit costs.** Let Cur_{ijkl} and $Cost_{ijkl}$ be the rate of cured infection cases and costs correspondingly over the population of the i th group using the j th screening test and being treated with k th and/or l th treatment regimen(s). So the corresponding number of cases cured and costs are $Pop_i \cdot Cur_{ijkl}$ and $Pop_i \cdot Cost_{ijkl}$ for group i. The Cur_{ijkl} under Option 1 ("Single screening test and single treatment for CT") is calculated as $Cur_{ijkl} = P_t(i) \cdot Sn_t(j) \cdot E_t(k) \cdot p_r$, where

Table 2. Sensitivity and specificity of test assays and effectiveness of treatment regimens for chlamydia and gonorrhea

	CT	GC
Test Sensitivity		
Pace 2 CT	0.716 (Black et al., 2002)	N/A
BD ProbeTec CT	0.928 (Van Der Pol et al., 2001)	N/A
Culture	N/A	0.848 (Martin et al., 2000)
Pace 2C Combo	0.716 (Black et al., 2002)	0.781 (Koumans et al., 1998)
BD ProbeTec CT/GC	0.928 (Van Der Pol et al., 2001)	0.966 (Van Der Pol et al., 2001)
APTIMA CT/GC	0.942 (Gaydos et al., 2003)	0.992 (Gaydos et al., 2003)
Test Specificity		
Pace 2 CT	0.995 (Black et al., 2002)	N/A
BD ProbeTec CT	0.981 (Van Der Pol et al., 2001)	N/A
Culture	N/A	1.000 (Martin et al., 2000)
Pace 2C Combo	0.995 (Black et al., 2002)	0.991 (Koumans et al., 1998)
BD ProbeTec CT/GC	0.981 (Van Der Pol et al., 2001)	0.994 (Van Der Pol et al., 2001)
APTIMA CT/GC	0.995 (Schachter et al., 2006)	0.995 (Schachter et al., 2006)
Treatment Effectiveness		
Doxycycline	0.92 (Geisler, 2007)	N/A
Azithromycin	0.95 (Geisler, 2007)	N/A
Ceftriaxone	N/A	0.988 (Newman et al., 2007)
Cefixime	N/A	0.975 (Newman et al., 2007)

p_r is the "probability of return for treatment" in Table 3. The corresponding $Cost_{ijkl}$ is calculated as

$$Cost_{ijkl} =$$
$$Bc(j) + Vc +$$
$$[P_t(i) \cdot Sn_t(j) + (1 - P_t(i)) \cdot (1 - Sp_t(j))] \cdot$$
$$(Dc_t(k) + Tc) \cdot p_r$$

For treatment,

$$P_t(i) \cdot Sn_t(j) + (1 - P_t(i)) \cdot (1 - Sp_t(j))$$

gives the probability of a person having a positive test result, where $P_t(i) \cdot Sn_t(j)$ is the probability of a person having CT infection and testing positively, and $(1 - P_t(i)) \cdot (1 - Sp_t(j))$ is the probability of a person not having CT infection but having a (false) positive test result. The

detailed calculations on Cur_{ijkl} and $Cost_{ijkl}$ for other options are in the Appendix B.

- **Objective function and constraints.** The objective function is to maximize the cured cases with available screening assays and treatment regimens for given patient groups.

$$Max \sum_{i,j,k,l} Pop_i \cdot Cur_{ijkl} \cdot x_i y_j z_{(k,l)} := \sum_{i=1}^{m} \sum_{j=1}^{r} \sum_{k=0}^{s} \sum_{l=0}^{t} Pop_i \cdot Cur_{ijkl} \cdot x_i y_j z_{(k,l)} \tag{1}$$

Subject to funding availability

$$\sum_{i,j,k,l} Pop_i \cdot Cost_{ijkl} \cdot x_i y_j z_{(k,l)} \leq b \tag{2}$$

Subject to funding availabilitywhich means the screening and treatment costs for identified

Table 3. Costs[1] related to CT and GC test and treatment and other parameters

	Baseline B
Test Cost	
Pace 2 CT	18.50[2] (Centers for Medicare and Medicaid Services, 2010)
BD ProbeTec CT	29.79[2] (Centers for Medicare and Medicaid Services, 2010)
GC Culture	9.26[2] (Centers for Medicare and Medicaid Services, 2010)
Pace 2C Combo[3]	35.16[2] (Centers for Medicare and Medicaid Services, 2010)
BD ProbeTec CT/GC	59.00[2] (Centers for Medicare and Medicaid Services, 2010)
APTIMA CT/GC	61.67[2] (Centers for Medicare and Medicaid Services, 2010)
Treatment Cost	
Doxycycline	8.12 (Thomson Healthcare, 2008)
Azithromycin	28.78 (Thomson Healthcare, 2008)
Ceftriaxone[4]	25.74 (Thomson Healthcare, 2008)
Cefixime	10.06 (Thomson Healthcare, 2008)
Test Visit Cost	14.00 (Howell, Quinn, Brathwaite, & Gaydos, 1998)
Treatment Visit Cost	28.43 (Begley, McGill, & Smith, 1989)
Prob. of return for treatment	0.86 (Bachmann, Richey, Waites, Schwebke, & Hook, 1999)

[1]All costs in 2006 US dollars (adjusted with medical CPI where needed) (Bureau of Labor Statistics, 2010). [2]Please also refer to (Association of Public Health Laboratories, 2002; Centers for Medicare and Medicaid Services, 2010; Howell, et al., 1998; Thomson Healthcare, 2008). [3]For the Pace 2C, a positive test (indicating either CT or GC, but not which organism) is followed by two separate supplemental tests. [4]For ceftriaxone, the baseline price includes the drug plus the fee for intramuscular injection (Centers for Medicare and Medicaid Services, 2010).

groups should be smaller than or equal to the annual available funding b to a clinic. Furthermore, according to the realistic assumption that the same screening assay and the same treatment must be applied for all patients served at the clinic, only one assay among the r screening assays will be used:

$$\sum_{j=1}^{r} y_j = 1 \qquad (3)$$

Only one treatment regimen for each infection among the s CT treatment regimens and t GC treatment regimens will be used:

$$\sum_{k=0}^{s}\sum_{l=0}^{t} z_{(k,l)} = 1 \qquad (4)$$

where k, l and $z_{(k,l)}$ are defined in treatment notations.

In our previous published mixed-integer programming (MIP) model, we used x_{ijk} as a binary variable to control the combination of group i, screening assays j, treatment k for single CT infections. In order to model the realistic assumption of applying same screening assay and the same treatment for all patients, we had to introduce two auxiliary binary variables to control the combinatorial relationships among constraints (Tao et al., 2004). Auxiliary binary variables representing the yes-or-no decisions are introduced to reduce the problem to a MIP model (Hillier & Lieberman, 2001). In the MIP model, auxiliary binary variables can be viewed as contingent decisions, i.e., decisions that depend upon previous decisions. While modeling single CT infections, these variables make the formulation tedious and limit our model on only two screening regimens and two treatment regimens. In this work, we keep the number of binary variables and simplify the formulation by defining x_i, y_j and $z_{(k,l)}$. Now, the new model is able to consider CT and GC infections together with more than two screening regimens and two treatment regimens.

Two-Step Branch-and-Bound Algorithm

The model (1)-(4) is a cubic binary programming problem. Except for exhaustive methods, there is no efficient algorithm to solve this problem (Hillier & Lieberman, 2001). The exhaustive (exact) algorithm runs in exponential time, which can only produce solutions for the problems with a small number of variables. To solve this model in general, approximation algorithms have to be used by commercial software applications. We do know that approximation algorithms generally are unable to distinguish between a local maximum and a global maximum (Hillier & Lieberman, 2001), but we don't know much these local maximum will deviate from a global maximum in this practice case. Therefore, knowing the global optimal solutions rather than approximations to the global optimal solutions (e.g., global maximum) is very important here. In this study, we define that *a global optimal solution to our model under a fixed budget is the strategy which guarantees the maximal value of cured cases*. Base on real-life data, we established a two-step algorithm to calculate global optimal solutions. In the first step, by using an exhaustive algorithm, we reduced the original model to several classic 0-1 knapsack problems which is an NP-hard problem in combinatorial optimization (Kellerer, Pferschy, & Pisinger, 2004). In the second step, we used the branch-and-bound method to solve each knapsack problem and select best strategy among each knapsack problem. The following details the algorithm.

Because Equations (3) and (4) show that there is only one possible j such that $y_j = 1$ and there is only one possible (k,l) such that $z_{(k,l)} = 1$, we initially identify how many combinatorial strategies for screening assays and treatment regimens exist in the model by using an exhaustive algorithm. In real-life data, there are 26 possible screening and treatment strategies. Option 1). Single screening test and single treatment for CT only. There are a total of 4 (= 2 · 2) combinations using a single screening test (Pace 2 CT or BD ProbeTec CT) and a single treatment for CT (doxycycline or azithromycin). Option 2). Single screening test and single treatment for GC only. Similar to Option 1, there are 2 combinations using the culture test and a single treatment for GC (ceftriaxone or cefixime). Option 3). Sequence screening tests that tested for CT and then GC if a positive CT result. There are a total of 8 (= 2 · 1 · 2 · 2) combinations: two screening assays for CT (Pace 2 CT or BD ProbeTec CT), one GC screening assay (culture), two CT treatment regimens (doxycycline or azithromycin) and two GC treatment regimens (ceftriaxone or cefixime). Option 4). Combo screening test for both CT and GC. There are a total of 12 (= 3 · 2 · 2) combinations: three combo screening assays (Pace 2C Combo, BD ProbeTec CT/GC, or APTIMA CT/GC), two treatments for CT (doxycycline or azithromycin) and two treatments for GC (ceftriaxone or cefixime).

After exhausted all possible strategies, the original model was decomposed into 26 classical 0-1 knapsack problems. In general, a 0-1 knapsack problem defined in the following way. Given a set of items, each with a weight and a value, determine the number of each item to include in a collection so that the total weight is less than a given limit and the total value is as large as possible (Hillier & Lieberman, 2001). As for our case, the 12 population groups are "items"; the costs $Pop_i \cdot Cost_{ijkl}$ are "weights"; the cured cases $Pop_i \cdot Cur_{ijkl}$ are "values", and the budget is a "given limit". We then applied the classical Horowitz-Sahni's branch-and-bound method (Martello & Toth, 1990) to find which group should be identified to go through the screening and treatment strategy. This method is further discussed in the Discussion section and Appendix C. After applied the method, we were able to record the corresponding numbers of the cured cases and the costs within each knapsack problem. These results are the optimal results for each of the 26 knapsack problems. Finally, the global optimal result to the whole model is reported as the one with maximum cured cases among the 26 optimal results.

The two-step branch-and-bound algorithm is implemented in Java. For comparison purposes, we applied the dynamic programming as an alternative method to the branch-and-bound method in the algorithm. The pseudocodes in Martello and Toth (1990, pp. 38-39) were used in this study. Furthermore, Excel Solver was applied to solve our original model as oppose to the two-step algorithm. The following computational results were run on an Intel Celeron M 1.6GHz processor and a RAM of 512MB.

RESULTS

Optimal strategy results under randomly selected budget levels are presented in Table 4. The two-step branch-and-bound algorithm has a faster running time and provides the global optimal results rather than the approximation solutions generated by the Solver's GRG2 algorithm, although Excel Solver can solve our original model directly. For example, at the budget level of $17,350, Solver's algorithm suggested to screen the group with a prevalence rate of 11.8% while the global optimal strategy screened the group with the highest prevalence rate of 15.6%. Using the optimal strategy calculated by two-step branch-and-bound algorithm, 10 more patients could be cured compared to Solver's algorithm. At the budget level of $30,000,

Solver's GRG2 algorithm recommended to treat CT alone with azithromycin. However, a better optimal strategy suggested that two more patients could be cured if we treat CT and GC together for the same groups. At the budget level of $100,000 and $200,000, Solver's GRG2 algorithm screened groups different from ours, and it also selected different treatment regimens. As the result, Solver's GRG2 algorithm cured two and five fewer patients respectively than our algorithm suggested. When the budget is low, the dynamic programming can identify the global optimal solution. However, when the budget is high, the dynamic program has a longer running time and it might run out of computer memory before it reaches its results.

DISCUSSION

The two-step branch-and-bound algorithm is our primary algorithm. It is an exact algorithm because both of first and second steps are exhaustive methods. In reality there are a limited number of combined screening and treatment regimens, the first step could be enumerated quickly. (There are only 26 combinations based on real-life data). In the second step, the Horowitz-Sahni's branch-and-bound method to each knapsack problem is also exhaustive (Martello & Toth, 1990). This method consists of a systematic enumeration of all at-risk population groups, where large subsets of candidate groups are discarded *en masse*, by using upper and lower estimated bounds of the cured cases being optimized. We selected this method because it is one of the most effective, structured and easiest to implement (Martello & Toth, 1990). Within each knapsack problem, the global optimal result could be calculated because the number of at-risk population groups is small according to a realistic division of patients (Tao et al., 2004). (There are only 12 groups based on real-life data.) The selection of the maximal number of cured cases among each optimal solution to the 26 knapsack problems guarantees

Table 4. Optimal strategy results for screening and treating 10,000 female patients for chlamydia and gonorrhea under the selected budget levels by three different algorithms

	Two-Step Algorithm		Solver's
	BnB[1]	DP[2]	GRG2[3]
Optimal Strategy for budget $17, 350			
Cured cases	42	42	32
Costs($)	17,348.92	17,348.92	16,941.28
Costs($) per case cured	413.07	413.07	529.42
Screening	Pace 2 CT	same	same
Treatment	DXC[4]	same	same
Running time (second)	<1	1	3
Optimal Strategy for budget $30, 000			
Cured cases	65	65	63
Costs($)	29,151.61	29,151.61	29,654.71
Costs($) per case cured	448.49	448.49	471.71
Screening	Pace 2 CT	same	same
Treatment	DXC+CFX[5]	same	ATM[6]
Running time (second)	<1	9	4
Optimal Strategy for budget $100,000			
Cured cases	198	198	196
Costs($)	97,389.52	97,389.52	98,864.24
Costs($) per case cured	491.87	491.87	504.41
Screening	BD ProbeTec CT	same	same
Treatment	DXC+CFIX[7]	same	ATM+CFX
Running time (second)	<1	44	1
Optimal Strategy for budget $200,000			
Cured cases	267	267	262
Costs($)	197,104.2	197,104.2	166,227.57
Costs($) per case cured	738.22	738.22	634.46
Screening	BD ProbeTec CT	same	same
Treatment	DXC+CFX	same	ATM+CFX
Running time (second)	<1	1334	4
Optimal Strategy for budget $500,000			
Cured cases	393	out of memory	393
Costs($)	476,323.83	n/a	476,323.83
Costs($) per case cured	1,212.02	n/a	1,212.02
Screening	BD ProbeTec CT	n/a	same
Treatment	ATM+CFX	n/a	same
Running time (second)	<1	n/a	1

[1]branch-and-bound method; [2]dynamic programming; [3]generalized reduced gradient method; [4]doxycycline; [5]ceftriaxone; [6]azithromycin; [7]cefixime.

the global optimal solution to the original model (1)-(4). In summary, based on real-life data, the global optimal solution is obtained because the algorithm is exhaustive and the complexity of the model is very reasonable.

As a general approach to the knapsack problem, dynamic programming is an alternative exact method (Martello et al., 2000) to the branch-and-bound method. It has been proposed to solve a HIV resource allocation model (Kaplan & Pollack, 1998) and epidemic control model (Blount, Galambosi, & Yakowitz, 1997). We think it is interesting to see how the dynamic programming performs in the real-life case controlling CT and GC infections. Therefore, we replaced the branch-and-bound method with dynamic programming. The dynamic programming method we used is based on the classical Bellman recursion (Bellman, 1957; Martello & Toth, 1990) due to its ease for implementation. The time and the space complexity of this method is $O(nc)$, where n is the number of population groups and c is the budget in our case. As the budget increases, the time and space consumption increase, limiting the performance of the algorithm (Table 4).

Microsoft Excel has been used in STD research (Lasry et al., 2008; Rauner et al., 2005; Tao et al., 2004). Excel Solver implemented the Generalized Reduced Gradient (GRG2) algorithm for optimizing nonlinear problems and it is an approximation algorithm (Microsoft, 2006). As a convenient commercial tool, Solver is used to solve the cubic binary model and its algorithm's computation complexity is not reported though.

In general, the complexity of the two-step branch-and-bound algorithm to the new model has an overall running time of $O(m \cdot n2^n)$, where m is the number of the realistic combinations of screening and treatment strategies satisfying conditions (3) and (4), and n is the number of population groups. For example, $m=26$ and $n=12$ in this real-life study. The first step runs in $O(m)$ time. The branch-and-bound method as the second step runs in $O(n2^n)$ time (Kellerer et al., 2004).

The complexity of the model increases as the choices of regimens and the partitions of population groups increases. Theoretically, these could be a potential computation limitation to solve the underlying model as opposed to the approximation algorithms. However, we are optimistic about the proposed algorithm for the following two reasons. First, in real-life m and n are fixed constants. The availability of regimens always determines the m for certain diseases. There are usually practical guidelines available at each clinic, regarding how to partite patients into n groups. The m and n in reality are small numbers. Second, for given realistic data, the new algorithm could calculate more accurate solutions.

Our finding highlights that the optimal outcomes and computation time could be significantly improved by our algorithm. The proposed cubic binary model could be widely used to manage budgets beyond the situation shown here with a fixed number of groups, screening assays and treatment regimens for CT and GC. It can be easily modified to solve the problem with different numbers of population groups, screening assays, and treatment regimens. It can be also modified to solve problems which have the characteristics of two or more major infections or diseases. For example, the model can be used to screen and treat patients for infectious diseases and chronic diseases.

There are still some improvements that could be done to the proposed model. In our current model, the side effect of the tests and treatments are not considered beyond the costs associated with treating false positive. For example, treating patients with false positive test results impose not only additional costs, but also medical side effects (such as gastrointestinal distress following azithromycin treatment) (Lau & Qureshi, 2002), which are difficult to value in monetary terms. Also, a false positive diagnosis can impose stress on a given patient and on her relationship with her sexual partner (Niccolai, Livingston, Teng, & Pettigrew, 2008; Shrier, Harris, & Beardslee, 2002).

For such concern, we could add some punishment components in the objective function. In other words, if there are too many mistreated cases, then a heavy punishment could be considered while selecting the optimal strategy.

We have restricted our work to one clinic. Government funding agencies, such as CDC, may need to optimize their funds for many clinics. Different clinics may use different screening and treatment regimens with more complicated constrains, which makes the optimization problem much more complicated. A future goal is to tackle this generalization problem.

CONCLUSION

We have designed a new mathematical model and the algorithm that can be used to identify the optimal strategies to screen and treat the two most common STDs in the US. By running on real-life data, this study shows that the optimal outcomes and computation time could be significantly improved by our algorithm, compared to other algorithms used in the existing software. Importantly, our algorithm always provides the global optimal solutions. In addition, our model and algorithm can be easily expanded to large number of population groups, screening assays, and treatment regimens, and more than two infections.

ACKNOWLEDGMENT

The authors would like to thank Dr. Charlotte Kent for her critical comments, Mr. Xin Wei for his initial work, Mr. Fasheng Qiu for his contribution on web-server, and Ms. Xue Wang for the fruitful discussion. The work was partially supported by NSF grant DMS-0070514, a CDC-GSU seed grant, and a GSU MBD fellowship.

REFERENCES

Association of Public Health Laboratories. (2002). *2001 Sexually Transmitted Diseases Laboratory Test Method Survey*. Retrieved from http://www.aphl.org/

Augenbraun, M., Bachmann, L., Wallace, T., Dubouchet, L., McCormack, W., & Hook, E. W. III. (1998). Compliance with doxycycline therapy in sexually transmitted diseases clinics. *Sexually Transmitted Diseases*, *25*(1), 1–4. doi:10.1097/00007435-199801000-00001

Bachmann, L. H., Richey, C. M., Waites, K., Schwebke, J. R., & Hook, E. W. III. (1999). Patterns of Chlamydia trachomatis testing and follow-up at a University Hospital Medical Center. *Sexually Transmitted Diseases*, *26*(9), 496–499. doi:10.1097/00007435-199910000-00002

Begley, C. E., McGill, L., & Smith, P. B. (1989). The incremental cost of screening, diagnosis, and treatment of gonorrhea and chlamydia in a family planning clinic. *Sexually Transmitted Diseases*, *16*(2), 63–67. doi:10.1097/00007435-198904000-00004

Bellman, R. (1957). *Dynamic programming*. Princeton, NJ: Princeton University Press.

Black, C. M., Marrazzo, J., Johnson, R. E., Hook, E. W. III, Jones, R. B., & Green, T. A. (2002). Head-to-head multicenter comparison of DNA probe and nucleic acid amplification tests for Chlamydia trachomatis infection in women performed with an improved reference standard. *Journal of Clinical Microbiology*, *40*(10), 3757–3763. doi:10.1128/JCM.40.10.3757-3763.2002

Blount, S., Galambosi, A., & Yakowitz, S. (1997). Nonlinear and dynamic programming for epidemic intervention. *Applied Mathematics and Computation*, *86*(2-3), 123–136. doi:10.1016/S0096-3003(96)00177-4

Brandeau, M. L., & Zaric, G. S. (2009). Optimal investment in HIV prevention programs: more is not always better. *Health Care Management Science, 12*(1), 27–37. doi:10.1007/s10729-008-9074-7

Bureau of Labor Statistics. (2010). *Consumer price index-all urban consumers*. Retrieved from http://www.bls.gov/cpi/

Centers for Disease Control and Prevention. (2010a). *Recommends screening of all sexually active women 25 and under.* Retrieved September 16, 2010, from http://www.cdc.gov/std/infertility/default.htm

Centers for Disease Control and Prevention. (2010b). *Sexually transmitted disease surveillance 2008.* Retrieved September 16, 2010, from http://www.cdc.gov/std/stats08/trends.htm

Centers for Medicare and Medicaid Services. (2010). *CMS programs and information.* Retrieved from http://www.cms.hhs.gov/

Dicker, L. W., Mosure, D. J., Levine, W. C., Black, C. M., & Berman, S. M. (2000). Impact of switching laboratory tests on reported trends in Chlamydia trachomatis infections. *American Journal of Epidemiology, 151*(4), 430–435.

Gaydos, C. A., Quinn, T. C., Willis, D., Weissfeld, A., Hook, E. W., & Martin, D. H. (2003). Performance of the APTIMA Combo 2 assay for detection of Chlamydia trachomatis and Neisseria gonorrhoeae in female urine and endocervical swab specimens. *Journal of Clinical Microbiology, 41*(1), 304–309. doi:10.1128/JCM.41.1.304-309.2003

Geisler, W. M. (2007). Management of uncomplicated Chlamydia trachomatis infections in adolescents and adults: evidence reviewed for the 2006 Centers for Disease Control and Prevention sexually transmitted diseases treatment guidelines. *Clinical Infectious Diseases, 44*, S77–S83. doi:10.1086/511421

Gift, T., Walsh, C., Haddix, A., & Irwin, K. L. (2002). A cost-effectiveness evaluation of testing and treatment of Chlamydia trachomatis infection among asymptomatic women infected with Neisseria gonorrhoeae. *Sexually Transmitted Diseases, 29*(9), 542–551. doi:10.1097/00007435-200209000-00009

Hillier, F. S., & Lieberman, G. J. (2001). *Introduction to operations research* (7th ed.). Boston, MA: McGraw-Hill.

Howell, M. R., Quinn, T. C., Brathwaite, W., & Gaydos, C. A. (1998). Screening women for chlamydia trachomatis in family planning clinics: the cost-effectiveness of DNA amplification assays. *Sexually Transmitted Diseases, 25*(2), 108–117. doi:10.1097/00007435-199802000-00008

Kaplan, E. H., & Pollack, H. (1998). Allocating HIV prevention resources. *Socio-Economic Planning Sciences, 4*, 257–263. doi:10.1016/S0038-0121(98)00002-0

Kellerer, H., Pferschy, U., & Pisinger, D. (2004). *Knapsack problems* (1st ed.). New York, NY: Springer.

Koumans, E. H., Johnson, R. E., Knapp, J. S., & St. Louis, M. E. (1998). Laboratory testing for Neisseria gonorrhoeae by recently introduced nonculture tests: a performance review with clinical and public health considerations. *Clinical Infectious Diseases, 27*(5), 1171–1180. doi:10.1086/514994

Lasry, A., Carter, M. W., & Zaric, G. S. (2008). S4HARA: System for HIV/AIDS resource allocation. *Cost Effectiveness and Resource Allocation, 6*, 1–19. doi:10.1186/1478-7547-6-7

Lasry, A., Richter, A., & Lutscher, F. (2009). Recommendations for increasing the use of HIV/AIDS resource allocation models. *BMC Public Health, 9*, S8. doi:10.1186/1471-2458-9-S1-S8

Lasry, A., Zaric, G. S., & Carter, M. W. (2007). Multi-level resource allocation for HIV prevention: A model for developing countries. *European Journal of Operational Research, 180*(2), 786–799. doi:10.1016/j.ejor.2006.02.043

Lau, C. Y., & Qureshi, A. K. (2002). Azithromycin versus doxycycline for genital chlamydial infections: a meta-analysis of randomized clinical trials. *Sexually Transmitted Diseases, 29*(9), 497–502. doi:10.1097/00007435-200209000-00001

Martello, S., Pisinger, D., & Toth, P. (2000). New trends in exact algorithms for the 0-1 knapsack problem. *European Journal of Operational Research, 123*(2), 325–332. doi:10.1016/S0377-2217(99)00260-X

Martello, S., & Toth, P. (1990). *Knapsack problems: algorithms and computer implementations* (Toth, P., Trans.). New York, NY: John Wiley & Sons.

Martin, D. H., Cammarata, C., Van Der Pol, B., Jones, R. B., Quinn, T. C., & Gaydos, C. A. (2000). Multicenter evaluation of AMPLICOR and automated COBAS AMPLICOR CT/NG tests for Neisseria gonorrhoeae. *Journal of Clinical Microbiology, 38*(10), 3544–3549.

Martin, D. H., Mroczkowski, T. F., Dalu, Z. A., McCarty, J., Jones, R. B., & Hopkins, S. J. (1992). A controlled trial of a single dose of azithromycin for the treatment of chlamydial urethritis and cervicitis. The Azithromycin for Chlamydial Infections Study Group. *The New England Journal of Medicine, 327*(13), 921–925. doi:10.1056/NEJM199209243271304

Microsoft. (2006). *Microsoft Excel Solver User's Guide for Windows.* Retrieved from http://support.microsoft.com/kb/82890

Miller, W. C., Ford, C. A., Morris, M., Handcock, M. S., Schmitz, J. L., & Hobbs, M. M. (2004). Prevalence of chlamydial and gonococcal infections among young adults in the United States. *Journal of the American Medical Association, 291*(18), 2229–2236. doi:10.1001/jama.291.18.2229

Newman, L. M., Moran, J. S., & Workowski, K. A. (2007). Update on the management of gonorrhea in adults in the United States. *Clinical Infectious Diseases, 44*, S84–S101. doi:10.1086/511422

Niccolai, L. M., Livingston, K. A., Teng, F. F., & Pettigrew, M. M. (2008). Behavioral intentions in sexual partnerships following a diagnosis of Chlamydia trachomatis. *American Journal of Preventive Medicine, 46*(2), 170–176. doi:10.1016/j.ypmed.2007.08.013

Rauner, M. S., Brailsford, S. C., & Flessa, S. (2005). Use of discrete-event simulation to evaluate strategies for the prevention of mother-to-child transmission of HIV in developing countries. *The Journal of the Operational Research Society, 56*(2), 222. doi:10.1057/palgrave.jors.2601884

Schachter, J., Chow, J. M., Howard, H., Bolan, G., & Moncada, J. (2006). Detection of Chlamydia trachomatis by nucleic acid amplification testing: our evaluation suggests that CDC-recommended approaches for confirmatory testing are ill-advised. *Journal of Clinical Microbiology, 44*(7), 2512–2517. doi:10.1128/JCM.02620-05

Sendi, P., & Al, M. J. (2003). Revisiting the decision rule of cost-effectiveness analysis under certainty and uncertainty. *Social Science & Medicine, 57*(6), 969–974. doi:10.1016/S0277-9536(02)00477-X

Shrier, L. A., Harris, S. K., & Beardslee, W. R. (2002). Temporal associations between depressive symptoms and self-reported sexually transmitted disease among adolescents. *Archives of Pediatrics & Adolescent Medicine, 156*(6), 599–606.

Tao, G., Abban, B. K., Gift, T. L., Chen, G., & Irwin, K. L. (2004). Applying a mixed-integer program to model re-screening women who test positive for C. trachomatis infection. *Health Care Management Science, 7*(2), 135–144. doi:10.1023/B:HCMS.0000020653.31862.23

Tao, G., Gift, T. L., Walsh, C. M., Irwin, K. L., & Kassler, W. J. (2002). Optimal resource allocation for curing Chlamydia trachomatis infection among asymptomatic women at clinics operating on a fixed budget. *Sexually Transmitted Diseases, 29*(11), 703–709. doi:10.1097/00007435-200211000-00014

Thomson Healthcare. (2008). *Drug Topics Red Book*. Montvale, NJ: Thomson Healthcare.

U.S. Preventive Services Task Force. (2005). *Screening for Gonorrhea*. Retrieved from http://www.uspreventiveservicestaskforce.org/uspstf/uspsgono.htm

Van Der Pol, B., Ferrero, D. V., Buck-Barrington, L., Hook, E. III, Lenderman, C., & Quinn, T. (2001). Multicenter evaluation of the BDProbeTec ET System for detection of Chlamydia trachomatis and Neisseria gonorrhoeae in urine specimens, female endocervical swabs, and male urethral swabs. *Journal of Clinical Microbiology, 39*(3), 1008–1016. doi:10.1128/JCM.39.3.1008-1016.2001

APPENDIX A

Useful Formula

Let $P_{g|t}(i)$ be the conditional probability of a CT patient in group i having GC and $P_{t|g}(i)$ be the conditional probability of a GC patient in group i having CT. From Bayes' law, we have $P_{t|g}(i) = \dfrac{P_t(i) \cdot P_{g|t}(i)}{P_g(i)}$.

Let $P_{g|\bar{t}}(i)$ be the conditional probability of GC infection in a patient without CT infection. Since $P_g(i) = P_t(i) \cdot P_{g|t}(i) + (1 - P_t(i)) \cdot P_{g|\bar{t}}(i)$, we have $P_{g|\bar{t}}(i) = \dfrac{P_g(i) - P_t(i) \cdot P_{g|t}(i)}{1 - P_t(i)}$ which is used to cal-

culate costs. Similarly, $P_{t|\bar{g}}(i)$ is calculated as $P_{t|\bar{g}}(i) = \dfrac{P_t(i) - P_g(i) \cdot P_{t|g}(i)}{1 - P_g(i)}$ in cost estimates.

APPENDIX B

Three Other Options Calculations: Single Screening and Treating for GC Only

$$Cur_{ijkl} = P_g(i) \cdot Sn_g(j) \cdot E_g(l) \cdot p_r$$

$$Cost_{ijkl} = Bc(j) + Vc + \left[P_g(i) \cdot Sn_g(j) + (1 - P_g(i)) \cdot (1 - Sp_g(j)) \right] \cdot (Dc_g(l) + Tc) \cdot p_r$$

Sequence screening tests that tested for CT and then GC if a positive CT result.

$$Cur_{ijkl} = P_t(i) \cdot Sn_t(j) \cdot E_t(k) \cdot p_r + P_t(i) \cdot Sn_t(j) \cdot P_{g|t}(i) \cdot Sn_g(j) \cdot E_g(l) \cdot p_r$$
$$+ (1 - P_t(i)) \cdot (1 - Sp_t(j)) \cdot P_{g|\bar{t}}(i) \cdot Sn_g(j) \cdot E_g(l) \cdot p_r$$

$P_t(i) \cdot Sn_t(j)$ gives the rate over the population of group i tested positively by using the j th CT screening test; $P_t(i) \cdot Sn_t(j) \cdot P_{g|t}(i) \cdot Sn_g(j) \cdot E_g(l) \cdot p_r$ gives the rate of the cured number of the GC patients infected by both of CT and GC and tested both positively. $(1 - P_t(i)) \cdot (1 - Sp_t(j))$ is the rate of those who are not infected with CT but who test positive. So $(1 - P_t(i)) \cdot (1 - Sp_t(j)) \cdot P_{g|\bar{t}}(i) \cdot Sn_g(j)$ calculates the percentage of patients who are in a "stroke of good luck" case. In this case, patients only have GC and were accidentally diagnosed as having CT with the j th test firstly and were caught with the second GC test finally, which in turn shows that $(1 - P_t(i)) \cdot (1 - Sp_t(j)) \cdot P_{g|\bar{t}}(i) \cdot Sn_g(j) \cdot E_g(l) \cdot p_r$ is the percentage of the cured number of GC patients in the case of the "stroke of good luck".

$$Cost_{ijkl} = Bc(j) + Vc + \left[P_t(i) \cdot Sn_t(j) + (1 - P_t(i)) \cdot (1 - Sp_t(j)) \right] \cdot \left[(Dc_t(k) + Tc) \cdot p_r + Bc(j) \right]$$
$$+ \left[P_t(i) \cdot Sn_t(j) \cdot P_{g|t}(i) + (1 - P_t(i)) \cdot (1 - Sp_t(j)) \cdot P_{g|\bar{t}}(i) \right] \cdot Sn_g(j) \cdot (Dc_g(l) + Tc) \cdot p_r$$

The term $Bc(j) + Vc + \left[P_t(i) \cdot Sn_t(j) + (1 - P_t(i)) \cdot (1 - Sp_t(j))\right] \cdot \left[(Dc_t(k) + Tc) \cdot p_r + Bc(j)\right]$ can be viewed as the sum of $Bc(j) + Vc + \left[P_t(i) \cdot Sn_t(j) + (1 - P_t(i)) \cdot (1 - Sp_t(j))\right] \cdot (Dc_t(k) + Tc) \cdot p_r$ and $\left[P_t(i) \cdot Sn_t(j) + (1 - P_t(i)) \cdot (1 - Sp_t(j))\right] \cdot Bc(j)$.

$Bc(j) + Vc + \left[P_t(i) \cdot Sn_t(j) + (1 - P_t(i)) \cdot (1 - Sp_t(j))\right] \cdot (Dc_t(k) + Tc) \cdot p_r$ has been previous explained in the subsection of "Number of cured cases and unit costs". $\left[P_t(i) \cdot Sn_t(j) + (1 - P_t(i)) \cdot (1 - Sp_t(j))\right] \cdot Bc(j)$ represents the rate over the population of GC testing costs for the patients testing positive for CT. $\left[P_t(i) \cdot Sn_t(j) \cdot P_{g|t}(i) + (1 - P_t(i)) \cdot (1 - Sp_t(j)) \cdot P_{g|\bar{t}}(i)\right]$ represents the rate over the population of those testing positive on CT and then positive on GC.

$\left[P_t(i) \cdot Sn_t(j) \cdot P_{g|t}(i) + (1 - P_t(i)) \cdot (1 - Sp_t(j)) \cdot P_{g|\bar{t}}(i)\right] \cdot Sn_g(j) \cdot (Dc_g(l) + Tc) \cdot p_r$ is the rate over the population of treatment costs for curing these patients with a positive GC test.

Combo screening test for both CT and GC.

$$Cur_{ijkl} = P_t(i) \cdot Sn_t(j) \cdot E_t(k) \cdot p_r + P_g(i) \cdot Sn_g(j) \cdot E_g(l) \cdot p_r$$

The sum of $Bc(j) + Vc + \left[P_t(i) \cdot Sn_t(j) + (1 - P_t(i)) \cdot (1 - Sp_t(j))\right] \cdot (Dc_t(k) + Tc) \cdot p_r$ and $Bc(j) + Vc + \left[P_g(i) \cdot Sn_g(j) + (1 - P_g(i)) \cdot (1 - Sp_g(j))\right] \cdot (Dc_g(l) + Tc) \cdot p_r$ give the basic count except the visit costs for the screening test is counted twice and the treatment costs for those testing positive on both CT and GC are counted twice. Subtracting the double counted numbers, we obtain the following.

$$Cost_{ijkl} = Bc(j) + Vc + \left[P_g(i) \cdot Sn_g(j) + (1 - P_g(i)) \cdot (1 - Sp_g(j))\right] \cdot (Dc_g(l) + Tc) \cdot p_r$$
$$+ \left[P_g(i) \cdot Sn_g(j) + (1 - P_g(i)) \cdot (1 - Sp_g(j))\right] \cdot (Dc_g(l) + Tc) \cdot p_r - P_t(i) \cdot P_{g|t}(i) \cdot Tc \cdot p_r$$

Note: For a combo assay, there is an additional cost which is calculated slightly different from the above formula (Thomson Healthcare, 2008). We added the extra costs to the previous formula and it is

$$Cost_{ijkl} = Bc(j) + Vc + \left[P_g(i) \cdot Sn_g(j) + (1 - P_g(i)) \cdot (1 - Sp_g(j))\right] \cdot (Dc_g(l) + Tc) \cdot p_r$$
$$+ \left[P_g(i) \cdot Sn_g(j) + (1 - P_g(i)) \cdot (1 - Sp_g(j))\right] \cdot (Dc_g(l) + Tc) \cdot p_r - P_t(i) \cdot P_{g|t}(i) \cdot Tc \cdot p_r$$
$$+ \left[P_t(i) \cdot Sn_t(j) + P_g(i) \cdot Sn_g(j) - P_t(i) \cdot P_{g|t}(i)\right] \cdot Ac(j)$$

APPENDIX C

The Horowitz-Sahni Branch-and-Bound Method

In general, this algorithm has two moves (Martello & Toth, 1990): "A forward move consists of inserting the largest possible set of new consecutive items into the current solutions. A backtracking move consists of removing the last inserted item from the current solution. Whenever a forward move is exhausted, the upper bound corresponding to the current solutions is computed and compared with the best solution so far, in order to check whether further forward moves could lead to a better one; if so, a new forward move is performed, otherwise, a backtracking follows." (p.30-31). In this algorithm, items initially are sorted according to decreasing rates of the values per unit weight. The pseudocodes (Martello & Toth, 1990) we used are: $\hat{x}_j$ =current solution; $\hat{z}$ =current solution value ($= \sum_{j=1}^{n} p_j \hat{x}_j$); $\hat{c}$ =current residual capacity ($= c - \sum_{j=1}^{n} w_j \hat{x}_j$); ($x_j$)=best solution so far; z = value of the best solution so far ($= \sum_{j=1}^{n} p_j x_j$).

```
input: n, c, p_j, w_j; output: z, x_j;
begin:
1:[initialize]
```
$z = 0$; $\hat{z} = 0$; $\hat{c} = c$; $p_{n+1} = 0$; $w_{n+1} = +\infty$; $j = 1$.
```
2:[compute upper bound U_1]
```
find $r = \min \left\{ i : \sum_{k=j}^{i} w_k > \hat{c} \right\}$; $u = \sum_{k=j}^{r-1} p_k + \left\lfloor (\hat{c} - \sum_{k=j}^{r-1} w_k) p_r / w_r \right\rfloor$;
```
if z ≥ ẑ + u then go to 5;
3:[perform a forward step]
```
while $w_j \leq \hat{c}$ do $\hat{c} = \hat{c} - w_j$; $\hat{z} = \hat{z} + p_j$; $\hat{x}_j = 1$; $j = j+1$;
```
if j ≤ n then x̂_j = 0; j = j+1;
if j < n then go to 2;
if j = n then go to 3;
4:[update the best solution so far]
```
if $\hat{z} > z$ then $z = \hat{z}$; for $k = 1$ to n do $x_k = \hat{x}_k$;
$j = n$;
if $\hat{x}_n = 1$ then $\hat{c} = \hat{c} + w_n$; $\hat{z} = \hat{z} - p_n$; $\hat{x}_n = 0$;
```
5:[backtrack]
```
find $i = \max \left\{ k < j : \hat{x}_k = 1 \right\}$;
```
if no such i then return;
```
$\hat{c} = \hat{c} + w_i$; $\hat{z} = \hat{z} - p_i$; $\hat{x}_i = 0$; $j = i+1$;
```
go to 2;
end.
```

This work was previously published in International Journal of Computational Models and Algorithms in Medicine, Volume 1, Issue 4, edited by Aryya Gangopadhyay, pp. 1-18, copyright 2010 by IGI Publishing (an imprint of IGI Global).

Chapter 15
Medical Outcome Prediction for Intensive Care Unit Patients

Simone A. Ludwig
North Dakota State University, USA

Stefanie Roos
Darmstadt University, Germany

Monique Frize
Carleton University, Canada

Nicole Yu
Carleton University, Canada

ABSTRACT

The rate of people dying from medical errors in hospitals each year is very high. Errors that frequently occur during the course of providing health care are adverse drug events and improper transfusions, surgical injuries and wrong-site surgery, suicides, restraint-related injuries or death, falls, burns, pressure ulcers, and mistaken patient identities. Medical decision support systems play an increasingly important role in medical practice. By assisting physicians in making clinical decisions, medical decision support systems improve the quality of medical care. Two approaches have been investigated for the prediction of medical outcomes: "hours of ventilation" and the "mortality rate" in the adult intensive care unit. The first approach is based on neural networks with the weight-elimination algorithm, and the second is based on genetic programming. Both approaches are compared to commonly used machine learning algorithms. Results show that both algorithms developed score well for the outcomes selected.

INTRODUCTION

A study of the health care system in the United States reported that at least 44,000 people, and perhaps as many as 98,000 people, die in hospitals each year as a result of medical errors, many of which could have been prevented. Medical errors can be defined as the failure of a planned action to be performed as intended or the use of the wrong action to achieve an aim. Problems that frequently occur during the course of providing health care are adverse drug events and improper transfusions,

DOI: 10.4018/978-1-4666-0282-3.ch015

surgical injuries and wrong-site surgery, suicides, restraint-related injuries or death, falls, burns, pressure ulcers, and mistaken patient identities. High error rates with serious consequences are most likely to occur in intensive care units, operating rooms, and emergency departments (Institute of Medicine, 1999).

Medical decision support systems play an increasingly important role in medical practice to address the above stated problems. By assisting physicians with making clinical decisions, medical decision support systems are expected to improve the quality of medical care (Wennber & Cooper, 1999).

Sim et al. (2001) define clinical or medical decision support systems as software designed to be a direct aid to clinical decision-making, where the characteristics of an individual patient are matched to a computerized clinical knowledge base; patient-specific assessments or recommendations are then presented to the clinician and/or the patient for a decision. Numerous medical decision support systems have been developed to assist medical practice. In 2001, Kaplan reviewed 27 clinical decision support systems reported in the literature (Kaplan, 2001), while Metaxiotis et al. (2000) list 13 well known systems developed for diagnosis, test result interpretation and knowledge management. The range of clinical decision support systems spans the realms of home health care, to enterprise-wide systems, to medical research laboratories. When developing a new CDSS, several factors need to be considered to increase the likelihood that it will be integrated into the health care delivery in a variety of clinical environments. These factors need to be applied at all stages of the development life cycle of the CDSS. The criteria for a successful deployment of a CDSS can be divided into three main areas: (i) The data entry and the decision algorithms; (ii) the human-computer interaction, which includes the data acquisition and the manner in which information is requested from the system; and its usability; (iii) the output of the CDSS, including

the format and type of information supplied (Frize et al., 2010).

The application of machine learning methods in medicine is the subject of considerable ongoing research, which mainly concentrates on modeling some of the human actions or thinking processes and recognizing diseases from a variety of input sources (e.g. cardiograms, CAT (Computed Axial Tomography) / MRI (Magnetic Resonance Imaging) / ultrasound scans, photomicrographs, etc.). Other application areas are knowledge discovery (Neves et al., 1999), and biomedical systems, which include genetics and DNA analysis. The use of machine learning has also been applied to biomedical science related systems. There is already a growing interest in the application of learning systems for the interpretation of gene expression data (Brown et al., 1999; Slonim et al., 2000).

In a medical diagnosis problem, what is needed is a set of examples that are representative of all the variations of the disease. The examples need to be selected very carefully if the system is to perform reliably and efficiently. However, development of machine learning systems for medical decision-making is not a trivial task. Difficulties include the acquisition, collection and organization of the data that will be used for training the system. This becomes a major problem, especially when the system requires large data sets over long periods of time, which in most cases is not available due to the lack of an efficient recording system, or because of privacy issues. Another difficulty arises when trying to automate some processes as not all of them can be automated due to ethical and safety issues. Deciding what could and needs to be automated directly influences the design and implementation of the learning system.

The aim of this paper is to compare two classifiers with other machine learning techniques for the prediction of medical outcomes, such as the hours of ventilation necessary for patients in the Intensive Care Unit (ICU), and the prediction on whether the patient is likely to survive. Our two classifiers developed are based on Artificial Neural Networks and Genetic Programming, which are compared to well-known classifiers.

The paper is structured as follows. The first section describes related work, in particular different classification models. The datasets and our two classifiers used for this investigation are described, as well as the other classifiers used to perform the comparison. The results are then provided and compared, and the conclusions and future work are presented.

RELATED WORK

Supervised classification is one of the tasks most frequently carried out in the area of medical informatics. The most prominent classification algorithms can be categorized into logic-based algorithms, neural network algorithms, statistical learning algorithms, instance-based learning algorithms and support-vector machine algorithms. A summary of all algorithms is given below.

There are two groups of learning-based models: decision trees and rule-based classifiers. Decision trees are trees that classify instances by sorting them based on feature values. Each node in a decision tree represents a feature in an instance to be classified, and each branch represents a value that the node can receive. Instances are classified starting at the root node and sorted based on their feature values. The most well-known algorithm is C4.5 (Quinlan, 1993). C4.5 is an extension of Quinlan's earlier ID3 algorithm (Quinlan, 1979).

Decision trees can be translated into a set of rules by creating a separate rule for each path from the root to a leaf in the tree (Quinlan, 1993). However, rules can also be directly induced from training data using a variety of rule-based algorithms. Classification rules represent each class by a disjunctive normal form relation. The goal is to construct the smallest rule-set that is consistent with the training data. A well-known rule-based

algorithm is RIPPER (Repeated Incremental Pruning to Produce Error Reduction) (Cohen, 1995).

Neural network approaches are based on the perceptron (Rosenblatt, 1962). A single-layer perceptron network consists of one or more artificial neurons in parallel. Each neuron in the layer provides one network output, and is usually connected to all of the external (or environmental) inputs. The perceptron learning algorithm works as follows. First, the weight and threshold values of the neuron are set to random values. Then, the input is presented. Afterwards, the output of the neuron is calculated, and the weights of the neurons are adjusted. These steps are repeated until a defined error criterion is satisfied. As perceptrons can only classify linearly separable sets of instances, multi-layered perceptrons were invented. A multi-layer neural network consists of large number of units jointed together in a pattern of connections. The pattern of connections is ordered into three layers: input, hidden and output layer. There are several algorithms with which the network can be trained; however, the most well-known and widely used learning algorithm to estimate the values of the weights is the Backpropagation algorithm (Bryson & Ho, 1969).

Statistical approaches are characterized by having an explicit underlying probability model, which provides a probability that an instance belongs in each class, rather than simply a classification. Bayesian networks are the most well known representative of statistical learning algorithms. A Bayesian network is a graphical model for probability relationships among a set of variables. The Bayesian network structure S is a directed acyclic graph (DAG) and the nodes in S are in one-to-one correspondence with the features X. The arcs represent causal influences among the features, which the lack of possible arcs in S encodes conditional interdependencies. Moreover, a feature is conditionally independent from its non-descendants given its parents. Typically, the task of learning a Bayesian network can be divided into two subtasks: first, the learning of the DAG structure of the network, and then the determination of its parameters (Jensen, 1996). Naive Bayesian network are very simple Bayesian networks, which are composed of DAG with only one parent (representing the unobserved node) and several children (corresponding to observed nodes) with a strong assumption of independence among child nodes in the context of their parent (Good, 1950).

Instance-based learning algorithms are lazy-learning algorithms (Mitchell, 1997), as they delay the induction or generalization process until classification is performed. Lazy-learning algorithms require less computation time during the training phase than eager-learning algorithms such as decision trees, neural and Bayes networks, but more computation time during the classification process. One of the most straightforward instance-based learning algorithms is the nearest neighbour (kNN) algorithm, which is based on the principle that the instances within a dataset generally exist in close proximity to other instances that have similar properties (Cover & Hart, 1967). If the instances are tagged with a classification label, then the value of the label of an unclassified instance can be determined by observing the class of its nearest neighbours. The kNN locates the k nearest instances to the query instance and determines its class by identifying the single most frequent class label.

Support vector machines (SVMs) is the newest commonly used supervised machine learning technique (Vapnik, 1995). SVMs revolve around the notion of a "margin" – either side of a hyperplane that separates two data classes. Maximizing the margin and thereby creating the largest possible distance between the separating hyperplane and the instances on either side of it has been shown to reduce an upper bound on the expected generalization error.

APPROACHES

For the classification of the medical ICU outcomes "death" and "hours of ventilation", our two approaches are investigated further by comparing them to the most common machine learning algorithms of WEKA. The datasets, evaluation measures, and classifiers are explained in detail below.

Dataset

In this study, there were two data sets from an adult intensive care unit, each having the following features:

- Age of the patient
- Chronic: 1 if illness is chronic, 0 otherwise
- Emergency case: 1 if it is an emergency, 0 otherwise
- Post operation: 1 if patient had an operation before, 0 otherwise
- Gender: 1 male, -1 female
- Body temperature
- MAP: mean arterial pressure
- Heart rate
- Respiratory rate
- FiO_2 (inspired oxygen)-concentration in blood
- PO_2 (partial pressure of oxygen) in blood
- pH-value (arterial)
- Na: serum sodium (mMol/L of blood)
- K: serum potassium (mMol/L of blood)
- Serum creatinine (mMol/L of blood)
- Hematocrit: (volume of red blood cells) / (volume of blood total)
- WBC: white blood cell count (total/mm^3 in 1000's)
- GCS: Glasgow Coma Score (level of consciousness)

One of the datasets contains data of the outcome "survival of patient", and the other contains the "hours of ventilation" needed by the patient. In the second case, the learning task is a classification into the classes "at most 8 hours of ventilation" and "more than 8 hours of ventilation". The complete data set contains 1491 entries with 18 features, 14 numerical, 4 boolean. The sets are divided into two smaller sets, according to one Boolean attribute, detailing whether the patient had an operation before coming to the ICU. In the following, the sets will be referred to as Mortality post-OP, Mortality non-OP, Ventilation post-OP and Ventilation non-OP. There are 884 entries for the post-OP case, 608 cases for non-OP patients; 12.50% of the non-OP patients' die, and 3.17% of the post-OPs. The prevalence of patients needing more than 8 hours of ventilation is 35.53% in the non-OP set, and 28.28% in the post-OP set. Table 1 shows the distribution of the data sets.

Evaluation Measures

The following measures are recorded: (1) sensitivity: the percentage of positives correctly identified (death or needing more than 8 hours of ventilation is considered 'positive'); (2) specificity: The percentage of negatives correctly identified; (3) CCR (Correct Classification Rate): percentage of correct predictions in total; (4) area under ROC (Receiver Operating Curve). The fitness function used for this study is the log-sensitivity:

$$logsens = -sensitivity^n * \log(1 - sensitivity * specificity) \tag{1}$$

WEKA Algorithms

The classifier of the open source machine-learning package called WEKA (Witten and Frank, 2005) will be compared to our two approaches. WEKA is a collection of machine learning algorithms for solving real-world data mining problems. Within WEKA there are several machine learning algorithms available for classification, which are neural networks, support vector machines, decision trees, Bayesian classifiers, and lazy learning methods. A set of the most common machine learning algorithms were chosen for this investigation and a brief description is provided below:

- BN: BN is a Bayes Network learning algorithm using various search algorithms and quality measures.
- IBk: K-nearest neighbours classifier, which can select an appropriate value of K based on cross-validation, and also performs distance weighting.
- J48: This algorithm, as explained earlier, contains the class for generating a pruned or unpruned C4.5 decision tree.
- JRip: This class implements a propositional rule learner RIPPER.
- K*: K* is an instance-based classifier, i.e. the class of a test instance is based upon the class of those training instances similar to it, as determined by some similarity function.
- MP: MP is a multilayer perceptron that uses backpropagation to classify instances. The nodes in this network are all sigmoid

Table 1. Distribution of data set split into 4 categories: ventilation non-OP, ventilation post-OP, mortality non-OP, and mortality post-OP

Data set	number of cases	mortality rate [%]	more than 8 hours of ventilation [%]
non-OP	608	12.50	35.53
post-OP	884	3.17	28.28

(except for when the class is numeric, in which case the output nodes become un-thresholded linear units).

- NB: Class for a Naive Bayes classifier using estimator classes. Numeric estimator precision values are chosen based on the analysis of the training data.

- SMO: Support vector machines are a set of related supervised learning methods that analyze data and recognize patterns, used for classification and regression analysis. SMO (Sequential minimal optimization) in particular implements the sequential minimal optimization algorithm for training a support vector classifier. This implementation globally replaces all missing values and transforms nominal attributes into binary ones. It also normalizes all attributes by default.

Neural Network with Weight-Elimination (NNWEA) Approach

The neural network implementation uses a weight-elimination algorithm, processing the data through the ANN and then applying the weight-elimination algorithm. Weight-elimination attempts to reduce small weights to zero (Frize et al., 1995, Ennett & Frize, 2003), effectively removing them from the neural network. This is essentially a form of pruning the network, which has been used to improve ANN classification results. The back-propagation portion updates the weights in order to maximize the log sensitivity value, an early stopping criterion used to balance sensitivity and specificity and slightly favor sensitivity (Ennett et al., 2002), given in Equation (1). Each ANN run is stopped when the best performance has been reached and maintained for the last 500 epochs. The ANN was set to create classifiers using between 3 and 11 hidden nodes. The best performing classifier was chosen from the nine classifiers. The process has been entirely automated (Rybchynski, 2005; Ennett et al., 2004).

The values are scaled between -1 and 1 by using a modified Z-score transformation equation. The fourteen input variables (as given in the dataset subsection) were normalized using Equation (2) where α' is the normalized value, α is the value, μ is the mean and σ is the standard deviation:

$$\alpha' = \frac{\alpha - \mu}{3 * \sigma} \tag{2}$$

Categorical variables (chronic, emergency surgery, sex) were given a value of -1 or 1. Once the variables were normalized, they were split into a training (46.0%), test (28%) and verification set (25%). Since the mortality dataset had a low prevalence of cases in both the post-OP (3.17%) and non-OP (12.50%) databases, we randomly re-sampled from this population in order to improve the performance of the ANN in terms of sensitivity (Ennett & Frize, 2000). For the post-OP dataset, the training set was raised to 5.06% of cases from the original 3.37%. For the verification sets for the outcome ventilation (that is, positive cases defined as "more than 8 hours of ventilation"), was randomly sampled to create ten different sets. The verification sets were used to measure the performance of the ANN and to determine the mean and standard deviation of the ANN performance. A satisfactory performance on the verification sets was indicative that the classifier generalizes well on new, unseen cases. Poor performance suggests overtraining of the network.

Automatic Genetic Programming (AGP) Approach

The origins of evolutionary computation reach back to the 50's of the last century. Genetic programming, in itself, was not considered until the middle of the 80's. The term first appeared in (Cramer, 1985), and the main development took place in the early and middle 90's, particularly through work by Koza (1992). Genetic programming uses the concepts of genetics and Darwinian natural selection to generate and evolve entire computer programs. Genetic programming largely resembles genetic algorithms in terms of its basic algorithm. The notions of mutation, reproduction (crossover) and fitness are essentially the same; however, genetic programming requires special attention when using those operations. While genetic algorithms are concerned with modifying fixed-length strings, usually associated with parameters to a function, genetic programming is concerned with actually creating and manipulating the (non-fixed length) structure of the program (or function). Therefore, genetic programming is more complex than genetic algorithms (Banzhaf et al., 1998) and works as follows. The solution is developed by first creating a number of initial programs, which are then recombined and changed in each evolution step. The set of programs is referred to as the population; any single program is an individual. Run of evolution is the term used to describe the whole process of finding a solution. Before starting an evolution, one has to define (at least) the following:

- Fitness measure/function: a function that evaluates how close a program is to the optimal solution. For the prognosis, the fitness value, as given by Equation (1), is to be minimized.
- Population size: the number of programs that are supposed to be used for evolving a solution.
- Function and terminal set: functions, constants, and variables the programs are allowed to use.
- Genetic operators: selection, crossover and mutation operators and the probability for using the later two. There are a variety of different selection, crossover and mutation operators available to choose from.
- Termination criterion: the evolution usually either ends if a sufficiently good solution is found, or if the maximum number of iterations is reached.

After setting these parameters, the initial population can be created. Unless one already has some idea about how the solution might look like, the programs are built randomly. Each evolution step works as follows: Until a certain percentage of the population size (crossover rate) is reached, new programs are constructed as follows: 2 programs are selected according to the chosen selection method. The programs are "crossed over", that means certain parts of them are swapped. In tree-based genetic programming, a subtree is selected in each program and the two subtrees are swapped. The remaining part of the new population consists of copied programs from the old population (reproduction is the term used for copying old programs) or newly created programs. With a certain probability, the mutation rate, an individual is changed. Mutation can have various forms, most commonly it only changes one function/terminal in a program to a different one. This process is repeated until the termination criterion is reached. The result of the run is usually the program with the best fitness value found during the whole evolution (Poli et al., 2010).

The Java Genetic Algorithms Package (JGAP) (JGAP, 2010) was chosen as the programming platform. JGAP is a Genetic Algorithms and Genetic Programming package written in Java. It is designed to require minimum effort to use, but is also designed to be highly modular. It provides basic genetic mechanisms that can be used to apply evolutionary principles to solve problems.

In order to achieve high accuracy measures such as sensitivity, specificity, CCR and ROC, the following approach was used to automatically fine-tune the GP approach. First, feature selection is performed, then different function sets are analyzed and afterwards the number of generations and population size are investigated.

In all experiments a crossover rate of 0.9 and a mutation rate of 0.1 is used, as well as a population of size 500 is evolved for 300 generations is used for the function set and feature selection. Per generation 10% of the new population is made up by randomly created new individuals, the maximal crossover depth is 12, maximal initial depth is 5, and the maximal number of nodes is 60.

Feature selection resulted in the following features chosen as GP operators as shown in Table 2. As can be seen, for each dataset different features were selected. The common features used for the ventilation datasets are FiO_2, respiratory rate and emergency case. The common features for the mortality datasets are MAP, serum creatinine and chronic.

Different function sets were tested. The function set with the highest CCR and ROC values consisted of the following: *addition, subtraction, multiplication, division, larger than, less than, if, logical and, logical or, power function, square root*. The reason why the function set worked best is because of the *if*, the *logical and*, and the *logical or*, as without these operators the evolved program only consists of one condition.

Population sizes of 500, 700 and 1000 are tested for 100, 200, 300 and 500 generations each. For all data sets the best fitness is indeed achieved for 1000 individuals and 500 generations: 1.493, which corresponds to an improvement of slightly more than 2.24%. Overall, a larger population size seems to have a higher impact than an increase in the number of generations.

EXPERIMENTS AND RESULTS

Tables 3 to 6 show the results of this investigation. The values of sensitivity, specificity, CCR and ROC value are shown for all algorithms tested. The first eight algorithms are run with WEKA, and the other two classifier implementations (NNWEA and AGP) are run independently. In order to assess these results, it is useful to follow a guideline that physician partners with the Carleton research group favor. For example, if a patient is predicted to live, but dies, this is considered worse than if a patient is predicted to die, but lives. In considering this guideline, we therefore need to ensure that

Table 2. Feature selection for GP approach

	Features
Ventilation non-OP	FiO_2, respiratory rate, GCS, PO_2, emergency case, body temperature, pH value, Na value
Ventilation post-OP	Respiratory rate, FiO_2, Na value, emergency case
Mortality non-OP	GCS, FiO_2, MAP, serum creatinine, age, chronic
Mortality post-OP	Emergency case, chronic, heart rate, gender, MAP, PO_2, serum creatinine

the specificity is close to or over 85%, and that the sensitivity is as high as possible, which means better than 65%.

The results below are judged according to this principle. The CCR is not that important to our clinician partners. For ROC, a value greater or equal to 0.80 shows fairly good discrimination ability. For ventilation, it is important to predict long-term use, as this will impact both the patient status and the planning of resources such as the availability of artificial ventilation machines.

As can be seen from Table 3, the AGP and the NNWEA approaches score best in considering a combination of sensitivity and specificity, and the ROC value is over 0.80. The AGP approach does a little better than the NNWEA on sensitivity and a little worse than the NNWEA for specificity. Neither approach reaches the optimal value of 0.85; however, as explained above, this is not very critical. These results can help to plan the use of ventilators in the ICU.

For the next dataset (see Table 4), the scores are as follows: K* ranks best in terms of sensitivity; AGP ranks highest in terms of specificity; the highest value of CCR is achieved by J48; and the ROC value is largest using BN. However, for the overall score, our two approaches meet the guideline and perform better than all other approaches.

Table 5 shows the results of the mortality dataset looking at non-OP patients. A sensitivity of 1 can be observed for SMO; however, the specificity is 0, which implies that the model

Table 3. Ventilation dataset – non-OP

	Sensitivity	Specificity	CCR	ROC
BN	0.793	0.759	0.781	0.853
IBk	0.823	0.560	0.729	0.693
J48	0.803	0.606	0.734	0.679
JRip	0.844	0.653	0.776	0.776
K*	0.911	0.338	0.707	0.772
MP	0.811	0.630	0.747	0.746
NB	0.809	0.690	0.766	0.834
SMO	0.844	0.588	0.753	0.716
NNWEA	0.840	0.750	0.760	0.820
AGP	0.913	0.693	0.772	0.803

specifically classified all unseen instances to one of the two classes (death). Therefore, SMO is not a good choice for this particular dataset. K* achieves the highest sensitivity, NNWEA achieves the highest specificity, CCR is highest using SMO, and the ROC value is largest using BN. For the overall performance, the NNWEA performs best, although more tuning would be needed to increase the specificity, although this would be slightly at the expense of the sensitivity.

The last table (Table 6) shows the same behavior of SMO. Besides that, again K* achieves a very high sensitivity value of 0.998. The highest values for specificity and ROC are achieved

by AGP and the highest CCR value is gained using BN. Here the best overall performing approach is the AGP, which meets the guideline.

In summary, looking at our two approaches, the values of all measures are very comparable, in particular for the two ventilation datasets. For the mortality datasets, much higher values for specificity are achieved by the WEKA algorithms, but sensitivity is fairly low for these approaches. The AGP approach scored best in quite a few categories, as did the NNWEA approach.

Table 4. Ventilation dataset – post-OP

	Sensitivity	Specificity	CCR	ROC
BN	0.910	0.820	0.884	0.934
IBk	0.869	0.548	0.778	0.693
J48	0.930	0.816	0.898	0.869
JRip	0.935	0.784	0.892	0.860
K*	0.952	0.408	0.798	0.841
MP	0.929	0.732	0.873	0.902
NB	0.897	0.680	0.836	0.898
SMO	0.938	0.726	0.878	0.835
NNWEA	0.920	0.860	0.880	0.930
AGP	0.906	0.882	0.890	0.894

Table 5. Mortality dataset – non-OP

	Sensitivity	Specificity	CCR	ROC
BN	0.925	0.368	0.855	0.852
IBk	0.912	0.329	0.839	0.610
J48	0.919	0.303	0.842	0.589
JRip	0.957	0.276	0.872	0.629
K*	0.959	0.237	0.868	0.762
MP	0.930	0.395	0.863	0.805
NB	0.838	0.579	0.806	0.826
SMO	1.000	0.000	0.875	0.500
NNWEA	0.520	0.820	0.690	0.800
AGP	0.921	0.737	0.760	0.829

CONCLUSION

Intensive care medicine most often involves rapid decision-making on the basis of a huge amount of information. ICU physicians often rely on conventional wisdom and personal experience to arrive at assessments and judgments. This requires an intuitive weighting of various factors to achieve an optimal balance between clinical situations that are often competing. There is increasing interest in computer-based decision support tools to automate aspects of the medical decision-making that takes place in complex clinical areas such as the ICU.

For the classification of the medical ICU outcomes "death" and "hours of ventilation", our two approaches (one based on Artificial Neural Networks and the other based on Genetic Programming) were investigated and found to perform better overall than most common machine learning algorithms of WEKA, given certain clinical expectations. As seen from the results of the experiments using the ICU datasets, our two approaches (NNWEA and AGP) are performing very well and are comparable to the algorithms provided by WEKA. In particular, the AGP and NNWEA approaches scored the highest values in some categories.

Table 6. Mortality dataset – post-OP

	Sensitivity	Specificity	CCR	ROC
BN	0.995	0.179	0.969	0.849
IBk	0.988	0.071	0.959	0.537
J48	0.984	0.107	0.956	0.585
JRip	0.987	0.143	0.960	0.567
K*	0.998	0.000	0.967	0.736
MP	0.987	0.071	0.958	0.704
NB	0.950	0.536	0.937	0.854
SMO	1.000	0.000	0.968	0.500
NNWEA	0.670	0.790	0.840	0.770
AGP	0.937	0.893	0.895	0.915

Future work includes further improvements and refinements to the algorithms, as well as the implementation of the algorithms into a classifier suite. This classifier suite would contain all available algorithms and a selection policy, which would run all classifiers, measuring their sensitivity, specificity, CCR and ROC values. Given user specified input on the importance of these four measures, a weighted approach would return the best classifier for a particular dataset. It is likely that this combined approach will increase the performance of a decision support system for critical care in estimating these two outcomes. Other outcomes could be added such as length of stay in the unit, and onset of sepsis for example. Another aspect which could be investigated in the future is to test our approaches with a large medical data set, collected from a different clinical environment, in order to validate them more thoroughly.

REFERENCES

Banzhaf, W., Nordin, P., Keller, R. E., & Francone, F. D. (1998). *Genetic programming: an introduction on the automatic evolution of computer programs and its applications.* San Francisco, CA: Morgan Kaufmann Publishers.

Brown, M. P. S., Grundy, W. N., Lin, D., Cristianini, N., Sugnet, C., Ares, M., & Haussler, D. (1999). *Support Vector Machine Classification of Microarray Gene Expression Data* (Tech. Rep. UCSC-CRL-99-09). Santa Cruz, CA: Department of Computer Science, University of California, Santa Cruz.

Bryson, A. E., & Ho, Y.-C. (1969). *Applied optimal control: optimization, estimation, and control.* New York, NY: Blaisdell Publishing Company and Xerox College Publishing.

Cohen, W. (1995). Fast Effective Rule Induction. In *Proceedings of, ICML-95,* 115–123.

Cover, T., & Hart, P. (1967). Nearest neighbor pattern classification. *IEEE Transactions on Information Theory, 13*(1), 21–27. doi:10.1109/TIT.1967.1053964

Cramer, N. L. (1985). A representation for the Adaptive Generation of Simple Sequential Programs. In J. Grefenstette (Ed.), *Proceedings of the International Conference on Genetic Algorithms and the Applications,* Pittsburgh, PA.

Ennett, C., & Frize, M. (2000). Selective Sampling to Overcome Skewed a Priori Probabilities with Neural Networks. In *Proceedings of the A.M.I.A. (American Medical Informatics Association) Annual Symposium,* Los Angeles, CA.

Ennett, C., & Frize, M. (2003). Weight-Elimination Neural Networks Applied to Coronary Surgery Mortality Prediction. *IEEE Transactions on Information Technology in Biomedicine, 7*(2), 86–92. doi:10.1109/TITB.2003.811881

Ennett, C. M., Frize, M., & Charette, E. (2004). Improvement and automation of artificial neural networks to estimate medical outcomes. *Medical Engineering & Physics, 26*(4), 321–328. doi:10.1016/j.medengphy.2003.09.005

Ennett, C. M., Frize, M., & Scales, N. (2002). Logarithmic-Sensitivity Index as a Stopping Criterion for Neural Networks. In *Proceedings of IEEE/EMBS* (Vol. 1, pp. 74-75).

Frize, M., Solven, F. G., Stevenson, M., Nickerson, B. G., Buskard, T., & Taylor, K. B. (1995, July). Computer-Assisted Decision Support Systems for Patient Management in an Intensive Care Unit. In *Proceedings of Medinfo95,* Vancouver, BC, Canada (pp. 1009-1012).

Frize, M., Weyand, S., & Bariciak, E. (2010, May). Suggested Criteria for Successful Deployment of a Clinical Decision Support System (CDSS). In *Proceedings of the MeMeA (Medical Measurements and Applications) Workshop,* Ottawa, ON, Canada (pp. 69-72).

Good, I. J. (1950). *Probability and the Weighing of Evidence*. London, UK: Charles Grin.

Institute of Medicine. (1999). *To Err Is Human: Building A Safer Health System*. Washington, DC: Author.

Jensen, F. (1996). *An Introduction to Bayesian Networks*. New York, NY: Springer.

JGAP. (2010). *Java Genetic Algorithms Package*. Retrieved from http://jgap.sourceforge.net

Kaplan, B. (2001). Evaluating informatics applications clinical decision support systems literature review. *International Journal of Medical Informatics, 64*, 15–37. doi:10.1016/S1386-5056(01)00183-6

Koza, J. R. (1992). *Genetic Programming: On the Programming of Computers by Means of Natural Selection*. Cambridge, MA: MIT Press.

Mextaxiotis, K., & Samouilidis, J.E. (2000). Expert systems in medicine: academic illusion or real power? *Information Management and Security*, 75-79.

Mitchell, T. (1997). *Machine Learning*. New York, NY: McGraw Hill.

Neves, J., Alves, V., Nelas, L., Romeu, A., & Basto, S. (1999). An Information System that Supports Knowledge Discovery and Data Mining in Medical Imaging. In *Proceedings of the ECCAI Advanced Course in Artificial Intelligence (ACAI) Workshop (W13) on Machine Learning in Medical Applications,* Chania, Greece.

Poli, R., Langdon, W. B., & McPhee, N. F. (2010). *A Field Guide to Genetic Programming*. Retrieved from http://www.gp-eld-guide.org.uk

Quinlan, J. R. (1979). Discovering rules by induction from large collections of examples. In Michie, D. (Ed.), *Expert Systems in the Microlectronic age* (pp. 168–201).

Quinlan, J. R. (1993). *C4.5: Programs for machine learning*. San Francisco, CA: Morgan Kaufmann Publishers.

Rosenblatt, F. (1962). *Priciples of Neurodynamics*. New York, NY: Spartan.

Rybchynski, D. (2005). *Design of an Artificial Neural Network Research Framework to Enhance the Development of Clinical Prediction Models*. Unpublished master's thesis, University of Ottawa, Ottawa, ON, Canada.

Sim, I., Gorman, P., Greenes, R., Hayes, R., Kaplan, B., & Lehmann, H. (2001). Clinical decision support systems for the practice of evidence-based medicine. *Journal of the American Medical Informatics Association, 8*(6), 527–534.

Slonim, D., Tamayo, P., Mesirov, J., Golub, T., & Lander, E. (2000). Class prediction and discovery using gene expression data. In *Proceedings of the 4th Annual International Conference on Computational Molecular Biology (RECOMB)*, Tokyo, Japan (pp. 263-272). Tokyo, Japan: Universal Academy Press.

Vapnik, V. (1995). *The Nature of Statistical Learning Theory*. Berlin, Germany: Springer Verlag.

Wennber, J., & Cooper, M. M. (1999). *The Dartmouth atlas of medical care in the United States: a report on the medicare program*. Chicago, IL: AHA Press.

This work was previously published in International Journal of Computational Models and Algorithms in Medicine, Volume 1, Issue 4, edited by Aryya Gangopadhyay, pp. 19-30, copyright 2010 by IGI Publishing (an imprint of IGI Global)

Chapter 16

Relevance of Mesh Dimension Optimization, Geometry Simplification and Discretization Accuracy in the Study of Mechanical Behaviour of Bare Metal Stents

Mariacristina Gagliardi
University of Pisa, Italy

ABSTRACT

In this paper, a set of analyses on the deployment of coronary stents by using a nonlinear finite element method is proposed. The author proposes a convergence test able to select the appropriate mesh dimension and a methodology to perform the simplification of structures composed of cyclically repeated units to reduce the number of degree of freedom and the analysis run time. A systematic study, based on the analysis of seven meshes for each model, is performed, gradually reducing the element dimension. In addition, geometric models are simplified considering symmetries; adequate boundary conditions are applied and verified based on the results obtained from analysis of the whole model.

INTRODUCTION

The implantation of a coronary stent in human patients in the treatment of the stenosis is a common clinical procedure (El-Menyar *et al.*, 2007; Goodney & Powell, 2008; Zeller, 2007). Stents are metallic cylindrical structures constituted of a cell-repeated pattern. Basing on cell pattern,

stents can be classified as slotted tubes, coil or mesh types (Xia *et al.*, 2007). These devices are rigid scaffolds used to maintain a diseased artery open after the implantation (Timmins, 2007). In order to foresee the mechanical behaviour of the structure and to quantify stresses and strains in the device after the application, computer simulations began to receive attention in the last years, when

DOI: 10.4018/978-1-4666-0282-3.ch016

a number of software tools, based on the Finite Element Method (FEM) were developed. In mechanics, the FEM is the most diffused simulation method, employed to study and predict the physical behaviour of bodies undergoing various external forces that involve complex phenomena like great displacements, large deformation or plasticity.

A large number of studies in literature reports the analysis of the mechanical behaviour of stent devices (Chua *et al.*, 2002; Chua *et al.*, 2004; Etave *et al.*, 2001). Finite Element (FE) models of the whole structure of the stent (Migliavacca *et al.*, 2005; Lally *et al.*, 2005), the half structure or a significant part were analyzed (Chua *et al.*, 2002; Kajzer *et al.*, 2005), taking or not into account the presence of the arterial wall. In addition, other computational models analysed effects of the stent on the blood flow (Lam *et al.*, 2008; LaDisa *et al.*, 2005; LaDisa *et al.*, 2006; Fung *et al.*, 2008).

FE computational analyses employ a mathematical model to describe the real behaviour of the structure being analyzed and a discrete model of the real structure by the use of finite elements. A FE analysis allows determining only an approximate numerical solution of the problem. In order to verify quality and reliability of the computational solution, the gathering of experimental and analytical data is required. However, FE packages generally report a great amount of warnings and errors that help the operator in the adjustment of the modelling process.

The choice of the mathematical model fulfilling to describe the object of the analysis depends on a theory that, in turn, is selected on object geometry, material properties constituting the object, as well as constraints and loads applied to the body. The accurate selection of the mathematical model minimizes the *modelling error*, or rather the error due to the difference between the mathematical function used to describe the theoretical behaviour and the physical property of the analyzed body. During the modelling process, a series of choices are generally made about, for example, the choice to model a thin structures with shell elements,

to simplify a body considering symmetries and to delete features unessential with respect of the whole structure. In addition, a predefined structural model, based on a small number of parameters, can schematize the mechanical behaviour of the employed materials. Furthermore, another important factor concerning the modelling procedure is the schematization of constraints and loads. The modelling error depends on these factors but is independent from the FE dimensions.

Finite elements are little but finite entities, with one, two or three dimensions, used to fill a structure with greater size. Discretisations (*meshes*) are *coarse* or *fine* basing on element size, furnishing solutions with different degrees of precision. From the degree of precision of the mesh arises the *finite-element discretization error*. Generally, a finer mesh allows obtaining results that are more accurate but decreasing the element dimensions an important increase in run time and hardware resource occurs. For this reason, the selection of the best element dimension is important in the optimization of a FE analysis. The selection of the element dimension derives from a systematic procedure that analyse the same problem by using different mesh dimensions and monitoring the trend of one or more interesting parameters in one or more nodal points. This systematic procedure is generally indicated as *convergence test*.

After the optimisation of the mesh size, it is suitable to simplify the problem and limit the number of degree of freedom in order to reduce the analysis time. The reduction of the geometry of the body represents one method of simplification. This procedure depends on the presence of symmetries of the whole structure and is not possible in all cases. When the simplification of the geometry can be performed, a fundamental step is represented by the identification of the symmetries and the choice of appropriate boundary conditions. This simplification procedure appears particularly important in problems where the whole structure being analyzed is composed of cyclically repeated units. In these cases, simplifications allow appreciably reducing the degrees of freedom of the analysis and then the calculation time.

The present work analyses both the optimization of the mesh dimension and the simplification of the geometry. The convergence test was carried out analyzing seven different mesh dimensions on three different geometries of commercial stents (Palmaz, Cypher and Multi-link Mini Vision). Results obtained with different meshes were compared and the convergence values of the numerical solutions were evaluated. It led to designate the best element dimensions for each geometry, in order to obtain results that are poorly affected by the discretisation error and, consequently, to reduce the analysis time. In addition, geometries were simplified analyzing the whole structure as well as two different simplified geometries for each device, comparing results to verify if the simplification process was correctly performed and if the boundary conditions, applied after the simplification of the structure were appropriate.

PROBLEM DESCRIPTION

The mechanical analysis of the deployment of a bare stent involves several different problems. The stent structure undergoes large deformations, changing its configuration with a nonlinear response. Furthermore, a nonlinear σ-ε relationship generally occurs when a material suffers large deformations or heavy loads. In the expansion of a balloon-expandable bare metal stent, in order to ensure the perviety of the blood vessel after the balloon deflation, a plastic deformation is necessary.

The numerical solution of a strongly nonlinear problem is possible only through an iterative numerical method.

To perform the optimization of two different procedures (the selection of the mesh dimension and the simplification of the geometry) it is necessary to have a standard method for the resolution of the problem in order to reach results not affected by the manual work of the operator. For this reason, the manual work was limited only to the migration of the parametric geometrical model from the CAD software to the FE software, used as pre-processor, solver and post-processor. A batch file, containing all the necessary command lines and the same numerical parameters for each analysis, automatically carried out the meshing procedure and the numerical solution, modifying only the mesh dimension in the case of the convergence test. It ensured the absence of errors of the operator.

In this work, loads were statically applied but the numerical method employed a discretisation of the load into a series of small increments. During the solving procedure, several numerical divergences occurred and dealt with the selection of the right solving scheme. On the other hand, in a systematic optimization procedure, it is important to minimize the divergence occurrences. This implies a careful choose of the solution control options. The description of the calculation algorithm and the explanation of the numerical parameters are following reported.

Constitutive Material Model

Stents were considered composed of AISI 316L stainless steel and a bilinear σ-ε curve (Equation 1) accurately schematizes its mechanical behaviour, described only by the Young modulus (E) in the linear elastic range, the first yield stress ($\sigma_{0,ys}$) and the tangent modulus (E_t) when plastic phenomena occurred. Mechanical parameters introduced into the mathematical model were (Gijsen *et al.*, 2008): $E_x = 193$ GPa, Poisson ratio $\nu = 0.27$, $\sigma_{0,ys} = 207$ MPa, $E_t = 692$ MPa (Feng *et al.*, 2008). The Von Mises plasticity criterion with isotropic hardening schematized the inelastic response of the material.

$$\sigma(\varepsilon) = if\left[\varepsilon < \varepsilon_{0,ys}, E \cdot \varepsilon, \sigma_{0,ys} + E_t \cdot \left(\varepsilon - \varepsilon_{0,ys}\right)\right]$$

(1)

Algorithm of Calculation

In the presence of large displacements and deformations and the nonlinearity due to the material plasticity, the use of a full Newton-Raphson (NR) mathematical method is advisable. The method provides to updates the stiffness matrix at each equilibrium iteration. The NR method convergence criterion generally consists of guarantying that the greater residual in the balance equations and the greater correction to any nodal unknown, evaluated during the current iteration, are sufficiently small. In the present work the condition to satisfy was that both residual force and moment were smaller than 0.005.

MATERIALS AND METHODS

In this work, three different commercial stent structures were considered: Palmaz, Cypher and Multi-link Mini Vision stents. The author performed this research only to reach a best understanding of the mechanical properties of different structures, characterized by different unit cells, and without any sponsor.

The geometries of the Cypher and the Multi-link Mini Vision stents present two different types of elements: tubular-like rings and bridging links. Rings have the specific function to scaffold the vessel after the stenting procedure and are the more stressed structures during the expansion of the device. Bridging links longitudinally connect rings in a flexible way and they are fundamental during the stent positioning, giving the appropriate flexibility to the structure. On this consideration, it is reasonable to identify a single unit of the stent, constituted of two rings and at least one longitudinal link that could be used to study the overall behaviour of the whole structure. Otherwise, the geometry of the Palmaz stent does not contain rings and the repetition of the typical closed cell constitutes the whole structure.

The machine used to carry out analyses was a desktop pc with a Intel® Core™ 2 Duo CPU T6600 (2.20 GHz) with 4 Gb of RAM.

3D Geometrical Models

Geometric data of stents were gathered from the web. Geometric models were obtained using the parametric Pro|ENGINEER WildFire 2.0 (Parametric Technology Corporation, Needham, MA).

Stent initial diameters, radial expansions and radial strains are reported in Table 1. Final diameter imposed was 3.1 mm; filament thickness was 0.1 mm.

Importing the Geometry

ANSYS 12.0 (ANSYS Inc., Canonsburg, PA) as pre-processor, solver and post-processor was used. FE models were prepared using the APDL package for a better control of all parameters.

CAD geometries were imported from Pro|ENGINEER to ANSYS previously saving the parametric CAD models in.igs format, then the ANSYS /AUX15 command and the IOPTN options were used to import the.igs file in the FE software. During the importing process, an automatic *merging procedure* was performed with a consideration tolerance equal to 75% of the shortest distance between the endpoints of the active lines. Small areas were deleted to avoid geometrical inconsistencies that could cause the aborting of the import process. During the importation, the software automatically created solids.

Table 1. Initial stent diameters and imposed constraints in terms of difference of diameter

Stent	Initial diameter [mm]	Δd [mm]	ε_r
Palmaz Stent	1.13	1.97	1.74
Cypher Stent	1.10	2.00	1.82
Multi-link Vision Stent	1.13	1.97	1.74

Element Attribution

Meshes of stents were composed of 10-nodes tetrahedral structural SOLID92 *h*-elements. Nodes associated to these elements have three degrees of freedom in the translations on *x*, *y* and *z* directions. These elements support large deflections and strains and several plasticity models could be associated. These elements have quadratic displacement behaviour and are suited to model irregular geometries.

Application of Loads and Constraints

FE analyses were performed applying a fixed radial displacement (different for the used geometries, as reported in Table 1) on the nodes lying onto the internal surface of the structures to reproduce the balloon inflation and the stent expansion.

The choice to expand the structures through the application of a nodal displacement was a strong simplification of the balloon inflation. Several studies analysed models of stent expansions by the inflation of a balloon, with different geometries (Kiousis *et al.*, 2009; Li *et al.*, 2009, Hall & Kasper, 2006; Takashima *et al.*, 2007; Wu *et al.*, 2007), paying a particular attention to the contact phenomena between the balloon and the stent occurring during this process. Other works (Migliavacca *et al.*, 2004; Holzapfel *et al.*, 2005; De Beule *et al.*, 2006; Migliavacca *et al.*, 2002) simulated the balloon inflation with the application of a pressure to the internal struts of the stent, reproducing accurately the stent deployment. A FE analysis including a balloon is necessary to model more accurately the expansion characteristics of a stent (De Beule *et al.*, 2008) like dogboning. When the aim of the research is the determination of the stresses within a stented vessel, it is appropriate to expand the stent to the same shape as that which would occur under the action of a balloon (Pericevic *et al.*, 2009) by the applica-

tion of a pressure. However, differences in the stent expansion were reported in a previous work (Gervaso *et al.*, 2008). Since the aim of this work was the optimisation of a model describing the free expansion of the bare stent and the biological tissues were not considered, the stent deployment was reproduced without considering other aspects and the simplified expansion, produced only by the application of nodal displacements, resulted adequate to the present work.

In order to prevent rigid body motions during the stent deployment, weak springs were manually generated using COMBIN14 elements. Two nodes with three degrees of freedom (translation on *x*, *y* and *z* plane) define COMBIN14 elements. The number of links generated depended on the analyzed structure. The number of weak springs added to make intrinsically hyperstatic the models is reported in Table 2. Applied links were generated as longitudinal springs setting the KEYOPT(3) on 0. The spring constant was $1 \cdot 10^{-3}$ N/mm.

Simplification of the Geometries

In order to reduce the degrees of freedom of the models and then to reduce errors related to the discretization and the calculation time, stent structures were simplified using geometric symmetries. Geometries showed periodicities in both longitudinal and circumferential directions. Structures could be decomposed into repeatable unit cells (the single mesh), obtaining a significant simplification of the geometry. After the geometry simplification, some boundary conditions allowed reproducing accurate results. Results obtained analysing simplified geometries needs to be verified comparing results with those obtained from the whole model. For this aim, in order to understand all numerical phenomena occurring during the deployment of the simplified structures, the simplification of the structures was tackled in two steps: in the first step, only one symmetry was considered and the starting model was halved, in

Table 2. Number of weak springs added to make hyperstatic the models

Device	Model	Number of cells	Number of weak springs
Palmaz stent	Whole structure	12	24
	Half-portion	6	12
	Unit cell	1	2
Cypher stent	Whole structure	6	12
	Half-portion	3	6
	Unit cell	1	2
Multi-link Mini Vision stent	Whole structure	4	8
	Half-portion	2	4
	Unit cell	1	2

the second step, only the fundamental structure of the stent (the unit cell) was studied. After every simplification, appropriate boundary conditions were applied and verified.

Three different geometries were constructed for each stent. All geometries constructed are reported in Figure 1.

Convergence Test

In order to carry out the convergence test, seven different meshes per geometry were generated. ANSYS automatically generates *smart* meshes with the command SMRTSIZE. In the present work, this command was used to define seven different size levels for the mesh, from the level 1 (finer) to the level 7 (coarser). In Table 3 the number of nodes and elements for each mesh are summarized.

An element shape test verified the quality of the meshes controlling three different parameters: aspect ratio, maximum corner angle and Jacobian ratio. In Table 4 the limit values used to perform the test are reported. All geometries passed the test.

In order to study the influence of the mesh on the results, three nodes for each mesh were selected and the plastic equivalent stress was monitored at selected nodes.

RESULTS AND DISCUSSION

Following, results obtained from convergence tests are summarised. Even if analyses were performed on all models, because results were very similar and important differences were not highlighted after geometry simplification, only results related to models A are reported.

Convergence Test

Palmaz Stent

In previous works (Xia *et al.*, 2007; Feng *et al.*, 2008; Dumolin & Cochelin, 2000) the sensitivity of the results by varying the element dimension was not considered. In the work of Narracott et al. (2007) this problem was studied but the convergence analysis was performed in a smaller range of element size obtaining results not affected by the mesh. The present work showed great differences of the results obtained by analyzing meshes composed of coarser elements. In particular, results obtained with meshes with element size level (ESL) from 1 to 5 were very similar and the percentage error due to the mesh dimension $\%\varepsilon_{mesh}$ (Equation 2) was always smaller than 1%. The equivalent plastic stress (NLSEPL, in the ANSYS notation) related to the Palmaz stent in three different nodes versus the number of nodes is reported in Figure 2a.

Results indicated that coarser meshes furnished results with $\%\varepsilon_{mesh}$ up to 5.5% in respect to meshes with ESL from 1 to 5 and then results were considered not reliable. In the ESL range from 1 to 5 important differences in analysis time occurred. A good compromise between quality of the solution, hardware resources consumption and

Figure 1. Geometries studied: whole structures (A), half-portions (B) and unit cells (C)

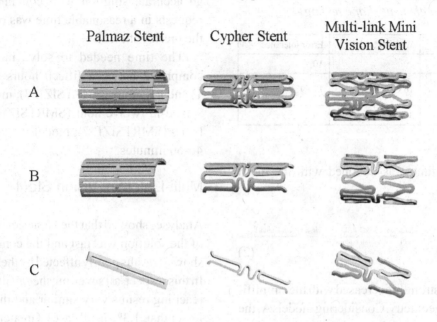

Table 3. Number of nodes and elements related to smart meshes for each studied model

Number of nodes									
	Palmaz			Cypher			Multi-link Mini Vision		
SMRTSIZE	A	B	C	A	B	C	A	B	C
1	425445	153484	22597	135488	116330	23443	304368	152192	77805
2	312723	129161	16836	119580	92444	20082	243663	122201	60145
3	271485	95535	14838	77685	72267	13546	189927	94281	46190
4	242030	85868	12276	59218	54992	10074	131525	65087	30273
5	166118	69422	10005	38212	40331	6331	82505	41118	20838
6	164796	68658	9942	36053	34387	6104	68951	34187	17317
7	120057	55193	7490	20775	23046	3395	42708	21231	10324
Number of elements									
	Palmaz Stent			Cypher Stent			Multi-link Mini Vision		
SMRTSIZE	A	B	C	A	B	C	A	B	C
1	273514	98085	13599	79267	71313	13750	190673	95236	48759
2	196917	82431	9834	69419	55928	11646	150720	75565	37030
3	169711	58875	8623	42972	43381	7519	115656	57227	28037
4	150676	52411	6997	31823	32492	5403	77594	38262	17602
5	99709	42036	5559	19369	23116	3181	46159	22980	11569
6	99388	41596	5498	18483	19403	3115	37813	18688	9470
7	70770	32939	3992	9720	12617	1548	22275	11030	5330

Table 4. Warning and error tolerances imposed to perform the element shape testing

	Warning tolerance	Error tolerance
Aspect ratio	20	10^6
Maximum corner angle	165°	179.9°
Jacobian ratio	30	10^3

analysis run-time was obtained with the mesh with ESL = 5.

$$\%\varepsilon_{mesh} = \frac{|\text{NLSEPL with mesh dimension } x - \text{NLSEPL in the mesh reference model}|}{\text{NLSEPL in the mesh reference model}} \cdot 100$$

(2)

Run time strongly decreased with the simplification of the geometry. Considering models A, the time needed to solve the models was comprised between five hours (SMRTSIZE 1) and two hours (SMRTSIZE 7); models B were solved in one hour (SMRTSIZE 1) or 20 minutes (SMRTSIZE 7); models C were fast solved in few minutes (5-10 minutes for all SMRTSIZEs).

Cypher Stent

A previous work (Mortier *et al.*, 2008) reports that the variation of the mesh dimension caused a variation in the results smaller than 1%. In the present analysis, the convergence of the solution for this device was very difficult and only meshes with ESL from 1 to 3 allowed obtaining results that could be considered not affected by the mesh dimensions. The variation in NLSEPL versus the number of nodes for this geometry is reported in Figure 2b. Considering finer meshes, the $\%\varepsilon_{mesh}$ assumed values smaller than 0.005% while errors in the results with coarser meshes, with reference of the finer meshes, were comprised in the range 2.2%-5.8% and then results could be considered not acceptable. A good compromise to obtain an accurate solution with contained hardware requests in a reasonable time was obtained with the mesh with ESL = 3.

The time needed to solve models A was comprised between fifteen hours (SMRTSIZE 1) and ten hours (SMRTSIZE 7); models B were solved in twelve hour (SMRTSIZE 1) or seven hours (SMRTSIZE 7); models C were solved in 40-60 minutes.

Multi-Link Mini Vision Stent

Analyses showed that the numerical convergence of the solution was fast and the convergence test showed results poorly affected by the element size. In this respect, all seven meshes analyzed allowed reaching results very similar and the $\%\varepsilon_{mesh}$ was lower than 1.3% in all cases. Greater errors (from 1% to 1.3%) were obtained considering results obtained using meshes with ESL = 6 and 7, in respect to finer meshes. For this reason, it could be considered acceptable analyzing this device with a mesh with ESL = 5, that allowed containing the percentage mesh error lower than 0.1%, limiting the analysis run time and the hardware resource requests. In Figure 2c it could be noted that values of NLSEPL obtained in three different nodes by varying the element size were very similar.

The time needed to solve models A was comprised between seven hours (SMRTSIZE 1) and four hours (SMRTSIZE 7); models B were solved in two hour (SMRTSIZE 1) or one hour (SMRTSIZE 7); models C were solved in 20-40 minutes.

Simplification of the Geometries

Three different geometries for each stent were analyzed to study the influence of the simplification of the structure. Meshes used in this analysis had ESL = 5 for Palmaz stent, ESL = 3 for Cypher stent and ESL = 5 for Multi-link Mini Vision stent.

Figure 2. NLSEPL [MPa] obtained at three nodes versus the number of nodes of the mesh in the Palmaz (a), Cypher (b) and Multi-link Mini Vision (c) stents

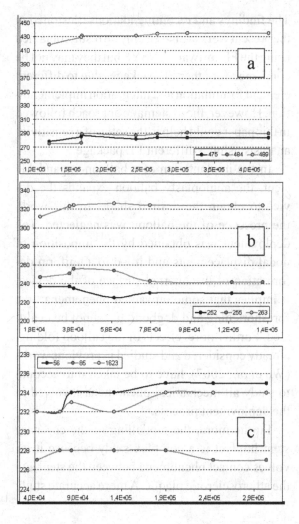

Palmaz Stent

The analysis of the results was performed comparing the maximum value of NLSEPL registered in the model. Each model showed the maximum value of NLSEPL in the same point of the structure, where the vertical joints link together the longitudinal elements. Results are reported in Table 5.

The whole model and the half-portion gave similar results while, from the analysis on the unit cell, registered values were generally different.

In this last case, the percentage error related to the simplification of the structure %ε_{geom} (Equation 3) was 2.24%.

$$\%\varepsilon_{geom} = \frac{|\text{Max NLSEPL in the whole model - Max NLSEPL in the model of interest}|}{\text{Max NLSEPL in the whole model}} \cdot 100$$

(3)

It could be due to the applied boundary conditions that are not suitable to describe accurately the behaviour of the cell with respect to the whole structure. A more accurate work (Xia *et al.*, 2007) described more in detail this aspect. However, the results obtained in the present work are comparable with those obtained in the above-mentioned reference paper.

This error related to the simplification of the structure has to be considered after the analysis in the interpretation of the results. The simplification introduces a small but not negligible error representing a further limitation of the computational study. Errors due to the simplification of the geometry evaluated for the models B and C are summarized in Table 5. In Figure 3 the NLSEPL distribution maps of all models are reported.

Table 5. Maximum value of NLSEPL registered in analysed models [MPa]

Palmaz Stent			
Model	A	B	C
Max NLSEPL	626	625	612
%ε_{geom}	-	0.16	2.24
Cypher Stent			
Model	A	B	C
Max NLSEPL	582	601	592
%ε_{geom}	-	3.26	1.72
Multi-link Mini Vision Stent			
Model	A	B	C
Max NLSEPL	552	557	555
%ε_{geom}	-	0.90	0.54

Cypher Stent

As previously described, it is reasonable to consider a single (open) unit of the stent, constituted of two portions of rings and one longitudinal link, to study the overall behaviour of the whole structure.

In Table 5 the maximum values of NLSEPL obtained for each model and the $\%\varepsilon_{geom}$ are reported. It could be notice that in both simplified geometries the evaluated error was not negligible. It could mean that simplified geometries are suitable only for a rough analysis and accurate results need to be obtained with the whole model.

In Figure 4 the NLSEPL distribution maps of all models are reported.

Multi-Link Mini Vision Stent

As discussed in the case of the Cypher stent, also the Multi-link Mini Vision stent showed a unit open cell, constituted of two portions of radial rings and one longitudinal link. In Table 5 the maximum values of NLSEPL and the $\%\varepsilon_{geom}$ are reported. In this case, evaluated errors were < 1% confirming that the simplification in this case can involve a good improvement in the FE analysis, introducing only small errors and allowing a significant reduction in number of equations to solve. In Figure 5 the NLSEPL distribution maps of all models are reported.

LIMITATIONS, USEFULNESS AND FURTHER DEVELOPMENT OF THE STUDY

The findings and recommendations illustrated in the present work are based only on results obtained using the FE software ANSYS but they may not be confirmed for other FE packages due to different element formulation and integration implementation. However, the systematic approach followed in this paper could help in the setup of a sensitivity analysis using a different FE package.

In the implantation of a balloon-expandable stent, the angioplasty balloon expands the device to obtain the desired shape. In this work, the presence of the balloon was neglected. The deployment was obtained by the imposition of nodal displacements and it led to a uniform deformation of the internal surface of the device. It implies that some unwanted phenomena, like foreshortening and dogboning, cannot be evaluated. Furthermore, effects of the balloon folding, already considered and studied in previous works (Wu *et al.*, 2007), have to be taken into account to study all mechanical phenomena involved in the deployment process.

Furthermore, the modelling of the coronary stent implant is a complex study because it involves contact phenomena between the stent and the atherosclerotic plaque. A more accurate study

Figure 3. NLSEPL obtained in the whole model (left), the half-portion (middle) and the unit cell (right) of the Palmaz Stent

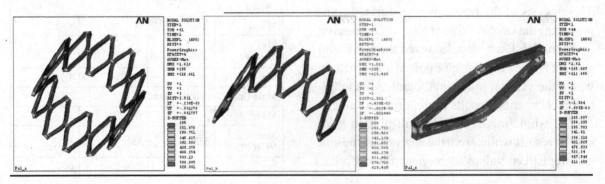

Figure 4. NLSEPL obtained in the whole model (left), the half-portion (middle) and the unit cell (right) of the Cypher Stent

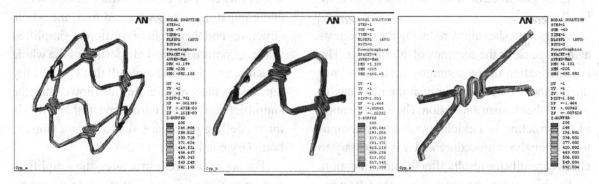

on the stent deployment process cannot neglect this aspect.

This study illustrates only how to quantify errors related to the modelling process and how to optimize the analysis minimizing the errors due to the modelling process. In addition, the proposed method is related only to the study the commercial stents considered in this paper but it could represent a starting point to improve the analysis of different devices under development and a basis for more advanced studies.

Further developments of the present study are a convergence test and the analysis of the influence of geometry simplifications considering the use of a balloon to expand the stent. Only when these results will be available, contact between stent and atherosclerotic plaque, which has a huge effect on the mesh sensitivity, will be analysed.

CONCLUSION

The aim of the present study was to outline some guidelines in the right choice and in the correct individuation of the mesh to perform computational analyses of bare coronary stents.

In the analysis of the mechanical behaviour of endovascular stents and the phenomena related to the stenting procedure, strong nonlinear phenomena, due to the plasticity of the materials and to the large displacements and deformations, occurred. For this reason, in order to simplify the analysis and to reduce the calculation time, it is important to optimize the problem with the best choice of the mesh dimensions. Generally, it is a common practice to use fine meshes to obtain more accurate results but with the increase of the requested resources, also introducing problems

Figure 5. NLSEPL obtained in the whole model (left), the half-portion (middle) and the unit cell (right) of the Multi-link Mini Vision Stent

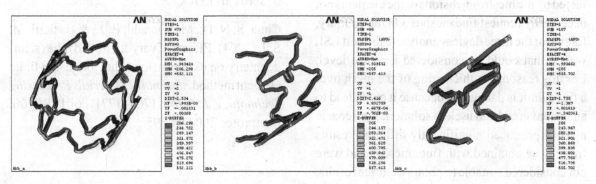

related to the convergence of the solution. This common practice could be not properly suitable in all cases.

Coarser meshes allow reducing these requests at the expense of the accuracy of the analysis. The right reduction of the geometry permits to limit the number of elements without the necessity to increase the element dimension. The simplification of the structure is a crucial event in the computational analysis procedure and it is necessary to check carefully the results after the simplification.

In this paper, two different aspects were considered, in particular: the effect of the mesh dimension and the simplification of the geometry.

The effect of the mesh dimension was studied through a convergence test, analyzing three different commercial devices (Palmaz stent, Cypher stent and Multi-link Mini Vision stent) and seven different meshes for each structure. Geometries were also simplified taking into account the geometric symmetries of the whole structure and a convergence test was also carried out on the simplified geometries.

The effect of the simplification of the structures was analyzed through the comparison of the results obtained with the seven meshes proposed. This comparison also allowed evaluating the accuracy in the application of the boundary conditions proposed after the simplification of the structures.

Results obtained after the convergence analysis showed that finer meshes introduced serious problems related to the convergence of the solution, especially in more complex structures with a greater number of nodes. Solutions poorly affected by the mesh dimensions of the elements not necessarily request fine meshes. On the contrary, for two of the three devices analyzed, the best ESL was 5, that could be considered a coarse level. For this reason, the thickening of the mesh over a fixed limit is dangerous because it could lead to an unconverged and useless solution. Very coarse meshes produced significantly different results from those obtained with finer meshes and were not considered suitable to obtain accurate results.

The effect of the simplification of the structure was evaluated on the considered devices, analyzing and comparing results obtained from the whole structures and then from two different simplified models, comprising the half-portion of the whole structure and the basic unit cell that is cyclically repeated in the structure. Results showed that the simplification process introduced further errors in the modelling procedure, related to not suitable boundary conditions.

Basing on different structures, the simplification errors were different. For example, the analysis of the half-portion of the Palmaz stent caused a smaller error while, considering the closed cell, the error was greater than 2%. It means that the operator can decide if the error could be considered acceptable or not.

Even if computational methods present a very high potential in the analysis of several engineering problems, the understanding of limitations of the modelling procedure and of the necessary level of accuracy is essential to reach comprehensible and plausible results without forgetting that, in any case, like in every science areas, the knowledge and sensibility of the operator is fundamental to obtain reasonable and proper results.

REFERENCES

Chua, S. N. D., MacDonald, B. J., & Hashmi, M. S. J. (2002). Finite-element simulation of stent expansion. *Journal of Materials Processing Technology, 120*, 335–340. doi:10.1016/S0924-0136(01)01127-X

Chua, S. N. D., MacDonald, B. J., & Hashmi, M. S. J. (2004). Effects of varying slotted tube (stent) geometry on its expansion behaviour using finite element method. *Journal of Materials Processing Technology, 155-156*, 1764–1771. doi:10.1016/j.jmatprotec.2004.04.395

De Beule, M., Mortier, P., Carlier, S. G., Verhegghe, B., Van Impe, R., & Verdonck, P. (2008). Realistic finite element-based stent design: the impact of balloon folding. *Journal of Biomechanics, 41*(2), 383–389. doi:10.1016/j.jbiomech.2007.08.014

De Beule, M., Van Impe, R., Verhegghe, B., Segers, P., & Verdonck, P. (2006). Finite element analysis and stent design: reduction of dogboning. *Technology and Health Care, 14*, 233–241.

Dumoulin, C., & Cochelin, B. (2000). Mechanical behaviour modelling of balloon-expandable stents. *Journal of Biomechanics, 33*(11), 1461–1470. doi:10.1016/S0021-9290(00)00098-1

El-Menyar, A. A., Al Suwaidi, J., & Holmes, D. R. (2007). Left main coronary artery stenosis: state-of-the-art. *Current Problems in Cardiology, 32*, 103–193. doi:10.1016/j.cpcardiol.2006.12.002

Etave, F., Finet, G., Boivin, M., Boyer, J., Rioufol, G., & Thollet, G. (2001). Mechanical properties of coronary stents determined by using finite element analysis. *Journal of Biomechanics, 34*(8), 1065–1075. doi:10.1016/S0021-9290(01)00026-4

Feng, J., Zihui, X., & Katsuhiko, S. (2008). On the finite element modelling of balloon-expandable stents. *Journal of the Mechanical Behavior of Biomedical Materials, 1*(1), 86–95. doi:10.1016/j.jmbbm.2007.07.002

Fung, G. S. K., Lam, S. K., Cheng, S. W. K., & Chow, K. W. (2008). On stent-graft models in thoracic aortic endovascular repair: A computational investigation of the hemodynamic factors. *Computers in Biology and Medicine, 38*, 484–489. doi:10.1016/j.compbiomed.2008.01.012

Gervaso, F., Capelli, C., Petrini, L., Lattanzio, S., Di Virgilio, L., & Migliavacca, F. (2008). On the effects of different strategies in modelling balloon-expandable stenting by means of finite element method. *Journal of Biomechanics, 41*(6), 1206–1212. doi:10.1016/j.jbiomech.2008.01.027

Gijsen, F. J. H., Migliavacca, F., Schievano, S., Socci, L., Petrini, L., & Thury, A. (2008). Simulation of stent deployment in a realistic human coronary artery. *Biomedical Engineering Online, 7*, 23. doi:10.1186/1475-925X-7-23

Goodney, P. P., & Powell, R. J. (2008). Carotid artery stenting: what have we learned from the clinical trials and registries and where do we go from here? *Annals of Vascular Surgery, 22*, 148–158. doi:10.1016/j.avsg.2007.10.002

Hall, G. J., & Kasper, E. P. (2006). Comparison of element technologies for modeling stent expansion. *Journal of Biomechanical Engineering, 128*, 751–756. doi:10.1115/1.2264382

Holzapfel, G. A., Stadler, M., & Gasser, T. C. (2005). Changes in the mechanical environment of stenotic arteries during interaction with stents: computational assessment of parametric stent designs. *Journal of Biomechanical Engineering, 127*, 166–180. doi:10.1115/1.1835362

Kajzer, W., Kaczmarek, M., & Marciniak, J. (2005). Biomechanical analysis of stent - oesophagus system. *Journal of Materials Processing Technology, 162-163*, 196–202. doi:10.1016/j.jmatprotec.2005.02.209

Kiousis, D. E., Wulff, A. R., & Holzapfel, G. A. (2009). Experimental studies and numerical analysis of the inflation and interaction of vascular balloon catheter-stent systems. *Annals of Biomedical Engineering, 37*(2), 315–330. doi:10.1007/s10439-008-9606-9

LaDisa, J. F., Olson, L. E., Hettrick, D. A., Warltier, D. C., Kersten, J. R., & Pagel, P. S. (2005). Axial stent strut angle influences wall shear stress after stent implantation: analysis using 3D computational fluid dynamics models of stent foreshortening. *Biomedical Engineering Online*, *4*, 59. doi:10.1186/1475-925X-4-59

LaDisa, J. F., Olson, L. E., Hettrick, D. A., Warltier, D. C., Kersten, J. R., & Pagel, P. S. (2006). Alterations in regional vascular geometry produced by theoretical stent implantation influence distributions of wall shear stress: analysis of a curved coronary artery using 3D computational fluid dynamics modelling. *Biomedical Engineering Online*, *5*, 40. doi:10.1186/1475-925X-5-40

Lally, C., Dolan, F., & Prendergast, P. J. (2005). Cardiovascular stent design and vessel stresses: a finite element analysis. *Journal of Biomechanics*, *38*(8), 1574–1581. doi:10.1016/j.jbiomech.2004.07.022

Lam, S. K., Fung, G. S. K., Cheng, S. W. K., & Chow, K. W. (2008). A computational study on the biomechanical factors related to stent-graft models in the thoracic aorta. *Medical & Biological Engineering & Computing*, *46*, 1129–1138. doi:10.1007/s11517-008-0361-8

Li, N., Zhang, H., & Ouyang, H. (2009). Shape optimization of coronary artery stent based on a parametric model. *Finite Elements in Analysis and Design*, *45*(6-7), 468–475. doi:10.1016/j.finel.2009.01.001

Migliavacca, F., Petrini, L., Colombo, M., Auricchio, F., & Pietrabissa, R. (2002). Mechanical behavior of coronary stents investigated through the finite element method. *Journal of Biomechanics*, *35*, 803–811. doi:10.1016/S0021-9290(02)00033-7

Migliavacca, F., Petrini, L., Massarotti, P., Schievano, S., Auricchio, F., & Dubini, G. (2004). Stainless and shape memory alloy coronary stents: a computational study on the interaction with the vascular wall. *Biomechanics and Modeling in Mechanobiology*, *2*, 205–217. doi:10.1007/s10237-004-0039-6

Migliavacca, F., Petrini, L., Montanari, V., Quagliana, I., Auricchio, F., & Dubini, G. (2005). A predictive study of the mechanical behaviour of coronary stents by computer modelling. *Medical Engineering & Physics*, *27*(1), 13–18. doi:10.1016/j.medengphy.2004.08.012

Mortier, P., De Beule, M., Carlier, S. G., Van Impe, R., Verhegghe, B., & Verdonck, P. (2008). Numerical Study of the Uniformity of Balloon-Expandable Stent Deployment. *Journal of Biomechanical Engineering*, *130*(2), 021018. doi:10.1115/1.2904467

Narracott, A. J., Lawford, P. V., Gunn, J. P. G., & Hose, D. R. (2007). Balloon folding affects the symmetry of stent deployment: Experimental and computational evidence. In *Proceedings of the 29th Annual International Conference of IEEE-EMBS, Engineering in Medicine and Biology Society, EMBC'07* (pp. 3069-3073).

Pericevic, I., Lally, C., Toner, D., & Kelly, D. J. (2009). The influence of plaque composition on underlying arterial wall stress during stent expansion: The case for lesion-specific stents. *Medical Engineering & Physics*, *31*(4), 428–433. doi:10.1016/j.medengphy.2008.11.005

Takashima, K., Kitou, T., Mori, K., & Ikeuchi, K. (2007). Simulation and experimental observation of contact conditions between stents and artery models. *Medical Engineering & Physics*, *29*, 326–335. doi:10.1016/j.medengphy.2006.04.003

Timmins, L. H., Moreno, M. R., Meyer, C. A., Criscione, J. C., Rachev, A., & Moore, J. E. (2007). Stented artery biomechanics and device design optimization. *Medical & Biological Engineering & Computing, 45*, 505–513. doi:10.1007/s11517-007-0180-3

Wu, W., Wang, W. Q., Yang, D. Z., & Qi, M. (2007). Stent expansion in curved vessel and their interactions: a finite element analysis. *Journal of Biomechanics, 40*, 2580–2585. doi:10.1016/j.jbiomech.2006.11.009

Xia, Z., Ju, F., & Sasaki, K. (2007). A general finite element analysis method for balloon expandable stents based on repeated unit cell (RUC) model. *Finite Elements in Analysis and Design, 43*, 649–658. doi:10.1016/j.finel.2007.01.001

Zeller, T. (2007). Current state of endovascular treatment of femoro-popliteal artery disease. *Vascular Medicine, 12*, 223–234. doi:10.1177/1358863X07079823

This work was previously published in International Journal of Computational Models and Algorithms in Medicine, Volume 1, Issue 4, edited by Aryya Gangopadhyay, pp. 31-45, copyright 2010 by IGI Publishing (an imprint of IGI Global).

Chapter 17
Home Blood Pressure Measurement:
A Review

Gurmanik Kaur
SLIET, India

Ajat Shatru Arora
SLIET, India

Vijender Kumar Jain
SLIET, India

ABSTRACT

Hypertension, the leading global risk factor for early mortality, cannot be detected or treated without accurate and practical methods of blood pressure (BP) measurement. Although home BP measurement has considerable popularity among patients, the lack of evidence needed to assure its place in modern clinical practice has hindered its widespread acceptance among physicians. This paper demonstrates that home BP measurement is more accurate than conventional clinic and ambulatory monitoring BP measurement and can be used effectively in clinical practice. On the basis of the data from different studies, it can be concluded that home BP measurement is an improvement over conventional clinic BP measurement. Home monitoring of BP is a convenient, accurate, and widely available option and may become the method of choice when diagnosing and treating hypertension. A paradigm shift is needed in BP measurement as evidence-based medicine suggests that clinic BP measurement should only be used for screening purposes.

INTRODUCTION

A few risk factors account for a large contribution to global loss of healthy life. Overall, 26% of the worldwide adult population had high BP i.e. hypertension (clinic BP ≥ 140 mmHg systolic and/or 90 mmHg diastolic) in 2000 and 29% are projected to have this condition in 2025 (Kearney, et al. 2005). Hypertension has been identified as the third most important cause for global burden of disease and as the leading global risk factor for mortality, accounting for over 7 million deaths

DOI: 10.4018/978-1-4666-0282-3.ch017

yearly (Ezzati et al., 2002). The risks of high BP are not only limited to those with severe hypertension, as there is a continuous relationship with cardiovascular risk even throughout the normal range of usual BP (down at least as far as 115/75 mmHg). Lowering of the systolic BP by only 10 mmHg, or lowering the diastolic BP by only 5 mmHg would, in the long term, be associated with a lower risk (about 40%) of stroke death and a lower risk (about 30%) of death from ischemic heart disease or other vascular causes throughout middle age (Lewington et al., 2002).

BP, however, cannot be prevented, detected, treated and controlled without accurate and practical methods of measurement. If proper methods are not used, inexact BP measurement can lead to poor diagnostic accuracy, unnecessary costs and therapy, and poor medical treatment. Despite several limitations, measurement of BP has until recently occurred primarily at the physician's office using a stethoscope and a conventional mercury sphygmomanometer. The technological advances during the past decade have provided novel options for measuring BP, such as home monitoring, which is becoming increasingly popular world-wide (Burton, 2006).

One of the reasons why home BP measurement has not received widespread acceptance in the minds of physicians, despite its considerable popularity with patients, is a lack of evidence needed to assure its place in modern clinical practice. This paper is planned to provide physicians and researchers with evidence that home BP measurement can be used effectively in clinical practice, and that it offers clear benefits compared with conventional clinic measurement.

HISTORY OF HOME BP MEASUREMENT

The standard method of indirect measurement of BP is based on the principle of arterial occlusion and BP detection by various techniques,

the first of which was palpation, described by Scipione Riva-Rocci in 1896. In 1905, Nikolai Korotkoff improved Riva-Rocci's method when he recognized that by placing a stethoscope over the brachial artery at the cubital fossa, distal to a Riva-Rocci cuff, tapping sounds could be heard as the cuff was deflated, caused by blood flowing back into the artery. Korotkoff concluded correctly that the appearance of the tapping sounds coincided with systolic BP and the disappearance of the sounds with diastolic BP (Korotkoff, 1905). The method of BP measurement invented by Korotkoff quickly received wide recognition and became a standard medical procedure. His technique has truly stood the test of time as it has been used for more than a century with practically no alterations (Booth, 1977).

Brown was the first to report that BP measured in the home was lower than that recorded by a doctor (Brown, 1930). Ayman and Goldshine proposed the concept of "self BP measurement" in 1940 and also concluded that BP measured at home was lower than clinic BP. They have also suggested that home BP monitoring was useful for (1) instructing the patients about their chronic diseases, (2) teaching physicians about the natural course of the disease and about factors that affect the disease, (3) learning the prognosis of disease, and (4) increasing the precision of determining the effectiveness of treatment, as all of these hypotheses are slowly being proved correct (Ayman, 1940).

MEASUREMENT OF HOME BP

Devices and Validation

Automated BP measuring devices are at present most commonly based on the oscillometric technique and on the use of stable electronic transducer. This implies that these devices quite accurately measure mean BP corresponding to the point of maximal oscillation of cuff air pressure during cuff deflation, and then calculate systolic and diastolic BP values. The latter procedure is carried out through proprietary algorithms, different for different devices and usually not made available by manufacturers. For this reason, the accuracy of the systolic and diastolic BP readings yielded by any of these systems has to be checked against conventional measurements performed in highly standardized conditions, according to one of the available protocols endorsed by American and/or European Hypertension Societies (Booth, 1977; Brown, 1930; Ayman, 1940; Mieke, 1997). The need for such a validation comes from the fact that accuracy is a mandatory requirement for all BP measurements (Booth, 1977) and from the general agreement that accuracy of any given BP measuring device should not be only based on claims from manufacturers, but should rather be supported by data from validation studies provided by independent investigators and published in peer-reviewed journals (Ayman, 1940).

Optimal Scheme for Home BP Measurement

The recommendations for performing home BP measurement do not vary in principle from those that apply to BP measurement in general: there should be a short period of rest before measurement, the arm should be supported with the cuff at the level of the heart, and a cuff of proper size should be used (Pickering et al., 2005; O'Brien et al., 2003).

The current European Hypertension Society guidelines recommend two measurements in the morning and two measurements in the evening for one week with the exclusion of measurements from the first day (O'Brien et al., 2003). However, the North American guidelines advise taking three readings on one occasion every morning and evening, but do not mention for how many days (Pickering et al., 2005). These conflicting guidelines only demonstrate that agreement on this matter has not yet been reached. Two meth-

ods have been used to define the most suitable schedule for home BP measurement, a statistical and a clinical approach (Parati et al., 2004).

In the statistical method, the criteria for defining the best frequency of home BP measurements should be based on (1) the reproducibility of home BP values obtained, (2) their stability over time, and (3) their relation to the average ambulatory BP values, the latter being considered the gold standard references (O'Brien et al., 2003; Mancia et al., 1993). Chatellier et al. concluded that the maximal reduction in the standard deviation in the difference between two mean BP values was obtained when each mean was defined by 30 measurements (three measurements for ten consecutive days). However, 80% of this maximal reduction was already obtained with mean values defined by 15 measurements (three measurements collected over five days) (Chatellier et al., 1995). This conclusion was supported by the results of the SMART study, which also showed that only a small decrease in the standard deviation of the mean difference in average home BP values between two sessions is achieved after six home BP measurements (Chatellier et al., 1996). Two studies by Stergiou et al. also concluded that at least 12 measurements taken on three days are needed for the reproducibility of home BP to be superior to that of office measurements (Stergiou et al., 1998, 2002). On the other hand, Brook reported that if the accuracy of the average home BP was determined by agreement with average ambulatory BP values, the total number of measurements and the total duration of monitoring were not important and that most benefits could be achieved by obtaining as few as two home BP measurements on one day (Brook, 2000).

Prognostic clinical data is, of course, a more suitable method than statistical methods for defining the best amount of BP measurements needed. Recent follow-up studies have shown that even two home BP measurements are able to predict the risk of cardiovascular events (Mancia et al., 2006; Ohkubo et al., 1998). However, only Ohkubo et al. have tried to identify the best frequency of home BP measurements based on prognostic data from the community-based Ohasama study (Ohkubo et al., 2004).

They reported that the predictive value for the risk of stroke increases progressively without any threshold if the number of measurements was increased from 1 to 14. In any case, whether the statistical or clinical approach is used for determining an optimal BP measurement schedule, it appears that the advantages of home BP measurement depend not only on the statistical advantages associated with the availability of repeated measurements, but also in obtaining information out of the clinical setting with even a few home BP measurements (Ohkubo et al., 2004; Stergiou et al. 2007).

DIAGNOSING HYPERTENSION WITH HOME BP

Reference Values for Home Blood Pressure Measurement

The association between BP and cardiovascular risk is continuous, without a threshold above which risk suddenly increases. However, clinical decisions must be based on diagnostic or operational thresholds. In this regard, there is an agreement that the thresholds currently applicable for conventional sphygmomanometry cannot be extrapolated to automated home BP measurements. Different methodological approaches may be used for the determination of threshold values, the most satisfactory of which is to relate BP thresholds to cardiovascular outcome, but there are limited data available for home BP measurement (Su et al., 2001; Zanchetti et al., 2001; Blacher et al., 1999). The threshold of 135/85 mmHg for home BP measurement is the same as that for mean daytime ambulatory BP measurements (Glen et al., 1996; Zanchetti et al., 2001).

Isolated Clinic ("White Coat") Hypertension

In 1983, Mancia used a continuous intra-arterial recorder to measure BP in the periods during which a doctor repeatedly measured BP by the cuff method [27]. He observed that in almost all normotensive and hypertensive subjects tested the doctor's arrival at the bedside induced immediate rises in systolic and diastolic BP peaking within 1–4 minutes. This was the first recognition of the phenomenon known as "white-coat effect". Mancia also demonstrated that the white-coat effect cannot be avoided by repeated measurements by a physician over a short time span, but can be reduced by over 40%, however, if BP measurements are performed by a nurse (Mancia et al., 1987). The white-coat effect leads to poor diagnostic accuracy and is one of the main shortcomings of clinic BP measurement. Some patients have a persistently elevated clinic BP while their ambulatory or home BP is within normal range. This condition is widely known as "white-coat hypertension" (Pickering et al., 1988), although the European Society of Hypertension (ESH) guidelines suggest a more descriptive term "isolated clinic hypertension" (ICH) be used.

ICH should be diagnosed whenever clinic BP is repeatedly $\geq$ 140/90 mmHg, while home BP is within normal range (< 135/85 mmHg). Its diagnosis can also be based on 24-hour mean and daytime BP, bearing in mind that subjects with ICH diagnosed with home BP may not be entirely the same group identified by ambulatory BP measurements (Stergiou et al., 1998; Sega et al., 2001). Automated serial BP measurement in a clinic setting has also been successfully used to identify patients with ICH, but no reference values exist yet for this method of measurement (Culleton et al., 2006). Depending on the definition of ICH and the characteristics of the study cohort, its prevalence can range from 11–17% in the general population (Sega et al., 2001; Bjorklund et al., 2002; Ohkubo et al., 2005) to 10–60% of the patients with elevated clinic BP (Pickering et al., 1988; Khattar et al., 1998; Martinez et al., 1999; Dolan et al., 2004; Verdecchia et al., 1994, 2001; Bobrie et al., 2004; Hozawa et al., 2002).

Masked Hypertension

Masked hypertension should be diagnosed whenever home BP or 24-hour mean/daytime ambulatory BP is ≥ 135/85 mmHg, while clinic BP is within normal range (< 140/90mmHg). Home-measured BP also appears to be an appropriate method for assessing masked hypertension, as similar proportions of subjects with masked hypertension are detected by ambulatory and home BP monitoring, although slight disagreement exists between the two methods (Stergiou et al., 2005).

The concept of masked hypertension, like ICH, has several weaknesses. Again, as for ICH, the major determinant for masked hypertension appears to be a BP level close to the diagnostic thresholds (Mancia et al., 2006; Mallion et al., 2006), and two studies that have examined the persistence of masked hypertension with repeated ambulatory measurement found reproducibility rates of only 38% and 72%, respectively (Ben-Dov et al., 2007; Lurbe et al., 2005). In 4 repeated home measurements performed on hypertensive patients, 50% had masked hypertension during the entire study, while only 2% consistently had masked hypertension on each visit (Verberk et al., 2007). Furthermore, the clinical significance of masked hypertension remains quite unclear as "unmasking" these masked patients would necessitate performing ambulatory or home BP monitoring on subjects who appear to have normal BP.

HOME BP AND THE MANAGEMENT OF HYPERTENSION

The two randomized, controlled trials have compared the use of home and clinic BP measurement for the adjustment of antihypertensive treatment. Both studies concluded that self-measurement leads to lower costs, less medication use than clinic BP measurement, and slightly poorer BP control, although with no differences in end-organ damage (Staessen et al., 2004; Verberk et al., 2007). From these results, one may be inclined to conclude that it is better to base antihypertensive treatment on clinic BP instead of on home BP measurement. However, both of these studies used the same target BP for clinic and home BP groups, although clinic BP is nearly always higher than home BP and 5 mmHg lower BP targets should be used for home measurement according to current guidelines (Pickering et al., 2005; O'Brien et al., 2005). This limitation, also acknowledged by Verberk et al. in their article, in these studies unsurprisingly leads to more intensive drug therapy and greater BP decreases in the clinic BP group and somewhat nullifies the results of these studies (Verberk et al., 2007).

Home measurement might also be cost-effective when compared with clinic BP measurement. A study of 430 patients randomized to either usual care or home monitoring in a closed model health maintenance organization found that the costs of care were 29% lower in the self-monitoring group, and BP was equally well controlled in both groups at the end of one year (Soghikian et al., 1992). A mathematical model based on the Japanese Ohasama study also proposed that the introduction of home BP measurement for the diagnosis and treatment of hypertension would effectively reduce costs (Funahashi et al., 2006).

ASSOCIATION WITH END-ORGAN DAMAGE AND PROGNOSTIC SIGNIFICANCE

In 1977, it was reported that the changes in electrocardiographic evidence of left ventricular hypertrophy (ECG-LVH) were related to the degree of BP control and correlated better with home BP than with clinic BP (Ibrahim et al., 1977). After this a few small studies with selected hypertensive patients have concluded that clinic BP shows very poor or no correlation at all with hypertension-induced end-organ damage whereas home BP correlates significantly with echocardiographic left ventricular mass, pulse wave velocity (PWV) and albumin excretion rate (Mule et al., 2002; Martinez et al., 2006; Stergiou et al., 2007; Calvo-Vargas et al., 2003). No association was found between home BP and PWV in two of these studies so the results are still slightly mixed, although the small selected study cohorts and ongoing antihypertensive treatment work as confounding factors (Martinez et al., 2006; Stergiou et al., 2007). On the other hand, one study with 239 treated hypertensive patients also concluded that very meticulously controlled clinic BP measured by a nurse could be as reliable as home BP in predicting end-organ damage (Jula et al., 1999). In any case, data on the association between end-organ damage and home BP from population-based studies remain very scarce as only two studies, one examining PWV and the other echocardiographic left ventricular mass, have concluded that home BP could predict end-organ damage better than clinic BP (Sega et al., 2001; Hara et al., 2007).

Until recently, no prognostic data have been available for home BP as a risk factor of cardiovascular morbidity and mortality. The results from two large population studies have recently been published, the community-based Ohasama and Pressioni Arteriose Monitorate E Loro Associazioni (PAMELA) studies. Results from the Ohasama study show that home BP has a stronger predictive power for strokes than clinic BP, and both studies have concluded that home BP is more closely associated with future cardiovascular mortality than clinic BP, even when only a few home measurements are used (Ohkubo et al., 1998, 2004; Sega et al., 2005). Elevated home BP also predicted cardiovascular events better than elevated clinic BP in a study with 4939 elderly treated hypertensives (Bobrie et al., 2004). One smaller population study with only 662 subjects and an 8-year follow-up did not find any prognostic superiority of home BP compared to clinic BP (Stergiou et al., 2007). Morning home BP and evening home BP seem to provide equally useful information for stroke risk (Asayama et al., 2006).

INDICATIONS FOR HOME BLOOD PRESSURE MEASUREMENT

Although home BP is starting to be used in almost every aspect of BP measurement from screening to follow-up, there are still some areas where it is particularly useful. Home BP measurement eliminates white-coat effect and allows the detection of ICH. It may also be used in virtually any patient in whom there is a suspicion that the clinic readings may be unrepresentative of the patients true BP. It should also be considered as a first option for a patient with resistant hypertension, further reducing the need for ambulatory monitoring, which cannot be performed in primary care and which is inconvenient for the patient. It can also be used for improving adherence to treatment in patients with poor compliance (Edmonds et al., 1985; Friedman et al. 1996). In clinical drug trials, the duration of action of an antihypertensive drug can be assessed by measuring BP a number of times each day over several weeks (Menard et al., 1994).

LIMITATIONS OF HOME BP MEASUREMENT

Besides the many advantages, HBPM also carries some limitations. The accuracy of some home monitors is inadequate, especially with wrist and finger monitors (Mancia et al., 2007; Pickering et al., 2005). Reporting bias is possible if the patient reports the BP readings him/herself (Mengden et al., 1998). BP measurements can easily be performed incorrectly. One study concluded that most patients with home monitors had never been informed by anyone of proper BP measurement techniques and that only about half of them knew how to place the cuff correctly, which led to poor measurement accuracy (Stryker et al., 2004). However, these shortcomings can often be avoided by following the current recommendations for home BP measurement (Pickering et al., 1996; O'Brien et al., 2003). The clinical use of home measurement should require the use of validated and calibrated home monitors and good patient training. Some guidelines also recommend using a home monitor with a printed or electronic report of the measurements, although this does not completely eliminate the possibility of reporting bias (O'Brien et al., 2003).

Home BP monitors use the oscillometric technique, which may yield results that differ substantially from BP readings taken with a sphygmomanometer. This is particularly true in elderly subjects and diabetics (Van Popele et al., 2000; Raptis et al., 1997). BP measuring devices also vary greatly in their ability to measure BP accurately in patients with arrhythmias, indicating that device should be validated independently in patients with arrhythmias (Stewart et al., 1995). Home BP also cannot be measured at night, which is possible with ambulatory BP measurement, although home BP devices with the capacity to perform measurements at predetermined times are coming to the market (Chonan et al., 2001). Some patient selection for home BP measurement may also be necessary because of its complexity as it still requires some instruction before the patients understand the procedure correctly. Furthermore, home BP measurement may induce anxiety in some patients, who might take an obsessional interest in BP.

CONCLUSION

It can be concluded that home BP measurement offers clear advantages not only over conventional clinic BP measurement, but also over ambulatory monitoring. Home BP measurement allows the identification of ICH patients with readings under standardized conditions, little measurement variability and good reproducibility. Home monitoring is a method preferred by patients that can lead to better BP control by increasing awareness of hypertension and compliance with drug treatment. Preliminary data, although mostly from small, selected hypertensive populations, show that home BP correlates better than clinic BP with target-organ damage. Early data of the prognostic superiority of home BP, when compared with clinic BP, also exist. There are, however, some shortcomings of home BP measurement, which can mostly be avoided with good patient training and by using only validated and calibrated home monitors. The worst birth pains of home BP measurement are over, but several aspects require further elucidation.

REFERENCES

Asayama, K., Ohkubo, T., Kikuya, M., Obara, T., Metoki, H., & Inoue, R. (2006). Prediction of stroke by home "morning" versus "evening" blood pressure values: the Ohasama study. *Hypertension, 48*, 737–743.

Ayman, D., & Goldshine, A. D. (1940). Blood pressure determinations by patients with essential hypertension: the difference between clinic and home readings before treatment. *The American Journal of the Medical Sciences, 200*, 465–474.

Ben-Dov, I. Z., Ben-Arie, L., Mekler, J., & Bursztyn, M. (2007). Reproducibility of white-coat and masked hypertension in ambulatory BP monitoring. *International Journal of Cardiology, 117*, 355–359.

Bjorklund, K., Lind, L., Vessby, B., Andren, B., & Lithell, H. (2002). Different metabolic predictors of white-coat and sustained hypertension over a 20-year follow-up period: a population based study of elderly men. *Circulation, 106*, 63–68.

Blacher, J., Asmar, R., Djane, S., London, G. M., & Safar, M. E. (1999). Aortic pulse wave velocity as a marker of cardiovascular risk in hypertensive patients. *Hypertension, 33*, 1111–1117.

Bobrie, G., Chatellier, G., Genes, N., Clerson, P., Vaur, L., & Vaisse, B. (2004). Cardiovascular prognosis of "masked hypertension" detected by blood pressure self-measurement in elderly treated hypertensive patients. *Journal of the American Medical Association, 291*, 1342–1349.

Booth, J. (1977). A short history of blood pressure measurement. *Proceedings of the Royal Society of Medicine, 70*, 793–799.

Brook, R. D. (2000). Home blood pressure: accuracy is independent of monitoring schedules. *American Journal of Hypertension, 13*, 625–631.

Brown, G. E. (1930). Daily and monthly rhythm in the blood pressure of a man with hypertension: a three-year study. *Annals of Internal Medicine, 3*, 1177–1189.

Burton, S. (2006). *The market for home-use digital blood-pressure monitors 2006 – worldwide.* Wellingborough, UK: In Medica.

Calvo-Vargas, C., Padilla-Rios, V., Meza-Flores, A., Vazquez-Linares, G., Troyo-Sanroman, R., Cerda, A. P., & Asmar, R. (2003). Arterial stiffness and blood pressure self-measurement with loaned equipment. *American Journal of Hypertension, 16*, 375–380.

Chatellier, G., Day, M., Bobrie, G., & Menard, J. (1995). Feasibility study of N-of-1 trials with blood pressure self-monitoring in hypertension. *Hypertension, 25*, 294–301.

Chatellier, G., Dutrey-Dupagne, C., Vaur, L., Zannad, F., Genes, N., Elkik, F., & Menard, J. (1996). Home self blood pressure measurement in general practice, The SMART study, Self measurement for the Assessment of the Response to Trandolapril. *American Journal of Hypertension, 9*, 644–652.

Chonan, K., Kikuya, M., Araki, T., Fujiwara, T., Suzuki, M., & Michimata, M. (2001). Device for the self-measurement of blood pressure that can monitor blood pressure during sleep. *Blood Pressure Monitoring, 6*, 203–205.

Culleton, B. F., McKay, D. W., & Campbell, N. R. (2006). Performance of the automated BpTRU measurement device in the assessment of white-coat hypertension and white-coat effect. *Blood Pressure Monitoring, 11*, 37–42.

Dolan, E., Stanton, A., Atkins, N., Den Hond, E., Thijs, L., & McCormack, P. (2004). Determinants of white-coat hypertension. *Blood Pressure Monitoring, 9*, 307–309.

Edmonds, D., Foerster, E., Groth, H., Greminger, P., Siegenthaler, W., & Vetter, W. (1985). Does self measurement of blood pressure improve patient compliance in hypertension? *Journal of Hypertension, 3*, S31–S34.

Ezzati, M., Lopez, A. D., Rodgers, A., Hoorn Vander, S., & Murra, C. J. (2002). Selected major risk factors and global and regional burden of disease. *Lancet, 360*, 1347–1360.

Friedman, R. H., Kazis, L. E., Jette, A., Smith, M. B., Stollerman, J., Torgerson, J., & Carey, K. (1996). A telecommunications system for monitoring and counseling patients with hypertension. Impact on medication adherence and blood pressure control. *American Journal of Hypertension, 9*, 285–292.

Funahashi, J., Ohkubo, T., Fukunaga, H., Kikuya, M., Takada, N., & Asayama, K. (2006). The economic impact of the introduction of home blood pressure measurement for the diagnosis and treatment of hypertension. *Blood Pressure Monitoring, 11*, 257–267.

Glen, S. K., Elliott, H. L., Curzio, J. L., Lees, K. R., & Reid, J. L. (1996). White-coat hypertension as a cause of cardiovascular dysfunction. *Lancet, 348*, 654–657.

Hara, A., Ohkubo, T., Kikuya, M., Shintani, Y., Obara, T., & Metoki, H. (2007). Detection of carotid atherosclerosis in individuals with masked hypertension and white-coat hypertension by self-measured blood pressure at home: the Ohasama study. *Journal of Hypertension, 25*, 321–327.

Hozawa, A., Ohkubo, T., Kikuya, M., Yamaguchi, J., Ohmori, K., & Fujiwara, T. (2002). Blood pressure control assessed by home, ambulatory and conventional blood pressure measurements in the Japanese general population: the Ohasama study. *Hypertension Research, 25*, 57–63.

Ibrahim, M. M., Tarazi, R. C., Dustan, H. P., & Gifford, R. W. Jr. (1977). Electrocardiogram in evaluation of resistance to antihypertensive therapy. *Archives of Internal Medicine, 137*, 1125–1129.

Jula, A., Puukka, P., & Karanko, H. (1999). Multiple clinic and home blood pressure measurements versus ambulatory blood pressure monitoring. *Hypertension, 34*, 261–266.

Kearney, P. M., Whelton, M., Reynolds, K., Muntner, P., Whelton, P. K., & He, J. (2005). Global burden of hypertension: analysis of worldwide data. *Lancet, 365*, 217–223.

Khattar, R. S., Senior, R., & Lahiri, A. (1998). Cardiovascular outcome in white-coat versus sustained mild hypertension: a 10-year follow-up study. *Circulation, 98*, 1892–1897.

Korotkoff, N. S. (1905). On the subject of methods of determining blood pressure (from the clinic of Prof. S.P. Fedorov). *Bulletin of the Imperial Military Medical Academy, 11*, 356–367.

Lewington, S., Clarke, R., Qizilbash, N., Peto, R., & Collins, R. (2002). Age-specific relevance of usual blood pressure to vascular mortality: a meta-analysis of individual data for one million adults in 61 prospective studies. *Lancet, 360*, 1903–1913.

Lurbe, E., Torro, I., Alvarez, V., Nawrot, T., Paya, R., Redon, J., & Staessen, J. A. (2005). Prevalence, persistence, and clinical significance of masked hypertension in youth. *Hypertension, 45*, 493–498.

Mallion, J. M., Clerson, P., Bobrie, G., Genes, N., Vaisse, B., & Chatellier, G. (2006). Predictive factors for masked hypertension within a population of controlled hypertensives. *Journal of Hypertension, 24*, 2365–2370.

Mancia, G., Bertinieri, G., Grassi, G., Parati, G., Pomidossi, G., & Ferrari, A. (1983). Effects of blood-pressure measurement by the doctor on patient's blood pressure and heart rate. *Lancet, 2*, 695–698.

Mancia, G., De Backer, G., Dominiczak, A., Cifkova, R., Fagard, R., & Germano, G. (2007). 2007 Guidelines for the Management of Arterial Hypertension: The Task Force for the Management of Arterial Hypertension of the European Society of Hypertension (ESH) and of the European Society of Cardiology (ESC). *Journal of Hypertension, 25*, 1105–1187.

Mancia, G., Di Rienzo, M., & Parati, G. (1993). Ambulatory blood pressure monitoring use in hypertension research and clinical practice. *Hypertension, 21*, 510–524.

Mancia, G., Facchetti, R., Bombelli, M., Grassi, G., & Sega, R. (2006). Long-term risk of mortality associated with selective and combined elevation in office, home, and ambulatory blood pressure. *Hypertension, 47*, 846–853.

Mancia, G., Parati, G., Pomidossi, G., Grassi, G., Casadei, R., & Zanchetti, A. (1987). Alerting reaction and rise in blood pressure during measurement by physician and nurse. *Hypertension, 9*, 209–215.

Martinez, M. A., Garcia-Puig, J., Martin, J. C., Guallar-Castillon, P., Aguirre de Carcer, A., & Torre, A. (1999). Frequency and determinants of white coat hypertension in mild to moderate hypertension: A primary care-based study. *American Journal of Hypertension, 12*, 251–259.

Martinez, M. A., Sancho, T., Garcia, P., Moreno, P., Rubio, J. M., & Palau, F. J. (2006). Home blood pressure in poorly controlled hypertension: relationship with ambulatory blood pressure and organ damage. *Blood Pressure Monitoring, 11*, 207–213.

Menard, J., Chatellier, G., Day, M., & Vaur, L. (1994). Self-measurement of blood pressure at home to evaluate drug effects by the trough: peak ratio. *Journal of Hypertension, 12*, S21–S25.

Mengden, T., Hernandez Medina, R. M., Beltran, B., Alvarez, E., Kraft, K., & Vetter, H. (1998). Reliability of reporting self-measured blood pressure values by hypertensive patients. *American Journal of Hypertension, 11*, 1413–1417.

Mieke, S. (1997). Substitute of simulators for human subjects. *Blood Pressure Monitoring, 2*, 251–256.

Mule, G., Caimi, G., Cottone, S., Nardi, E., Andronico, G., & Piazza, G. (2002). Value of home blood pressures as predictor of target organ damage in mild arterial hypertension. *Journal of Cardiovascular Risk, 9*, 123–129.

O'Brien, E., Asmar, R., Beilin, L., Imai, Y., Mallion, J. M., & Mancia, G. (2003). European Society of Hypertension recommendations for conventional, ambulatory and home blood pressure measurement. *Journal of Hypertension, 21*, 821–848.

O'Brien, E., Asmar, R., Beilin, L., Imai, Y., Mancia, G., & Mengden, T. (2005). Practice guidelines of the European Society of Hypertension for clinic, ambulatory and self blood pressure measurement. *Journal of Hypertension, 23*, 697–701.

Ohkubo, T., Asayama, K., Kikuya, M., Metoki, H., Hoshi, H., & Hashimoto, J. (2004). How many times should blood pressure be measured at home for better prediction of stroke risk? Ten-year follow-up results from the Ohasama study. *Journal of Hypertension, 22*, 1099–1104.

Ohkubo, T., Imai, Y., Tsuji, I., Nagai, K., & Kato, J., ikuchi, N. K., et al. (1998). Home blood pressure measurement has a stronger predictive power for mortality than does screening blood pressure measurement: a population-based observation in Ohasama, Japan. *Journal of Hypertension, 16*, 971–975.

Ohkubo, T., Kikuya, M., Metoki, H., Asayama, K., Obara, T., & Hashimoto, J. J. (2005). Prognosis of "masked" hypertension and "white-coat" hypertension detected by 24-h ambulatory blood pressure monitoring 10-year follow-up from the Ohasama study. *Journal of the American College of Cardiology, 46*, 508–515.

Parati, G., & Stergiou, G. (2004). Self blood pressure measurement at home: how many times? *Journal of Hypertension, 22*, 1075–1079.

Pickering, T. (1996). Recommendations for the use of home (self) and ambulatory blood pressure monitoring, American Society of Hypertension Ad Hoc Panel. *American Journal of Hypertension, 9*, 1–11.

Pickering, T. G., Hall, J. E., Appel, L. J., Falkner, B. E., Graves, J., & Hill, M. N. (2005). Recommendations for blood pressure measurement in humans and experimental animals: part 1: Blood pressure measurement in humans: a statement for professionals from the Subcommittee of Professional and Public Education of the American Heart Association Council on High Blood Pressure Research. *Circulation, 111*, 697–716.

Pickering, T. G., James, G. D., Boddie, C., Harshfield, G. A., Blank, S., & Laragh, J. H. (1988). How common is white coat hypertension? *Journal of the American Medical Association, 259*, 225–228.

Raptis, A. E., Spring, M. W., & Viberti, G. (1997). Comparison of blood pressure measurement methods in adult diabetics. *Lancet, 349*, 175–176.

Sega, R., Facchetti, R., Bombelli, M., Cesana, G., Corrao, G., Grassi, G., & Mancia, G. (2005). Prognostic value of ambulatory and home blood pressures compared with office blood pressure in the general population - Follow-up results from the Pressioni Arteriose Monitorate e Loro Associazioni (PAMELA) study. *Circulation, 111*, 1777–1783.

Sega, R., Trocino, G., Lanzarotti, A., Carugo, S., Cesana, G., & Schiavina, R. (2001). Alterations of cardiac structure in patients with isolated office, ambulatory, or home hypertension: Data from the general population (Pressione Arteriose Monitorate E Loro Associazioni [PAMELA] Study). *Circulation, 104*, 1385–1392.

Soghikian, K., Casper, S. M., Fireman, B. H., Hunkeler, E. M., Hurley, L. B., Tekawa, I. S., & Vogt, T. M. (1992). Home blood pressure monitoring, Effect on use of medical services and medical care costs. *Medical Care, 30*, 855–865.

Staessen, J. A., Den Hond, E., Celis, H., Fagard, R., Keary, L., Vandenhoven, G., & O'Brien, E. T. (2004). Antihypertensive treatment based on blood pressure measurement at home or in the physician's office: a randomized controlled trial. *Journal of the American Medical Association, 291*, 955–964.

Stergiou, G. S., Argyraki, K. K., Moyssakis, I., Mastorantonakis, S. E., Achimastos, A. D., Karamanos, V. G., & Roussias, L. G. (2007). Home blood pressure is as reliable as ambulatory blood pressure in predicting target-organ damage in hypertension. *American Journal of Hypertension, 20*, 616–621.

Stergiou, G. S., Baibas, N. M., Gantzarou, A. P., Skeva, I. I., Kalkana, C. B., Roussias, L. G., & Mountokalakis, T. D. (2002). Reproducibility of home, ambulatory, and clinic blood pressure: implications for the design of trials for the assessment of antihypertensive drug efficacy. *American Journal of Hypertension, 15*, 101–104.

Stergiou, G. S., Baibas, N. M., & Kalogeropoulos, P. G. (2007). Cardiovascular risk prediction based on home blood pressure measurement: the Didima study. *Journal of Hypertension, 25*, 1590–1596.

Stergiou, G. S., & Parati, G. (2007). The optimal schedule for self-monitoring of blood pressure by patients at home. *Journal of Hypertension, 25*, 1992–1997.

Stergiou, G. S., Salgami, E. V., Tzamouranis, D. G., & Roussias, L. G. (2005). Masked hypertension assessed by ambulatory blood pressure versus home blood pressure monitoring: is it the same phenomenon? *American Journal of Hypertension, 18*, 772–778.

Stergiou, G. S., Skeva, I. I., Zourbaki, A. S., & Mountokalakis, T. D. (1998). Self-monitoring of blood pressure at home: how many measurements are needed? *Journal of Hypertension, 16,* 725–731.

Stergiou, G. S., Zourbaki, A. S., Skeva, I. I., & Mountokalakis, T. D. (1998). White coat effect detected using self-monitoring of blood pressure at home: comparison with ambulatory blood pressure. *American Journal of Hypertension, 11,* 820–827.

Stewart, M. J., Gough, K., & Padfield, P. L. (1995). The accuracy of automated blood pressure measuring devices in patients with controlled atrial fibrillation. *Journal of Hypertension, 13,* 297–300.

Stryker, T., Wilson, M., & Wilson, T. W. (2004). Accuracy of home blood pressure readings: monitors and operators. *Blood Pressure Monitoring, 9,* 143–147.

Su, T. C., Jeng, J. S., Chien, K. L., Sung, F. C., Hsu, H. C., & Lee, Y. T. (2001). Hypertension status is the major determinant of carotid atherosclerosis: a community-based study in Taiwan. *Stroke, 32,* 2265–2271.

Van Popele, N. M., Bos, W. J., de Beer, N. A., Van Der Kuip, D. A., Hofman, A., Grobbee, D. E., & Witteman, J. C. (2000). Arterial stiffness as underlying mechanism of disagreement between an oscillometric blood pressure monitor and a sphygmomanometer. *Hypertension, 36,* 484–488.

Verberk, W. J., Kroon, A. A., Lenders, J. W., Kessels, A. G., van Montfrans, G. A., & Smit, A. J. (2007). Self-measurement of blood pressure at home reduces the need for antihypertensive drugs: a randomized, controlled trial. *Hypertension, 50,* 1019–1025.

Verberk, W. J., Thien, T., Kroon, A. A., Lenders, J. W., van Montfrans, G. A., Smit, A. J., & De Leeuw, P. W. (2007). Prevalence and persistence of masked hypertension in treated hypertensive patients. *American Journal of Hypertension, 20,* 1258–1265.

Verdecchia, P., Palatini, P., Schillaci, G., Mormino, P., Porcellati, C. C., & Pessina, A. C. (2001). Independent predictors of isolated clinic ('white-coat') hypertension. *Journal of Hypertension, 19,* 1015–1020.

Verdecchia, P., Porcellati, C., Schillaci, G., Borgioni, C., Ciucci, A., & Battistelli, M. (1994). Ambulatory blood pressure, An independent predictor of prognosis in essential hypertension. *Hypertension, 24,* 793–801.

Zanchetti, A., Crepaldi, G., Bond, M. G., Gallus, G. V., Veglia, F., & Ventura, A. (2001). Systolic and pulse blood pressures (but not diastolic blood pressure and serum cholesterol) are associated with alterations in carotid intima-media thickness in the moderately hypercholesterolaemic hypertensive patients of the Plaque Hypertension Lipid Lowering Italian Study, PHYLLIS study group. *Journal of Hypertension, 19,* 79–88.

This work was previously published in International Journal of Computational Models and Algorithms in Medicine, Volume 1, Issue 4, edited by Aryya Gangopadhyay, pp. 46-56, copyright 2010 by IGI Publishing (an imprint of IGI Global).

Compilation of References

Aggarwal, C. C., & Yu, P. S. (2004). *A Condensation Approach to Privacy Preserving Data Mining*. Paper presented at the 9th International Conference on Extending Database Technology (pp. 183-199).

Aggarwal, C. C., Han, J., Wang, J., & Yu, P. S. (2003). *A framework for clustering evolving data streams*. Paper presented at the 29th International Conference on Very Large Data Bases (VLDB'03), Berlin.

Aggarwal, C. C., Han, J., Wang, J., & Yu, P. S. (2004, August 31 - September 3, 2004). *A framework for projected clustering of high dimensional data streams*. Paper presented at the 30th International Conference on Very Large Data Bases (VLDB'04), Toronto, Canada.

Agirre, E., Ansa, O., Hovy, E., & Martinez, D. (2000). Enriching very large ontologies using the WWW. In *Proceedings of ECAI Workshop on Ontology Learning*, Berlin.

Agrawal, D., & Aggarwal, C. (2001). *On the design and quantification of privacy preserving data mining algorithms*. Paper presented at the 20th ACM SIGMOD SIGACT-SIGART Symposium on Principles of Database Systems (pp. 247-255).

Agrawal, R., & Srikant, R. (1994). Fast algorithms for mining association rules. In *Proceedings of the 20th International Conference on Very Large Data Bases (VLDB)* (pp. 487-499). Santiago, Chile.

Agrawal, R., & Srikant, R. (2000). *Privacy preserving data mining*. Paper presented at the 2000 ACM SIGMOD Conference on Management of Data (pp. 439-450).

Agrawal, R., & Srikant, R. (2000). Privacy-preserving data mining. In *Proceedings of the 2000 ACM SIGMOD Conference on Management of Data* (pp. 439-450).

Agrawal, R., Evmfimievski, A., & Srikant, R. (2003). Information sharing across private databases. In *Proceedings of ACM SIGMOD International Conference on Management of Data*, San Diego, California.

Agrawal, R., & Srikant, R. (2000). Privacy-preserving data mining. *SIGMOD Record*, *29*(2), 439–450. doi:10.1145/335191.335438

Akbani, R., Kwek, S., & Japkowicz, N. (2004). Applying support vector machines to imbalanced datasets. *Lecture Notes in Computer Science*, *3201*, 39–50.

Alani, H., & Brewster, C. (2005). Ontology Ranking based on the Analysis of Concept Structure. In *Proceedings of the Third International Conference on Knowledge Capture (K-Cap)* (pp. 51-58), Banff, Alberta, Canada.

Ali, T., & Stanley, W. (2007). *Shackelford's Surgery of the alimentary tract* (6th ed., p. 802).

Alshalalfa, M., Alhajj, R., & Rokne, J. (2008). Combining Singular Value Decomposition and t-test into Hybrid Approach for Significant Gene Extraction from Microarray Data. In *Proceedings of the 8th IEEE International Conference on BioInformatics and BioEngineering (BIBE)* (pp. 1-6). Washington, DC: IEEE.

American Heart Association. (2010). *Metabolic Syndrome*. Retrieved July 13, 2010, from http://www.americanheart.org/presenter.jhtml?identifier=4756

American Heart Association. (2010). *Statistical fact sheet risk factors 2010 update*. Retrieved July 13, 2010, from http://www.americanheart.org/downloadable/heart/1260809371480FS15META10.pdf

An, Y. J. (2008). *Ontology Learning for the Semantic Deep Web*. Doctoral dissertation, New Jersey Institute of technology. Retrieved from NJIT eTD: The New Jersey Institute of Technology's electronic Theses & Dissertations Web site: http://library1.njit.edu/etd/2000s/2008/njit-etd2008-027/njit-etd2008-027.html

Anderson, R. (1996). A security policy model for clinical information systems. In Proceedings of the IEEE Symposium on Security and Privacy. Oakland, CA: IEEE Press.

Anton, I., Eart, J. B., Vail, M. W., Jain, N., Gheen, C. N., & Frink, J. M. (2007). HIPAA's effect on web site privacy policies. IEEE Security and Privacy, 5(1), 45–52. doi:10.1109/MSP.2007.7doi:10.1109/MSP.2007.7

An, Y. J., Huang, K.-C., & Geller, J. (2006). Naturalness of Ontology Concepts for Rating Aspects of the Semantic Web. *Communications of the International Information Management Association, 6*(3), 63–76.

Asayama, K., Ohkubo, T., Kikuya, M., Obara, T., Metoki, H., & Inoue, R. (2006). Prediction of stroke by home "morning" versus "evening" blood pressure values: the Ohasama study. *Hypertension, 48*, 737–743.

Ascribe Newswire: Health. (2008). *Study in 7,000 Men and Women Ties Obesity, Inflammatory Proteins to Heart Failure Risk; Obesity-Related Inflammation Also Pegged as Catalyst in Metabolic Syndrome* (p. 3). Health Source - Consumer Edition.

Association of Public Health Laboratories. (2002). *2001 Sexually Transmitted Diseases Laboratory Test Method Survey*. Retrieved from http://www.aphl.org/

Asuman, D. (2006). Artemis: Deploying semantically enriched Web services in the healthcare domain. *Information Systems, 31*(4), 321–339. doi:10.1016/j.is.2005.02.006

Atallah, M. J., Elmagarmid, A. K., Ibrahim, M., & Verykios, V. S. (1999). *Disclosure Limitation of Sesitive Rules*. Paper presented at the IEEE Knowledge and Data Engineering Workshop (pp. 45-52).

Atallah, M. J., Kerschbaum, F., & Du, K. (2003). Secure and private sequence comparisons. In *Proceedings 2d. ACM Workshop on Privacy in the Electronic Society (WPES)* (pp. 39-44). Washington, DC.

Atallah, M., Bertino, E., Elmagarmid, A., Ibrahim, M., & Verikyos, V. (1999, November). Disclosure Limitations of Sensitive Rules. In *Proceedings of IEEE Knowledge and Data Engineering Workshop* (pp. 45-52), Chicago, Illinois.

Atallah, M., Elmongui, H. G., Deshpande, V., & Schwartz, L. B. (2003, June 24-27). *Secure Supply-Chain Protocols*. In IEEE International Conference on E-Commerce (pp. 293-302), Newport Beach, California.

Ateniese, G., Fu, K., Green, M., & Hohenberger, S. (2006). Improved proxy re-encryption schemes with applications to secure distributed storage. [TISSEC]. *ACM Transactions on Information and System Security, 9*(1), 1–30. doi:10.1145/1127345.1127346

Augenbraun, M., Bachmann, L., Wallace, T., Dubouchet, L., McCormack, W., & Hook, E. W. III. (1998). Compliance with doxycycline therapy in sexually transmitted diseases clinics. *Sexually Transmitted Diseases, 25*(1), 1–4. doi:10.1097/00007435-199801000-00001

Ayman, D., & Goldshine, A. D. (1940). Blood pressure determinations by patients with essential hypertension: the difference between clinic and home readings before treatment. *The American Journal of the Medical Sciences, 200*, 465–474.

Azzalini, A., & Valle, A. D. (1996). The multivariate skew-normal distribution. *Biometrika, 83*(4), 715–726. doi:doi:10.1093/biomet/83.4.715

Baader, F., Calvanese, D., McGuinness, D., Nardi, D., & Patel-Schneider, P. F. (Eds.). (2003). *The Description Logic Handbook: Theory, Implementation, and Applications*. Cambridge: Cambridge University Press.

Babcock, B., Babu, S., Datar, M., Motwani, R., & Widom, J. (2002, June 3-6, 2002). *Models and issues in data stream systems*. Paper presented at the 21st ACM SIGMOD-SIGACT-SIGART Symposium on Principles of Database Systems (ACM PODS'02), Madison, WI.

Bachmann, L. H., Richey, C. M., Waites, K., Schwebke, J. R., & Hook, E. W. III. (1999). Patterns of Chlamydia trachomatis testing and follow-up at a University Hospital Medical Center. *Sexually Transmitted Diseases, 26*(9), 496–499. doi:10.1097/00007435-199910000-00002

Ball, M. J., Smith, C., & Bakalar, R. S. (2007). Personal Health Records: Empowering Consumers. *Journal of Healthcare Information Management, 21*(1).

Baneyx, B., Charlet, J., & Jaulent, M.-C. (2005). Building Medical Ontologies Based on Terminology Extraction from Texts: An Experimentation in Pneumology. *Studies in Health Technology and Informatics, 116*, 659–664.

Banzhaf, W., Nordin, P., Keller, R. E., & Francone, F. D. (1998). *Genetic programming: an introduction on the automatic evolution of computer programs and its applications*. San Francisco, CA: Morgan Kaufmann Publishers.

Barbará, D. (2002). Requirements for clustering data streams. *ACM SIGKDD Explorations Newsletter, 3*(2), 23–27. doi:doi:10.1145/507515.507519

Barnsley, M. F., Devaney, R. L., Mandlebrot, B. B., Peitgen, H., Saupe, D., & Voss, R. F. (1988). *The Science of Fractal Images*. New York: Springer-Verlag. doi:10.1007/978-1-4612-3784-6

Bartschat, W. E. A. (2006). Surveying the rhio landscape. a description of current rhio models with a focus on patient identiˉcation. *Journal of American Health Information Management Association, 77*(1), 64A–64D.

Bayardo, R. J., & Agrawal, R. (2005). Data privacy through optimal k-anonymization. In *ICDE '05: Proceedings of the 21st International Conference on Data Engineering* (pp. 217-228) Washington, DC: IEEE Press.

Bayardo, R. J., & Agrawal, R. (2005). *Data Privacy through Optimal k-Anonymization*. Paper presented at the ICDE (pp. 217-228).

Begley, C. E., McGill, L., & Smith, P. B. (1989). The incremental cost of screening, diagnosis, and treatment of gonorrhea and chlamydia in a family planning clinic. *Sexually Transmitted Diseases, 16*(2), 63–67. doi:10.1097/00007435-198904000-00004

Bellman, R. (1957). *Dynamic programming*. Princeton, NJ: Princeton University Press.

Ben-Dov, I. Z., Ben-Arie, L., Mekler, J., & Bursztyn, M. (2007). Reproducibility of white-coat and masked hypertension in ambulatory BP monitoring. *International Journal of Cardiology, 117*, 355–359.

Bethencourt, J., Sahai, A., & Waters, B. (2007). Ciphertext-policy attribute-based encryption. In D. Shands (Ed.), *Proceedings of the 28th IEEE Symposium on Security and Privacy* (pp. 321-334). Oakland, CA: Citeseer.

Bhatti, R., & Grandison, T. (2007). Towards Improved Privacy Policy Coverage in Healthcare Using Policy Refinement. In *Proceedings of the 4th VLDB Workshop on Secure Data Management*. Vienna, Austria: Springer Verlag.

BioChemWeb.org. (2010). Genes & Gene Expression. *The Virtual Library of Biochemistry and Cell Biology*. BioChemWeb.org.

Bjorklund, K., Lind, L., Vessby, B., Andren, B., & Lithell, H. (2002). Different metabolic predictors of white-coat and sustained hypertension over a 20-year follow-up period: a population based study of elderly men. *Circulation, 106*, 63–68.

Blacher, J., Asmar, R., Djane, S., London, G. M., & Safar, M. E. (1999). Aortic pulse wave velocity as a marker of cardiovascular risk in hypertensive patients. *Hypertension, 33*, 1111–1117.

Black, C. M., Marrazzo, J., Johnson, R. E., Hook, E. W. III, Jones, R. B., & Green, T. A. (2002). Head-to-head multicenter comparison of DNA probe and nucleic acid amplification tests for Chlamydia trachomatis infection in women performed with an improved reference standard. *Journal of Clinical Microbiology, 40*(10), 3757–3763. doi:10.1128/JCM.40.10.3757-3763.2002

Blaze, M., Bleumer, G., & Strauss, M. (1998). Divertible protocols and atomic proxy cryptography. In K. Nyberg (Ed.), *Proceeding of Eurocrypt 1998* (Vol. 1403 of LNCS) (pp. 127-144). New York: Springer Verlag.

Blobel, B. (2004). Authorisation and Access Control for Electronic Health Record systems. *International Journal of Medical Informatics, 73*(3), 251–257. doi:10.1016/j.ijmedinf.2003.11.018

Blount, S., Galambosi, A., & Yakowitz, S. (1997). Nonlinear and dynamic programming for epidemic intervention. *Applied Mathematics and Computation, 86*(2-3), 123–136. doi:10.1016/S0096-3003(96)00177-4

Bobrie, G., Chatellier, G., Genes, N., Clerson, P., Vaur, L., & Vaisse, B. (2004). Cardiovascular prognosis of "masked hypertension" detected by blood pressure self-measurement in elderly treated hypertensive patients. *Journal of the American Medical Association, 291*, 1342–1349.

Boneh, D., & Boyen, X. (2004). Efficient selective-id secure identity-based encryption without random oracles. In C. Cachin & J. Camenisch (Eds.), *Proceedings of Eurocrypt 2004* (Vol. 3027 of LNCS) (pp. 223-238). New York: Springer Verlag.

Boneh, D., & Franklin, M. K. (2001). Identity-based encryption from the weil pairing. In J. Kilian (Ed.), *Proceedings of Crypto 2001* (Vol. 2139 of LNCS) (pp. 213-229). New York: Springer Verlag.

Booth, J. (1977). A short history of blood pressure measurement. *Proceedings of the Royal Society of Medicine, 70*, 793–799.

Brachman, R. J. (1992). Reducing CLASSIC to practice: Knowledge Representation Theory Meets Reality. In *Proceedings of the Third International Conference on the Principles of Knowledge Representation and Reasoning (KR-92)* (pp. 247-258).

Bragge, T., Tarvainen, M. P., & Karjalainen, P. A. (2004). *High-resolution QRS detection algorithm for sparsely sampled ECG recordings* (Tech. Rep. No. 1/2004). Kuopio, Finland: University of Kuopio, Department of Applied Physics.

Brandeau, M. L., & Zaric, G. S. (2009). Optimal investment in HIV prevention programs: more is not always better. *Health Care Management Science, 12*(1), 27–37. doi:10.1007/s10729-008-9074-7

Braun, R., & Rowe, W. (2009). Needles in the haystack: identifying individuals present in pooled genomic data. *PLOS Genetics, 5*(10), e1000668. doi:10.1371/journal.pgen.1000668

Breiman, L. (1996). Bagging Predictors. *Machine Learning, 24*(2), 123–140. doi:10.1007/BF00058655

Breiman, L. (2001). Random Forests. *Machine Learning, 45*(1), 5–32. doi:10.1023/A:1010933404324

Brewster, C., Ciravegna, F., & Wilks, Y. (2002). User-Centred Onlology Learning for Knowledge Management. In *Proceedings of the 7th International Workshop on Applications of Natural Language to Information Systems*.

Brewster, C., Ciravegna, F., & Wilks, Y. (2003). Background and Foreground Knowledge in Dynamic Ontology Construction: Viewing Text as Knowledge Maintenance. In *Proceedings of the Semantic Web Workshop (SIGIR)*. Retrieved from AKT EPrint Archiveat Web site: http://eprints.aktors.org/307/

Brinegar, C., Zhang, H., Wu, Y. L., Foley, L. M., Hitchens, T. K., Ye, Q., et al. (2009). Real-Time Cardiac MRI using Prior Spatial-Spectral Information. In *Proceedings of the Annual International Conference of the IEEE Engineering in Medicine and Biology Society (EMBC)* (pp. 4383-4386). Washington, DC: IEEE.

Brockwell, A. E., Kass, R. E., & Schwartz, A. B. (2007). Statistical Signal Processing and the Motor Cortex. []. Washington, DC: IEEE.]. *Proceedings of the IEEE, 95*, 881–898. doi:10.1109/JPROC.2007.894703

Brook, R. D. (2000). Home blood pressure: accuracy is independent of monitoring schedules. *American Journal of Hypertension, 13*, 625–631.

Brooks, P. M. (2006, November). The burden of musculoskeletal disease--a global perspective. *Clinical Rheumatology, 25*(6), 778–781. doi:10.1007/s10067-006-0240-3

Brown, M. P. S., Grundy, W. N., Lin, D., Cristianini, N., Sugnet, C., Ares, M., & Haussler, D. (1999). *Support Vector Machine Classification of Microarray Gene Expression Data* (Tech. Rep. UCSC-CRL-99-09). Santa Cruz, CA: Department of Computer Science, University of California, Santa Cruz.

Brown, G. E. (1930). Daily and monthly rhythm in the blood pressure of a man with hypertension: a three-year study. *Annals of Internal Medicine, 3*, 1177–1189.

Brun, M., Sima, C., Hua, J., Lowey, J., Carroll, B., & Suh, E. (2007). Model-based evaluation of clustering validation measures. *Pattern Recognition, 40*(3), 807–824. doi:doi:10.1016/j.patcog.2006.06.026

Bryson, A. E., & Ho, Y.-C. (1969). *Applied optimal control: optimization, estimation, and control.* New York, NY: Blaisdell Publishing Company and Xerox College Publishing.

Brzycki, M. (2010). AF Q & A. *American Fitness, 28,* 15–15.

Bunn, P., & Ostrovsky, R. (2007). Secure two-party k-means clustering. In P. Ning (Ed.), *Proceedings of the 14th ACM conference on Computer and communications security* (pp. 486-497). New York: ACM.

Bureau of Labor Statistics. (2010). *Consumer price index-all urban consumers.* Retrieved from http://www.bls.gov/cpi/

Burgun, A., & Bodenreider, O. (2001). Mapping the UMLS Semantic Network into General Ontologies. In *Proceedings of American Medical Informatics Association (AMIA) Annual Symposium* (pp. 81-85).

Burton, S. (2006). *The market for home-use digital blood-pressure monitors 2006 – worldwide.* Wellingborough, UK: In Medica.

Byers, S., Cranor, L. F., & Kormann, D. (2003). Automated Analysis of P3P-enabled web sites. In *proceedings of the International Conference on Electronic Commerce* (pp. 326-338). Pittsburgh, Philadelphia, USA: ACM Press.

Caestecker, J., & Straus, J. (2007, December 23). *Upper Gastrointestinal Bleeding: Surgical Perspective.eMedicine.* Retrieved from http:/ www.emedicine.com/ MED/ topic3566.htm

Cales, P., Zabotto, B., & Meskens, C. (1990). Gastro-esophageal endoscopic features in cirrhosis. Observer variability, in there associations and relationship to hepatic dysfunction. *Gastroenterology, 98,* 186.

Calvo-Vargas, C., Padilla-Rios, V., Meza-Flores, A., Vazquez-Linares, G., Troyo-Sanroman, R., Cerda, A. P., & Asmar, R. (2003). Arterial stiffness and blood pressure self-measurement with loaned equipment. *American Journal of Hypertension, 16,* 375–380.

Castano, S., & Antonellis, V. D. (1999). A Discovery-Based Approach to Database Ontology Design. *Distributed and Parallel Databases - Special Issue on Ontologies and Databases. 7*(1), 67-98.

Center for Disease Control (CDC). *(1997).* NHANES III: Series 11 Data Files. *Retrieved May 30, 2009, from* http://www.cdc.gov/nchs/nhanes/nh3data.htm#1a

Centers for Disease Control and Prevention (CDC). (1996). Prevalence and impact of arthritis by race and ethnicity-United States. *MMWR Morb Mortal Wkly, 45,* 373–378.

Centers for Disease Control and Prevention. (2010a). *Recommends screening of all sexually active women 25 and under.* Retrieved September 16, 2010, from http://www.cdc.gov/std/infertility/default.htm

Centers for Disease Control and Prevention. (2010b). *Sexually transmitted disease surveillance 2008.* Retrieved September 16, 2010, from http://www.cdc.gov/std/stats08/trends.htm

Centers for Medicare and Medicaid Services. (2010). *CMS programs and information.* Retrieved from http://www.cms.hhs.gov/

Chan, C.-L., Chen, C. W., & Liu, B. J. (2008). Discovery of association rules in metabolic syndrome related diseases. In *Proceedings of the IEEE International Joint Conference on Neural Networks (IJCNN 2008)* (pp. 856-862). Washington, DC: IEEE.

Chang, C.-C., & Lin, C.-J. (2009). *LIBSVM: A library for support vector machines.* Software available at http://www.csie.ntu.edu.tw/~cjlin/libsvm/.

Chang, R. F., Wu, W. J., Moon, W. K., & Chen, D. R. (2003). Improvement in breast tumor discrimination by support vector machines and speckle-emphasis texture analysis. *Ultrasound in Medicine & Biology, 29*(5), 679–686. PubMed doi:10.1016/S0301-5629(02)00788-3

Chang, R. F., Wu, W. J., Moon, W. K., & Chen, D. R. (2005). Automatic ultrasound segmentation and morphology based diagnosis of solid breast tumors. *Breast Cancer Research and Treatment, 89*(2), 179–185. PubMed doi:10.1007/s10549-004-2043-z

Chaovalit, P., & Gangopadhyay, A. (2007). *A method for clustering time series using connected components.* Paper presented at the 17th Annual Workshop on Information Technologies and Systems (WITS'07), Montreal, Canada.

Chatellier, G., Day, M., Bobrie, G., & Menard, J. (1995). Feasibility study of N-of-1 trials with blood pressure self-monitoring in hypertension. *Hypertension, 25,* 294–301.

Chatellier, G., Dutrey-Dupagne, C., Vaur, L., Zannad, F., Genes, N., Elkik, F., & Menard, J. (1996). Home self blood pressure measurement in general practice, The SMART study, Self measurement for the Assessment of the Response to Trandolapril. *American Journal of Hypertension*, *9*, 644–652.

Chawla, N. V., Japkowicz, N., & Kotcz, A. (2004). Editorial: special issue on learning from imbalanced data sets. *ACM SIGKDD Explorations Newsletter*, *6*(1), 1–6. doi:10.1145/1007730.1007733

Chen, C. M., Chou, Y. H., Han, K. C., Hung, G. S., Tiu, C. M., Chiou, H. J., et al. (2003). Breast lesions on sonograms: computer-aided diagnosis with nearly setting-independent features and artificial neural networks. *Radiology*, *226*(2), 504–514. PubMed doi:10.1148/radiol.2262011843

Chen, D. R., Chang, R. F., Chen, C. J., Ho, M. F., Kuo, S. J., Chen, S. T., et al. (2005). Classification of breast ultrasound images using fractal feature. *Clinical Imaging*, *29*(4), 235–245. PubMed doi:10.1016/j.clinimag.2004.11.024

Chen, D. R., Chang, R. F., Huang, Y. L., Chou, Y. H., Tiu, C. M., & Tsai, P. P. (2000). Texture analysis of breast tumors on sonograms. *Seminars in Ultrasound, CT, and MR*, *21*(4), 308–316. PubMed doi:10.1016/S0887-2171(00)90025-8

Chen, D. R., Chang, R. F., Kuo, W. J., Chen, M. C., & Huang, Y. L. (2002). Diagnosis of breast tumors with sonographic texture analysis using wavelet transform and neural networks. *Ultrasound in Medicine & Biology*, *28*(10), 1301–1310. PubMed doi:10.1016/S0301-5629(02)00620-8

Chen, L. (2007). An interpretation of identity-based cryptography. In A. Aldini & R. Gorrieri (Eds.), *Foundations of Security Analysis and Design, IV FOSAD 2006/2007 Tutorial Lectures* (Vol. 4677 of LNCS) (pp. 183-208). New York: Springer Verlag.

Chen, X., & Wasikowski, M. (2008). *FAST: a roc-based feature selection metric for small samples and imbalanced data classification problems.*

Chen, Y., & Tu, L. (2007, August 12-15, 2007). *Density-based clustering for real-time stream data.* Paper presented at the 13th International Conference on Knowledge Discovery and Data Mining (SIGKDD'07), San Jose, CA.

Chen, Z.-Y., & Liu, G.-H. (2005). *Quantitative Association Rules Mining Methods with Privacy-preserving.* Paper presented at the Sixth International Conference on. Parallel and Distributed Computing, Applications and Technologies, PDCAT.

Chen, D. R., Chang, R. F., & Huang, Y. L. (1999). Computer-aided diagnosis applied to US of solid breast nodules by using neural networks. [PubMed]. *Radiology*, *213*, 407–412.

Cheung, L., & Newport, C. (2007). Provably secure ciphertext policy ABE. In P. Ning (Ed.), *Proceedings of the 14th ACM Conference on Computer and Communications Security* (pp. 456–465). New York: ACM.

Chonan, K., Kikuya, M., Araki, T., Fujiwara, T., Suzuki, M., & Michimata, M. (2001). Device for the self-measurement of blood pressure that can monitor blood pressure during sleep. *Blood Pressure Monitoring*, *6*, 203–205.

Chua, S. N. D., MacDonald, B. J., & Hashmi, M. S. J. (2002). Finite-element simulation of stent expansion. *Journal of Materials Processing Technology*, *120*, 335–340. doi:10.1016/S0924-0136(01)01127-X

Chua, S. N. D., MacDonald, B. J., & Hashmi, M. S. J. (2004). Effects of varying slotted tube (stent) geometry on its expansion behaviour using finite element method. *Journal of Materials Processing Technology*, *155-156*, 1764–1771. doi:10.1016/j.jmatprotec.2004.04.395

Chun, S. A., & Geller, J. (2008). Evaluating Ontologies based on the Naturalness of their Preferred Terms. In *Proceedings of the 41st Annual Hawaii International Conference on System Sciences (HICSS 2008)* (p. 238).

Church, G., & Heeney, C. (2009). Public access to genome-wide data: five views on balancing research with privacy and protection. *PLOS Genetics*, *5*(10), e1000665. doi:10.1371/journal.pgen.1000665

Cimino, J. J. (1998). Desiderata for controlled medical vocabularies in the twenty-first century. *Methods of Information in Medicine*, *37*(4-5), 394–403.

Cimino, J. J. (2006). In defense of the Desiderata. *Journal of Biomedical Informatics*, *39*(3), 299–306. doi:10.1016/j.jbi.2005.11.008

Clifton, C., Doan, A., Elmagarmid, A., Kantarcioglu, M., Schadow, G., Suciu, D., & Vaidya, J. (2004). Privacy preserving data integration and sharing. In *Proceedings of The 9th ACM SIGMOD Workshop on Research Issues in Data Mining and Knowledge Discovery (DMKD'2004)*.

Clifton, C. (2001). Using Sample Size to Limit Exposure to Data Mining. *Journal of Computer Security*, *8*(4), 281–307.

Cohen, W. (1995). Fast Effective Rule Induction. In. *Proceedings of, ICML-95*, 115–123.

Colomb, R. M. (2002, November). *Quality of Ontologies in Interoperating Information Systems*. Retrieved from the Institute of Cognitive Science and Technology, Laboratory for Applied Ontology Web site: http://www.loa-cnr.it/Papers/ISIB-CNR-TR-18-02.pdf

Commission on Classification and Terminology of the International League Against Epilepsy (1989). Proposal for revised classification of epilepsies and epileptic syndromes. *Epilepsia, 30*(4, August), 389-399.

Commission on Classification and Terminology of the International League Against Epilepsy. (1981). Proposal for revised clinical and electroencephalographic classification of epileptic seizures. *Epilepsia, 22*, 489–501. doi:10.1111/j.1528-1157.1981.tb06159.x

Costa, L. D. F. D., & Cesar, R. M. (2000). *Shape analysis and classification: theory and practise* (1st ed.). Boca Raton, FL: CRC Press Inc.

Cover, T., & Hart, P. (1967). Nearest neighbor pattern classification. *IEEE Transactions on Information Theory*, *13*(1), 21–27. doi:10.1109/TIT.1967.1053964

Cowley, M. (2006, January 8). *Electrodes, leads & wires: A practical guide to ecg monitoring and recording*. Retrieved August 15, 2010, from www.mikecowley.co.uk/leads.htm

Cramer, N. L. (1985). A representation for the Adaptive Generation of Simple Sequential Programs. In J. Grefenstette (Ed.), *Proceedings of the International Conference on Genetic Algorithms and the Applications*, Pittsburgh, PA.

Cranor, L., Langheinrich, M., Marchiori, M., Presler-Marshall, M., & Reagle, J. (2002). The Platform for Privacy Preferences 1.0 specifications. *W3C Recommendation*. Retrieved November 27, 2009 from http://www.w3.org/TR/P3P/

Cuellar, R. E., Gavaler, J., & Alexander, A. (1990). Gastrointestinal Hemorrhage. *Archives of Internal Medicine*, *150*, 1381. doi:doi:10.1001/archinte.150.7.1381

Culleton, B. F., McKay, D. W., & Campbell, N. R. (2006). Performance of the automated BpTRU measurement device in the assessment of white-coat hypertension and white-coat effect. *Blood Pressure Monitoring, 11*, 37–42.

Cycorp. (2005). *OpenCyc Version 0.9*. Retrieved from http://www.opencyc.org/releases/

D'Amico, G., Pagliaro, L., & Bosch, J. (1995). The treatment of portal hypertension: A meta-analytic review. *Hepatology (Baltimore, Md.)*, *22*, 332–354.

Dagradi, A. E., & Weingarten, A. J. F. (1979). Failure of endoscopy to establish a source of upper gastrointestinal bleeding. *The American Journal of Gastroenterology*, *72*, 395–402.

Dasseni, E., Verikyos, V., Elmagarmid, A., & Bertino, E. (2001, April). *Hiding Association Rules by Using Confidence and Support*. In proceedings of the 4th Information Hiding Workshop (pp. 369-383), Pittsburgh, PA.

De Beule, M., Mortier, P., Carlier, S. G., Verhegghe, B., Van Impe, R., & Verdonck, P. (2008). Realistic finite element-based stent design: the impact of balloon folding. *Journal of Biomechanics*, *41*(2), 383–389. doi:10.1016/j.jbiomech.2007.08.014

De Beule, M., Van Impe, R., Verhegghe, B., Segers, P., & Verdonck, P. (2006). Finite element analysis and stent design: reduction of dogboning. *Technology and Health Care, 14*, 233–241.

DeRisi, J. L., & Iyer, V. R. (1997). Exploring the metabolic and genetic control of gene expression on a genomic scale. *Science*, *278*(5338), 680–686. doi:10.1126/science.278.5338.680

Dicker, L. W., Mosure, D. J., Levine, W. C., Black, C. M., & Berman, S. M. (2000). Impact of switching laboratory tests on reported trends in Chlamydia trachomatis infections. *American Journal of Epidemiology, 151*(4), 430–435.

Dieng-Kuntz, R., Minier, D., Růžička, M., Corby, F., Corby, O., & Alamarguy, L. (2006). Building and using a medical ontology for knowledge management and cooperative work in a health care network. *Computers in Biology and Medicine, 36*(7-8), 871–892. doi:10.1016/j.compbiomed.2005.04.015

Dietterich, T. G. (1998). Approximate statistical tests for comparing supervised classification learning algorithms. *Neural Computation, 10*(7), 1895–1923. doi:10.1162/089976698300017197

Dietterich, T. G. (2000). Ensemble methods in machine learning. *Lecture Notes in Computer Science, 1857*, 1–15. doi:10.1007/3-540-45014-9_1

Ding, L., Finin, T., Joshi, A., Pan, R., Cost, R., Peng, Y., et al. (2004). Swoogle: a search and metadata engine for the semantic web. In *Proceedings of the 13th ACM Conference on Information and Knowledge Management* (pp. 652-659).

Dolan, E., Stanton, A., Atkins, N., Den Hond, E., Thijs, L., & McCormack, P. (2004). Determinants of white-coat hypertension. *Blood Pressure Monitoring, 9*, 307–309.

Domingos, P., & Hulten, G. (2000). *Mining high-speed data streams.* Paper presented at the 6th International Conference on Knowledge Discovery and Data Mining (SIGKDD'00).

Domingos, P., & Hulten, G. (2001, May 20). *Catching up with the data: research issues in mining data streams.* Paper presented at Workshop on Research Issues in Data Mining and Knowledge Discovery (DMKD 2001), Santa Barbara, CA.

Drukker, K., Giger, M. L., Horsh, K., Kupinski, M. A., & Vyborny, C. J. (2002). Computerized lesion detection on breast ultrasound. *Medical Physics, 29*(7), 1438–1446. PubMed doi:10.1118/1.1485995

Dumoulin, C., & Cochelin, B. (2000). Mechanical behaviour modelling of balloon-expandable stents. *Journal of Biomechanics, 33*(11), 1461–1470. doi:10.1016/S0021-9290(00)00098-1

Eapen, B. R. (2008). ONTODerm - A domain ontology for dermatology. *Dermatology Online Journal, 14*(6:16).

Edmonds, D., Foerster, E., Groth, H., Greminger, P., Siegenthaler, W., & Vetter, W. (1985). Does self measurement of blood pressure improve patient compliance in hypertension? *Journal of Hypertension, 3*, S31–S34.

ElGamal, T. (1985). A public key cryptosystem and a signature scheme based on discrete logarithms. In G. R. Blakley & D. Chaum (Eds.), *Proceedings of Crypto 1984* (Vol. 196 of LNCS) (pp. 10-18). New York: Springer Verlag.

Elkan, C., & Noto, K. (2008). *Learning classifiers from only positive and unlabeled data.*

El-Menyar, A. A., Al Suwaidi, J., & Holmes, D. R. (2007). Left main coronary artery stenosis: state-of-the-art. *Current Problems in Cardiology, 32*, 103–193. doi:10.1016/j.cpcardiol.2006.12.002

Engström, G., Gerhardsson, de Verdier., M., Rollof., J., Nilsson, P.M., & Lohmander, L.S. (2009). C-reactive protein, metabolic syndrome and incidence of severe hip and knee osteoarthritis. A population-based cohort study. *Osteoarthritis and Cartilage, 17*(2), 168–173. doi:10.1016/j.joca.2008.07.003

Ennett, C. M., Frize, M., & Scales, N. (2002). Logarithmic-Sensitivity Index as a Stopping Criterion for Neural Networks. In *Proceedings of IEEE/EMBS* (Vol. 1, pp. 74-75).

Ennett, C., & Frize, M. (2000). Selective Sampling to Overcome Skewed a Priori Probabilities with Neural Networks. In *Proceedings of the A.M.I.A. (American Medical Informatics Association) Annual Symposium*, Los Angeles, CA.

Ennett, C. M., Frize, M., & Charette, E. (2004). Improvement and automation of artificial neural networks to estimate medical outcomes. *Medical Engineering & Physics, 26*(4), 321–328. doi:10.1016/j.medengphy.2003.09.005

Ennett, C., & Frize, M. (2003). Weight-Elimination Neural Networks Applied to Coronary Surgery Mortality Prediction. *IEEE Transactions on Information Technology in Biomedicine*, 7(2), 86–92. doi:10.1109/TITB.2003.811881

Estabrooks, A., Jo, T., & Japkowicz, N. (2004). A multiple resampling method for learning from imbalanced data sets. *Computational Intelligence*, 20(1), 18–36. doi:10.1111/j.0824-7935.2004.t01-1-00228.x

Etave, F., Finet, G., Boivin, M., Boyer, J., Rioufol, G., & Thollet, G. (2001). Mechanical properties of coronary stents determined by using finite element analysis. *Journal of Biomechanics*, 34(8), 1065–1075. doi:10.1016/S0021-9290(01)00026-4

Evfimevski, A., Gehrke, J., & Srikant, R. (2003). *Limiting privacy breaches in privacy preserving data mining*. Paper presented at the 22nd ACM SIGMOD-SIGACT-SIGART Symposium on Principles of Database Systems, San Diego, CA.

Evfimevski, A., Srikant, R., Agrawal, R., & Gehrke, J. (2002). *Privacy preserving mining of association rules*. Paper presented at the 8th ACM SIGKDD International Conference on Knowledge Discovery and Data Mining (KDD'02) (pp. 217-228).

Ezzati, M., Lopez, A. D., Rodgers, A., Hoorn Vander, S., & Murra, C. J. (2002). Selected major risk factors and global and regional burden of disease. *Lancet*, 360, 1347–1360.

Federal Register. (2002, August 14). Standard for Privacy of Individually Identifiable Health Information. *Federal Register*, 67(157), 53181–53273.

Felson, T. D. (2004, October). Risk factors for osteoarthritis: understanding joint vulnerability. *Clinical Orthopaedics and Related Research*, (427), S16–S21. doi:10.1097/01.blo.0000144971.12731.a2

Feng, J., Zihui, X., & Katsuhiko, S. (2008). On the finite element modelling of balloon-expandable stents. *Journal of the Mechanical Behavior of Biomedical Materials*, 1(1), 86–95. doi:10.1016/j.jmbbm.2007.07.002

Findlay, D. M. (2007). Vascular pathology and osteoarthritis. *Rheumatology*, 46, 1763e8. Oxford

Finin, T., Sachs, J., & Parr, C. S. (2007). Finding Data, Knowledge, and Answers on the Semantic Web. In *Proceedings of the 20th International FLAIRS Conference* (pp. 2-7).

Fisher, R. S., van Emde Boas, W., Blume, W., Elger, C., Genton, P., & Lee, P. (2005). Epileptic seizures and epilepsy: definitions proposed by the International League Against Epilepsy (ILAE) and the International Bureau for Epilepsy (IBE). *Epilepsia*, 46, 470–472. doi:10.1111/j.0013-9580.2005.66104.x

Flugsrud, G.B., Nordsletten, L., Espehaug, B., Havelin, L.I., Engeland, A., & Meyer, H.E. (2006). The impact of body mass index on later total hip arthroplasty for primary osteoarthritis: a cohort study in 1.2 million persons. *Arthritis Rheum*, 54, 802e7.

Forman, G. (2003). An extensive empirical study of feature selection metrics for text classification. *Journal of Machine Learning Research*, 3, 1289–1305. doi:10.1162/153244303322753670

Frahling, G., & Sohler, C. (2006). A fast k-means implementation using corsets. In N. Amenta and O. Cheong, editors. In *Proceedings of the twenty-second annual symposium on Computational geometry* (pp. 135-143). New York: ACM.

Freund, Y. S., R. E. (1999). A short introduction to boosting. *Journal of Japanese Society for Artificial Intelligence*, 14(5), 771–780.

Friedman-Hill, E. (2003). *Jess in Action: Rule-Based Systems in Java*: Manning Publications.

Friedman, J., Hastle, T., & Tibshirani, R. (2000). Additive logistic regression: a statistical view of boosting. *Annals of Statistics*, 28(2), 337–407. doi:10.1214/aos/1016218223

Friedman, R. H., Kazis, L. E., Jette, A., Smith, M. B., Stollerman, J., Torgerson, J., & Carey, K. (1996). A telecommunications system for monitoring and counseling patients with hypertension. Impact on medication adherence and blood pressure control. *American Journal of Hypertension*, 9, 285–292.

Frize, M., Solven, F. G., Stevenson, M., Nickerson, B. G., Buskard, T., & Taylor, K. B. (1995, July). Computer-Assisted Decision Support Systems for Patient Management in an Intensive Care Unit. In *Proceedings of Medinfo95,* Vancouver, BC, Canada (pp. 1009-1012).

Frize, M., Weyand, S., & Bariciak, E. (2010, May). Suggested Criteria for Successful Deployment of a Clinical Decision Support System (CDSS). In *Proceedings of the MeMeA (Medical Measurements and Applications) Workshop,* Ottawa, ON, Canada (pp. 69-72).

Funahashi, J., Ohkubo, T., Fukunaga, H., Kikuya, M., Takada, N., & Asayama, K. (2006). The economic impact of the introduction of home blood pressure measurement for the diagnosis and treatment of hypertension. *Blood Pressure Monitoring, 11,* 257–267.

Fung, G. S. K., Lam, S. K., Cheng, S. W. K., & Chow, K. W. (2008). On stent-graft models in thoracic aortic endovascular repair: A computational investigation of the hemodynamic factors. *Computers in Biology and Medicine, 38,* 484–489. doi:10.1016/j.compbiomed.2008.01.012

Gabriel, S. E., Crowson, C. S., & O'Fallon, W. M. (1999). Co morbidity in arthritis. *The Journal of Rheumatology, 26,* 2475–2479.

Gama, J., Rodrigues, P., & Aguilar-Ruiz, J. (2007). An overview on learning from data streams. *New Generation Computing, 25,* 1–4. doi:doi:10.1007/s00354-006-0001-5

Garstang, S. V., & Stitik, T. P. (2006). Osteoarthritis: epidemiology, risk factors and pathophysiology. *American Journal of Physical Medicine & Rehabilitation, 85*(11Suppl), S2–S11. doi:10.1097/01.phm.0000245568.69434.1a

Gastaut, H. (1970). Clinical and electroencephalographical classification of epileptic seizures. *Epilepsia, 11,* 102–113. doi:10.1111/j.1528-1157.1970.tb03871.x

Gaydos, C. A., Quinn, T. C., Willis, D., Weissfeld, A., Hook, E. W., & Martin, D. H. (2003). Performance of the APTIMA Combo 2 assay for detection of Chlamydia trachomatis and Neisseria gonorrhoeae in female urine and endocervical swab specimens. *Journal of Clinical Microbiology, 41*(1), 304–309. doi:10.1128/JCM.41.1.304-309.2003

Geisler, W. M. (2007). Management of uncomplicated Chlamydia trachomatis infections in adolescents and adults: evidence reviewed for the 2006 Centers for Disease Control and Prevention sexually transmitted diseases treatment guidelines. *Clinical Infectious Diseases, 44,* S77–S83. doi:10.1086/511421

Gelber, A.C., Hochberg, M.C., Mead, L.A., Wang, N.Y., Wigley, F.M., & Klag, M.J. (1999). Body mass index in young men and the risk of subsequent knee and hip osteoarthritis. *Am J Med, 107,* 542e8

Gervaso, F., Capelli, C., Petrini, L., Lattanzio, S., Di Virgilio, L., & Migliavacca, F. (2008). On the effects of different strategies in modelling balloon-expandable stenting by means of finite element method. *Journal of Biomechanics, 41*(6), 1206–1212. doi:10.1016/j.jbiomech.2008.01.027

Gift, T., Walsh, C., Haddix, A., & Irwin, K. L. (2002). A cost-effectiveness evaluation of testing and treatment of Chlamydia trachomatis infection among asymptomatic women infected with Neisseria gonorrhoeae. *Sexually Transmitted Diseases, 29*(9), 542–551. doi:10.1097/00007435-200209000-00009

Gijsen, F. J. H., Migliavacca, F., Schievano, S., Socci, L., Petrini, L., & Thury, A. (2008). Simulation of stent deployment in a realistic human coronary artery. *Biomedical Engineering Online, 7,* 23. doi:10.1186/1475-925X-7-23

Glen, S. K., Elliott, H. L., Curzio, J. L., Lees, K. R., & Reid, J. L. (1996). White-coat hypertension as a cause of cardiovascular dysfunction. *Lancet, 348,* 654–657.

Gligorov, R., Aleksovski, Z., Kate, W., & Harmelen, F. (2007). Using Google Distance to Weight Approximate Ontology Matches. In *16th International World Wide Web Conference* (pp. 767-775).

Goethals. B. (n.d.). http://www.adrem.ua.ac.be/~goethals/software. Last accessed on 05/19/09.

Golab, L., & Özsu, M. T. (2003). Issues in data stream management. *SIGMOD Record, 32*(2), 5–14. doi:doi:10.1145/776985.776986

Goldberg, D. E. (1989). *Genetic algorithms in search, optimization & machine learning.* Reading, MA: Addison Wesley.

Goldreich, O. (1997). On the foundations of modern cryptography. In *Proceedings of the Advances in Cryptology (Crypto '97)* (Vol. 1294, pp. 46-74).

Goldreich, O. (2004). *The Foundations of Cryptography* (Vol. 2), chapter General Cryptographic Protocols. Cambridge, UK: Cambridge University Press.

Goldreich, O., Micali, S., & Wigderson, A. (1987). How to play any mental game - a completeness theorem for protocols with honest majority. In *Proccedings of the 19th ACM Symposium on the Theory of Computing* (pp. 218-229).

Goll, J., Rajagopala, S. V., Shiau, S. C., Wu, H., Lamb, B. T., & Uetz, P. (2008). MPIDB: the microbial protein interaction database. *Bioinformatics (Oxford, England)*, *24*(15), 1743–1744. doi:10.1093/bioinformatics/btn285

Good, I. J. (1950). *Probability and the Weighing of Evidence*. London, UK: Charles Grin.

Goodney, P. P., & Powell, R. J. (2008). Carotid artery stenting: what have we learned from the clinical trials and registries and where do we go from here? *Annals of Vascular Surgery*, *22*, 148–158. doi:10.1016/j.avsg.2007.10.002

Google. (2008). *Google Health*. Retrieved September 15, 2009 from http://www.google.com/health

Goyal, V., Pandey, O., Sahai, A., & Waters, B. (2006). Attribute-based encryption for fine-grained access control of encrypted data. In A. Juels (Ed.), *Proceedings of the 14th ACM Conference on Computer and Communications Security* (pp. 89-98). New York: ACM.

Graber, M. A., D'Alessandro, D. M., & Johnson-West, J. (2002). Reading level of privacy policies on internet health web sites. *Journal of Family Practice*.

Graham, G. S., & Denning, P. J. (1971). Protection: principles and practice. In *Proceedings of the November 16-18, 1971, Fall Joint Computer Conference* (pp. 417–429).

Green, M., & Ateniese, G. (2007). Identity-based proxy re-encryption. In J. Katz & M. Yung (Eds.), *Proceedings of Applied Cryptography and Network Security* (Vol. 4521 of LNCS) (pp. 288-306). New York: Springer Verlag.

Gruber, T. R. (1993). Toward principles for the design of ontologies used for knowledge sharing. In *Proceedings of International Workshop on Formal Ontology*, Padova, Italy. Retrieved from Web site: http://www-ksl.stanford.edu/knowledge-sharing/papers/README.html#onto-design

Grundy, S., Brewer, H. B., Cleeman, J., Smith, S., & Lenfant, C. (2004). Definition of metabolic syndrome. In *Proceedings of the NHLBI/AHA Conference* (Vol. 24, pp. 13-18). Retrieved August 1, 2010, from http://circ.ahajournals.org/cgi/content/full/109/3/433

Grundy, S.M., Cleeman, J.I., Daniels, S.R., Donato, K.A., Eckel, R.H., Franklin, B.A., Gordon, J.D., Krauss, M.R., Savage, J.P., Smith, C. S., Spertus, A.J., & Fernando, C. (2005). Diagnosis and management of the metabolic syndrome. An American Heart Association/National Heart, Lung and Blood Institute Scientific Statement. Executive Summary. *Circulation*, *112*, 2735e52.

Guetlein, M. (2006). Large scale attribute selection using wrappers.

Guha, S., Meyerson, A., Mishra, N., Motwani, R., & O'Callaghan, L. (2003). Clustering data streams: Theory and practice. *IEEE Transactions on Knowledge and Data Engineering*, *15*(3), 515–528. doi:doi:10.1109/TKDE.2003.1198387

Gupta, P. K., & Fleisher, D. E. (1993). Nonvariceal upper gastrointestinal bleeding. *The Medical Clinics of North America*, *77*(5), 973–1012.

Hackl, H., & Sanchez Cabo, F. (2004). Analysis of DNA microarray data. *Current Topics in Medicinal Chemistry*, *4*(13), 1357–1370. doi:10.2174/1568026043387773

Halkidi, M., Batistakis, Y., & Vazirgiannis, M. (2002b). Clustering Validity Checking Methods: Part II. *SIGMOD Record*, *31*, 19–27. doi:doi:10.1145/601858.601862

Hall, M. A. (1998). *Correlation-based feature subset selection for machine learning*. Unpublished dissertation/thesis, University of Waikato, Hamilton, New Zealand.

Hall, G. J., & Kasper, E. P. (2006). Comparison of element technologies for modeling stent expansion. *Journal of Biomechanical Engineering*, *128*, 751–756. doi:10.1115/1.2264382

Han, J., & Kamber, M. (2006). Data Mining: Concepts and Techniques (2nd ed.), Morgan Kaufmann.

Hand, D. J., Mannila, H., & Smyth, P. (2001). *Principles of Data Mining.* MIT Press.

Hara, A., Ohkubo, T., Kikuya, M., Shintani, Y., Obara, T., & Metoki, H. (2007). Detection of carotid atherosclerosis in individuals with masked hypertension and white-coat hypertension by self-measured blood pressure at home: the Ohasama study. *Journal of Hypertension, 25,* 321–327.

Hashizume, M., Kitano, S., Yamaga, H., Wada, H., & Sugimachi, K. (2005). Eradication of oesophageal varices recurring after portal non-decompressive surgery by injection sclerotherapy. *British Journal of Surgery, 7,* 940–943.

Hearst, M. A. (1992). Automatic Acquisition of Hyponyms form Large Text Corpora. *Proceedings of, COLING-92,* 539–545.

Heathfield, H. (1999). The rise and 'fall' of expert systems in medicine. *Expert Systems: International Journal of Knowledge Engineering and Neural Networks, 16*(3), 183–188. doi:10.1111/1468-0394.00107

Helmick, C., Felson, D., Lawrence, R., Gabriel, S., Hirsch, R., & Kwoh, C. K. (2008). National Arthritis Data Workgroup. Estimates of the Prevalence of Arthritis and Other Rheumatic conditions in the United States. *Arthritis and Rheumatism, 58*(1), 15–25. doi:10.1002/art.23177

Hernandez, C., Sancho, J. J., Belmonte, M. A., Sierra, C., & Sanz, F. (1994). Validation of the medical expert system RENOIR. *Computers and Biomedical Research, an International Journal, 27*(6), 456–471. doi:10.1006/cbmr.1994.1034

Hewitt, J., & O'Connor, M. (2002). Connecting care through EMPIs. *Journal of American Health Information Management Association, 73*(10).

Hillier, F. S., & Lieberman, G. J. (2001). *Introduction to operations research* (7th ed.). Boston, MA: McGraw-Hill.

HIMSS. (2009). *Privacy and Security Toolkit.* Retrieved November 27, 2009 from http://www.himss.org/CPRI-Toolkit/html/4.11.html

HIPAA. (2000). The health insurance portability and accountability act of 1996. Technical Report Federal Register 65 FR 82462, Department of Health and Human Services, Office of the Secretary.

Hochhauser, M. (2001). *Lost in the fine print: Readability of financial privacy notices.* Retrieved November 27, 2009 from http://www.privacyrights.org/ar/GLB-Reading.htm

Holzapfel, G. A., Stadler, M., & Gasser, T. C. (2005). Changes in the mechanical environment of stenotic arteries during interaction with stents: computational assessment of parametric stent designs. *Journal of Biomechanical Engineering, 127,* 166–180. doi:10.1115/1.1835362

Homer, N., & Szelinger, S. (2008). Resolving individuals contributing trace amounts of DNA to highly complex mixtures using high-density SNP genotyping microarrays. *PLOS Genetics, 4*(8), e1000167. doi:10.1371/journal.pgen.1000167

Hong, D., & Mohaisen, A. (2010). Augmented Rotation-Based Transformation for Privacy-Preserving Data Clustering. *Etri Journal, 32*(3), 351–361. doi:10.4218/etrij.10.0109.0333

Horrocks, I., Patel-Schneider, P. F., Boley, H., Tabet, S., Grosof, B., & Dean, M. (2004). SWRL: A Semantic Web Rule Language Combining OWL and RuleML. Retrieved May, 2008, from http://www.w3.org/Submission/2004/SUBM-SWRL-20040521/

Horrocks, I., Patel-Schneider, P. F., Bechhofer, S., & Tsarkov, D. (2005). OWL rules: A proposal and prototype implementation *Web Semantics: Science. Services and Agents on the World Wide Web, 3*(1), 23–40. doi:10.1016/j.websem.2005.05.003

Horsch, K., Giger, M. L., Venta, L. A., & Vyborny, C. J. (2002). Computerized diagnosis of breast lesions on ultrasound. *Medical Physics, 29*(2), 157–164. PubMed doi:10.1118/1.1429239

Howe, D. K. (2008). Big Problems. *American Fitness, 26,* 16–16.

Howell, M. R., Quinn, T. C., Brathwaite, W., & Gaydos, C. A. (1998). Screening women for chlamydia trachomatis in family planning clinics: the cost-effectiveness of DNA amplification assays. *Sexually Transmitted Diseases, 25*(2), 108–117. doi:10.1097/00007435-199802000-00008

Hozawa, A., Ohkubo, T., Kikuya, M., Yamaguchi, J., Ohmori, K., & Fujiwara, T. (2002). Blood pressure control assessed by home, ambulatory and conventional blood pressure measurements in the Japanese general population: the Ohasama study. *Hypertension Research, 25*, 57–63.

Hsu, C. H., & Chen, C. C. (2007). Svd-based projection for face recognition. In *Proceedings of the IEEE International Conference on Electro/Information Technology* (pp. 600-603). Washington, DC: IEEE.

Huang, Y. L., Chen, D. R., Jiang, Y. R., Kuo, S. J., Wu, H. K., & Moon, W. K. (2008). Computer-aided diagnosis using morphological features for classifying breast lesions on ultrasound. *Ultrasound Obstet. Gynecol.*

Huang, Y. L., & Chen, D. R. (2005). Support vector machines in sonography application to decision making in the diagnosis of breast cancer. *Journal of Clinical Imaging, 29*, 179–184. doi:10.1016/j.clinimag.2004.08.002

Ibrahim, M. M., Tarazi, R. C., Dustan, H. P., & Gifford, R. W. Jr. (1977). Electrocardiogram in evaluation of resistance to antihypertensive therapy. *Archives of Internal Medicine, 137*, 1125–1129.

Ibraimi, L., Tang, Q., Hartel, P., & Jonker, W. (2009). Efficient and provable secure ciphertext-policy attribute-based encryption schemes. In F. Bao, H. Li, & G. Wang (Eds.), *Proceedings of Information Security Practice and Experience* (Vol. 5451 of LNCS) (pp. 1-12). New York: Springer Verlag.

IHE. (2006). *The Patient Care Coordination Technical Framework: Basic Patient Privacy Consents, Supplement 2005-2006*. Retrieved November 27, 2009 from http://www.ihe.net/Technical_Framework/upload/IHE_PCC_TF_BPPC_Basic_Patient_Privacy_Consents_20060810.pdf

Institute of Medicine. (1999). *To Err Is Human: Building A Safer Health System*. Washington, DC: Author.

Ivan, A., & Dodis, Y. (2003). Proxy cryptography revisited. In C. Neuman (Ed.), *Proceedings of the Network and Distributed System Security Symposium*. Citeseer.

Jagannathan, G., & Wright, R. N. (2005). Privacy-preserving distributed k-means clustering over arbitrarily partitioned data. In *Proceedings of the eleventh ACM SIGKDD international conference on Knowledge discovery in data mining*, Chicago (pp. 593-599). New York: ACM.

Jagannathan, G., & Pillaipakkamnatt, K. (2010). Communication-Efficient Privacy-Preserving Clustering. *Trans. Data Privacy, 3*(1), 1–25.

Jain, A. K., Murty, M. N., & Flynn, P. J. (1999). Data Clustering: a review. [CSUR]. *ACM Computing Surveys, 31*, 264–323. doi:10.1145/331499.331504

Jakobsson, M. (1999). On quorum controlled asymmetric proxy re-encryption. In H. Imai & Y. Zheng (Eds.), *Proceedings of Public Key Cryptography* (Vol. 1560 of LNCS) (pp. 112–121). New York: Springer Verlag.

Japanese Ministry of Internal Affairs, Communications Information, and Communications Policy. (2003). *Personal data protection law*. Retrieved November 27, 2009 from http://www.kantei.go.jp/jp/it/privacy/houseika/hourituan/index.html

Jensen, C., Potts, C., & Jensen, C. (2005). Privacy practices of Internet users: Self reports versus observed behaviour. *International Journal of Human-Computer Studies, 63*, 203–227. doi:10.1016/j.ijhcs.2005.04.019

Jensen, F. (1996). *An Introduction to Bayesian Networks*. New York, NY: Springer.

JGAP. (2010). *Java Genetic Algorithms Package*. Retrieved from http://jgap.sourceforge.net

Joachims, T. (1998). Text categorization with Support Vector Machines: Learning with many relevant features. *In* Proc of Tenth European Conference on Machine Learning (ECML-98).

Joachims, T. (1999). *Making large-Scale SVM Learning Practical*. Advances in Kernel Methods - Support Vector Learning. MIT-Press.

John, G. H., & Pat Langley, P. (1995, 1995). *Estimating continuous distributions in Bayesian classifiers*. Paper presented at the Proceedings of the Eleventh Conference on Uncertainty in Artificial Intelligence, San Mateo, CA.

Joo, S., Yang, Y. S., Moon, W. K., & Kim, H. C. (2004). Computer-aided diagnosis of solid breast nodules: use of an artificial neural network based on multiple sonographic features. *IEEE Transactions on Medical Imaging, 23*(10), 1292–1300. PubMed doi:10.1109/TMI.2004.834617

Jula, A., Puukka, P., & Karanko, H. (1999). Multiple clinic and home blood pressure measurements versus ambulatory blood pressure monitoring. *Hypertension, 34*, 261–266.

Kajzer, W., Kaczmarek, M., & Marciniak, J. (2005). Biomechanical analysis of stent - oesophagus system. *Journal of Materials Processing Technology, 162-163*, 196–202. doi:10.1016/j.jmatprotec.2005.02.209

Kalfoglou, Y., & Hu, B. (2006, May). Issues with evaluating and using publicly available ontologies, In *Proceedings of the Fourth International Evaluation of Ontologies for the Web Workshop* (EON2006), Edinburgh, UK.

Kantarcioglu, M., & Clifton, C. (2004). Privacy-preserving distributed mining of association rules on horizontally partitioned data. *IEEE Transactions on Knowledge and Data Engineering, 16*(9), 1026–1037. doi:10.1109/TKDE.2004.45

Kaplan, B. (2001). Evaluating informatics applications clinical decision support systems literature review. *International Journal of Medical Informatics, 64*, 15–37. doi:10.1016/S1386-5056(01)00183-6

Kaplan, E. H., & Pollack, H. (1998). Allocating HIV prevention resources. *Socio-Economic Planning Sciences, 4*, 257–263. doi:10.1016/S0038-0121(98)00002-0

Kargupta, H., Datta, S., Wang, Q., & Sivakumar, K. (2003). Random data perturbation techniques and privacy preserving data mining. *Knowledge and Information Systems, 7*(4), 387–414. doi:10.1007/s10115-004-0173-6

Karjoth, G., Schunter, M., & Waidner, M. (2002). Platform for Enterprise Privacy Practices: Privacy-enabled management of customer data. In *Proceedings of the International Workshop on Privacy Enhancing Technologies*. San Francisco, California, USA: Springer Verlag.

Kaufman, L., & Rousseeuw, P. J. (1990). *Finding Groups in Data: An Introduction to Cluster Analysis*. New York: Wiley.

Kearney, P. M., Whelton, M., Reynolds, K., Muntner, P., Whelton, P. K., & He, J. (2005). Global burden of hypertension: analysis of worldwide data. *Lancet, 365*, 217–223.

Keles, A., & Keles, A. (2008). ESTDD: Expert system for thyroid diseases diagnosis. *Expert Systems with Applications, 34*(1), 242–246. doi:10.1016/j.eswa.2006.09.028

Kellerer, H., Pferschy, U., & Pisinger, D. (2004). *Knapsack problems* (1st ed.). New York, NY: Springer.

Kelman, C., Bass, A., & Holman, C. (2002). Research use of linked health data - a best practice protocol. [PubMed]. *Australian and New Zealand Journal of Public Health, 26*, 251–255.

Khattar, R. S., Senior, R., & Lahiri, A. (1998). Cardiovascular outcome in white-coat versus sustained mild hypertension: a 10-year follow-up study. *Circulation, 98*, 1892–1897.

Kiousis, D. E., Wulff, A. R., & Holzapfel, G. A. (2009). Experimental studies and numerical analysis of the inflation and interaction of vascular balloon catheter-stent systems. *Annals of Biomedical Engineering, 37*(2), 315–330. doi:10.1007/s10439-008-9606-9

Knublauch, H., Fergerson, R. W., Noy, N. F., & Musen, M. A. (2009). *The Prot'eg'e OWL Plugin: An Open Development Environment for Semantic Web Applications* [Electronic Version]. Retrieved May 2009 from http://protege.stanford.edu/plugins/owl/publications/ISWC2004-protege-owl.pdf.

Komarek, P., & Moore, A. (2005). *Making logistic regression a core data mining tool: A practical investigation of accuracy, speed, and simplicity* (pp. 685-688). Institute, Carnegie Mellon University.

Korochina, I. E., & Bagirova, G. G. (2007). Metabolic syndrome and a course of osteoarthritis. *Terapevticheskii Arkhiv, 79*, 13–20.

Korotkoff, N. S. (1905). On the subject of methods of determining blood pressure (from the clinic of Prof. S.P. Fedorov). *Bulletin of the Imperial Military Medical Academy, 11*, 356–367.

Koumans, E. H., Johnson, R. E., Knapp, J. S., & St. Louis, M. E. (1998). Laboratory testing for Neisseria gonorrhoeae by recently introduced nonculture tests: a performance review with clinical and public health considerations. *Clinical Infectious Diseases*, *27*(5), 1171–1180. doi:10.1086/514994

Koza, J. R. (1992). *Genetic Programming: On the Programming of Computers by Means of Natural Selection.* Cambridge, MA: MIT Press.

Kratnov, A. E., Kuryleva, K. V., & Kratnov, A. A. (2007). Association between primary osteoarthrosis and metabolic syndrome according to data from arthroscopic and cytochemical studies. [Mosk]. *Klinicheskaia Meditsina*, *84*(6), 42–46.

Kraus, V. B. (1997). Pathogenesis and treatment of osteoarthritis. *Adv Rheumatol*, *81*, 85–112.

Kuhnast, C., & Neuhauser, M. (2008). A note on the use of the non-parametric Wilcoxon-Mann-Whitney test in the analysis of medical studies. *German Medical Science*, *6*.

Kuznar, W. (2009). Diabetes found to protect against prostate cancer. *Urology Times*, *37*, 8.

LaDisa, J. F., Olson, L. E., Hettrick, D. A., Warltier, D. C., Kersten, J. R., & Pagel, P. S. (2005). Axial stent strut angle influences wall shear stress after stent implantation: analysis using 3D computational fluid dynamics models of stent foreshortening. *Biomedical Engineering Online*, *4*, 59. doi:10.1186/1475-925X-4-59

LaDisa, J. F., Olson, L. E., Hettrick, D. A., Warltier, D. C., Kersten, J. R., & Pagel, P. S. (2006). Alterations in regional vascular geometry produced by theoretical stent implantation influence distributions of wall shear stress: analysis of a curved coronary artery using 3D computational fluid dynamics modelling. *Biomedical Engineering Online*, *5*, 40. doi:10.1186/1475-925X-5-40

Lally, C., Dolan, F., & Prendergast, P. J. (2005). Cardiovascular stent design and vessel stresses: a finite element analysis. *Journal of Biomechanics*, *38*(8), 1574–1581. doi:10.1016/j.jbiomech.2004.07.022

Lam, S. K., Fung, G. S. K., Cheng, S. W. K., & Chow, K. W. (2008). A computational study on the biomechanical factors related to stent-graft models in the thoracic aorta. *Medical & Biological Engineering & Computing*, *46*, 1129–1138. doi:10.1007/s11517-008-0361-8

Lasry, A., Carter, M. W., & Zaric, G. S. (2008). S4HARA: System for HIV/AIDS resource allocation. *Cost Effectiveness and Resource Allocation*, *6*, 1–19. doi:10.1186/1478-7547-6-7

Lasry, A., Richter, A., & Lutscher, F. (2009). Recommendations for increasing the use of HIV/AIDS resource allocation models. *BMC Public Health*, *9*, S8. doi:10.1186/1471-2458-9-S1-S8

Lasry, A., Zaric, G. S., & Carter, M. W. (2007). Multi-level resource allocation for HIV prevention: A model for developing countries. *European Journal of Operational Research*, *180*(2), 786–799. doi:10.1016/j.ejor.2006.02.043

Lau, C. Y., & Qureshi, A. K. (2002). Azithromycin versus doxycycline for genital chlamydial infections: a meta-analysis of randomized clinical trials. *Sexually Transmitted Diseases*, *29*(9), 497–502. doi:10.1097/00007435-200209000-00001

Lawrence, R. C., Helmick, C. G., Arnett, F. C., Deyo, R. A., Felson, D. T., & Giannini, E. H. (1998). Estimates of the prevalence of arthritis and selected musculoskeletal disorders in the United States. *Arthritis and Rheumatism*, *43*, 778–779. doi:10.1002/1529-0131(199805)41:5<778::AID-ART4>3.0.CO;2-V

Lebrec, D., & Defleury, R. B. (1980). Portal hypertension, size of esophageal varices and risk of gastrointestinal bleeding in alcoholic cirrhosis. *Gastroenterology*, *79*, 1139.

Lee, S., & Hayes, M. (2004). Properties of the singular value decomposition for efficient data clustering. *IEEE Signal Processing Letters*, *11*(11), 862–866. doi:10.1109/LSP.2004.833513

Lee, Y., & Geller, J. (2005). Semantic Enrichment for Medical Ontologies. *Journal of Biomedical Informatics*, *39*(2), 209–226. doi:10.1016/j.jbi.2005.08.001

Leonardo, T., Maria, C. P., & Angelo, Z. (2008). Endoscopic finding in pts with UGI bleeding clinically classified in three risk groups prior to endoscopy. *World Journal of Gastroenterology, 14*(32), 5046–5050. doi:doi:10.3748/wjg.14.5046

Levine, B. A. (1987). Stress ulcer. *Problems in General Surgery, 4*, 208–222.

Lewington, S., Clarke, R., Qizilbash, N., Peto, R., & Collins, R. (2002). Age-specific relevance of usual blood pressure to vascular mortality: a meta-analysis of individual data for one million adults in 61 prospective studies. *Lancet, 360*, 1903–1913.

Lewis, D. (1983). New Work for a Theory of Universals. *Australasian Journal of Philosophy, 61*, 343–377. doi:10.1080/00048408312341131

Li, J., Zhu, W., Wang, X., de Santi, S., & de Leon, M. J. (2005). Bayesian Applications to Longitudinal Analysis on Medical Data with Discrete Outcomes. In Proceedings of the *27th Annual International Conference of the Engineering in Medicine and Biology Society (IEEE-EMBS)* (pp. 1204-1207). Washington, DC: IEEE.

Li, N., Li, T., & Venkatasubramanian, S. (2007). T-closeness: Privacy beyond k-anonymity and l-diversity. In *Proceedings of the ICDE* (pp. 106-115).

Li, N., Yu, T., & Anton, A. I. (2003). *A Semantics-based Approach to Privacy Languages* (Tech. Rep.). Center of Education and Research in Information Assurance and Security. Retrieved November 27, 2009 from http://www4.ncsu.edu/~tyu/pubs/p3p-csse06.pdf

Liang, X., Cao, Z., Lin, H., & Shao, J. (2009). Attribute based proxy re-encryption with delegating capabilities. In W. Li, W. Susilo, & U. Tupakula (Eds.), *Proceedings of the 4th International Symposium on Information, Computer, and Communications Security* (pp. 276-286). New York: ACM.

Liao, T. W. (2005). Clustering of time series data - a survey. *Pattern Recognition, 38*(11), 1857–1874. doi:doi:10.1016/j.patcog.2005.01.025

Liebowitz, J. (1997). *The Handbook of Applied Expert Systems*. Boca Raton, FL: CRC Press.

Lin, J.-L., & Liu, J. Y.-C. (2007). Privacy preserving itemset mining through fake transactions http://doi.acm.org/10.1145/1244002.1244092. In *Proceedings of the ACM symposium on Applied computing* (pp. 375-379), Seoul, Korea: ACM Press.

Li, N., Zhang, H., & Ouyang, H. (2009). Shape optimization of coronary artery stent based on a parametric model. *Finite Elements in Analysis and Design, 45*(6-7), 468–475. doi:10.1016/j.finel.2009.01.001

Lindell, Y., & Pinkas, B. (2002). Privacy preserving data mining. *Journal of Cryptology, 15*(3), 177–206. doi:doi:10.1007/s00145-001-0019-2

Liu, K., Kargupta, H., & Ryan, J. (2006). Random projection-based multiplicative data perturbation for privacy preserving distributed data mining. *IEEE Transactions on Knowledge and Data Engineering, 18*(1), 92–106. doi:10.1109/TKDE.2006.14

Liu, W., Yang, L., & Hanzo, L. (2009). Svd-assisted multiuser transmitter and multiuser detector design for MIMO systems. *IEEE Transactions on Vehicular Technology, 58*, 1016–1021. doi:10.1109/TVT.2008.927728

Li, X. B., & Sarkar, S. A. (2006). Tree-Based Data Perturbation Approach for Privacy-Preserving Data Mining. *IEEE Transactions on Knowledge and Data Engineering, 18*(9), 1278–1283. doi:10.1109/TKDE.2006.136

Longstreth, G. F. (1995). Epidemiology of Hospitalization for acute upper gastrointestinal hemorrhage: A population based study. *The American Journal of Gastroenterology, 90*(2), 206–210.

Lu, Y.-H., & Huang, Y. (2005, August 18-21). *Mining data streams using clustering*. Paper presented at the 4th International Conference on Machine Learning and Cybernatics, Guangzhou, China.

Lüders, H., Acharya, J., Baumgartner, C., Benbadis, S., Bleasel, A., & Burgess, R. (1998). Semiological seizure classification. *Epilepsia, 39*, 1006–1013. doi:10.1111/j.1528-1157.1998.tb01452.x

Lurbe, E., Torro, I., Alvarez, V., Nawrot, T., Paya, R., Redon, J., & Staessen, J. A. (2005). Prevalence, persistence, and clinical significance of masked hypertension in youth. *Hypertension, 45*, 493–498.

Lussier, Y., & Bodenreider, O. (2007). Clinical Ontologies for Discovery Applications. In C. J. O. Baker & K.-H. Cheung (Eds.), *SEMANTIC WEB Revolutionizing Knowledge Discovery in the Life Sciences* (pp. 101-121). NY,USA: Springer.

Machanavajjhala, A., Kifer, D., Gehrke, J., & Venkitasubramaniam, M. (2007). L-diversity: Privacy beyond k-anonymity. *ACM Trans. Knowl. Discov. Data, 1*(1), 3. doi:doi:10.1145/1217299.1217302

Maedche, A., & Staab, S. (2000). Mining Ontologies from Text. *Proceedings of EKAW-2000, Springer Lecture Notes in Artificial Intelligence (LNAI-1937)* (pp. 189-202), Juan-Les-Pins, France.

Maetzel, A., Li, L. C., Pencharz, J., Tomlinson, F., & Bombardier, C. (2004). The economic burden associated with osteoarthritis, rheumatoid arthritis, and hypertension: A comparative study. *Annals of the Rheumatic Diseases, 63*(4), 395–401. doi:10.1136/ard.2003.006031

Mahner, M., & Kary, M. (1997). What exactly are genomes, genotypes and phenotypes? And what about phenomes? *Journal of Theoretical Biology, 186*(1), 55–63. doi:10.1006/jtbi.1996.0335

Mallat, S. G. (1989). A theory for multiresolution signal decomposition: The wavelet representation. *IEEE Transactions on Pattern Analysis and Machine Intelligence, 11*(7), 674–693. doi:10.1109/34.192463

Mallion, J. M., Clerson, P., Bobrie, G., Genes, N., Vaisse, B., & Chatellier, G. (2006). Predictive factors for masked hypertension within a population of controlled hypertensives. *Journal of Hypertension, 24*, 2365–2370.

Mambo, M., & Okamoto, E. (1997). Proxy Cryptosystems: Delegation of the power to decrypt ciphertexts. *IEICE Transactions on Fundamentals of Electronics, Communications and Computer Science, 80*(1), 54–63.

Mancia, G., Bertinieri, G., Grassi, G., Parati, G., Pomidossi, G., & Ferrari, A. (1983). Effects of blood-pressure measurement by the doctor on patient's blood pressure and heart rate. *Lancet, 2*, 695–698.

Mancia, G., De Backer, G., Dominiczak, A., Cifkova, R., Fagard, R., & Germano, G. (2007). 2007 Guidelines for the Management of Arterial Hypertension: The Task Force for the Management of Arterial Hypertension of the European Society of Hypertension (ESH) and of the European Society of Cardiology (ESC). *Journal of Hypertension, 25*, 1105–1187.

Mancia, G., Di Rienzo, M., & Parati, G. (1993). Ambulatory blood pressure monitoring use in hypertension research and clinical practice. *Hypertension, 21*, 510–524.

Mancia, G., Facchetti, R., Bombelli, M., Grassi, G., & Sega, R. (2006). Long-term risk of mortality associated with selective and combined elevation in office, home, and ambulatory blood pressure. *Hypertension, 47*, 846–853.

Mancia, G., Parati, G., Pomidossi, G., Grassi, G., Casadei, R., & Zanchetti, A. (1987). Alerting reaction and rise in blood pressure during measurement by physician and nurse. *Hypertension, 9*, 209–215.

Mandelbaum, B., & Waddell, D. (2005, February). Etiology and pathophysiology of osteoarthritis. *Orthopedics, 28*(2Suppl), s207–s214.

Martello, S., Pisinger, D., & Toth, P. (2000). New trends in exact algorithms for the 0-1 knapsack problem. *European Journal of Operational Research, 123*(2), 325–332. doi:10.1016/S0377-2217(99)00260-X

Martello, S., & Toth, P. (1990). *Knapsack problems: algorithms and computer implementations* (Toth, P., Trans.). New York, NY: John Wiley & Sons.

Martin, J. G. (2005). Subproblem Optimization by Gene Correlation with Singular Value Decomposition. In H. Beyer (Ed.), *Proceedings of the 2005 conference on Genetic and evolutionary computation* (pp. 1507-1514). New York: ACM.

Martin, D. H., Cammarata, C., Van Der Pol, B., Jones, R. B., Quinn, T. C., & Gaydos, C. A. (2000). Multicenter evaluation of AMPLICOR and automated COBAS AMPLICOR CT/NG tests for Neisseria gonorrhoeae. *Journal of Clinical Microbiology, 38*(10), 3544–3549.

Martin, D. H., Mroczkowski, T. F., Dalu, Z. A., McCarty, J., Jones, R. B., & Hopkins, S. J. (1992). A controlled trial of a single dose of azithromycin for the treatment of chlamydial urethritis and cervicitis. The Azithromycin for Chlamydial Infections Study Group. *The New England Journal of Medicine, 327*(13), 921–925. doi:10.1056/NEJM199209243271304

Martinez, M. A., Garcia-Puig, J., Martin, J. C., Guallar-Castillon, P., Aguirre de Carcer, A., & Torre, A. (1999). Frequency and determinants of white coat hypertension in mild to moderate hypertension: A primary care-based study. *American Journal of Hypertension, 12,* 251–259.

Martinez, M. A., Sancho, T., Garcia, P., Moreno, P., Rubio, J. M., & Palau, F. J. (2006). Home blood pressure in poorly controlled hypertension: relationship with ambulatory blood pressure and organ damage. *Blood Pressure Monitoring, 11,* 207–213.

Massimo, G., Federico, B., & Giovanna, L. (1994). Survival after endoscopic sclerotherapy for esophageal varices in cirrhotics. *The American Journal of Gastroenterology,* 1815–1822.

Ma, T., Yao, R., Shao, Y., & Zhou, R. (2009). A SVD-Based Method to Assess the Uniqueness and Accuracy of Spect Geometrical Calibration. *IEEE Transactions on Medical Imaging, 28,* 1929–1939. doi:10.1109/TMI.2009.2025696

Mathworks. (2007). *Analyzing Illumina Bead Summary Gene Expression Data.* Retrieved from http://www.mathworks.com/matlabcentral/fx_files/16171/1/content/illuminageneexpdemo.html

Matsuo, T. (2007). Proxy re-encryption systems for identity-based encryption. In T. Takagi, T. Okamoto, E. Okamoto, & T. Okamoto (Eds.), *Proceedings of Pairing-Based Cryptography - Pairing 2007* (Vol. 4575 of LNCS) (pp. 247-267). New York: Springer Verlag.

McCray, A. T., Burgun, A., & Bodenreider, O. (2001). Aggregating UMLS Semantic Types for Reducing Conceptual Complexity. In [London, UK.]. *Proceedings of Medinfo, 2001,* 171–175.

McDonald, A., Reeder, R., Kelley, P., & Cranor, L. (2009). Comparative Study of Online Privacy Policies and Formats. In *Proceedings of the Annual Privacy Enhancing Technology Symposium (PETS) (LNCS Vol. 5672).* Seattle, Washington, USA.

Menard, J., Chatellier, G., Day, M., & Vaur, L. (1994). Self-measurement of blood pressure at home to evaluate drug effects by the trough: peak ratio. *Journal of Hypertension, 12,* S21–S25.

Mengden, T., Hernandez Medina, R. M., Beltran, B., Alvarez, E., Kraft, K., & Vetter, H. (1998). Reliability of reporting self-measured blood pressure values by hypertensive patients. *American Journal of Hypertension, 11,* 1413–1417.

Menon, S., & Sarkar, S. (2007). Minimizing Information Loss and Preserving Privacy. *Management Science, 53*(1), 101–116. doi:10.1287/mnsc.1060.0603

Menon, S., Sarkar, S., & Mukherjee, S. (2005). Maximizing Accuracy of Shared Databases when Concealing Sensitive Patterns. *Information Systems Research, 16*(3), 256–270. doi:10.1287/isre.1050.0056

Mextaxiotis, K., & Samouilidis, J.E. (2000). Expert systems in medicine: academic illusion or real power? *Information Management and Security,* 75-79.

Microsoft. (2006). *Microsoft Excel Solver User's Guide for Windows.* Retrieved from http://support.microsoft.com/kb/82890

Microsoft. (2007). *HealthVault Connection Center.* Retrieved September 15, 2009 from http://www.healthvault.com/

Mieke, S. (1997). Substitute of simulators for human subjects. *Blood Pressure Monitoring, 2,* 251–256.

Migliavacca, F., Petrini, L., Colombo, M., Auricchio, F., & Pietrabissa, R. (2002). Mechanical behavior of coronary stents investigated through the finite element method. *Journal of Biomechanics, 35,* 803–811. doi:10.1016/S0021-9290(02)00033-7

Migliavacca, F., Petrini, L., Massarotti, P., Schievano, S., Auricchio, F., & Dubini, G. (2004). Stainless and shape memory alloy coronary stents: a computational study on the interaction with the vascular wall. *Biomechanics and Modeling in Mechanobiology, 2,* 205–217. doi:10.1007/s10237-004-0039-6

Migliavacca, F., Petrini, L., Montanari, V., Quagliana, I., Auricchio, F., & Dubini, G. (2005). A predictive study of the mechanical behaviour of coronary stents by computer modelling. *Medical Engineering & Physics, 27*(1), 13–18. doi:10.1016/j.medengphy.2004.08.012

Mihalcea, R., & Moldovan, D. I. (1999). An Automatic Method for Generating Sense Tagged Corpora. In *Proceedings of American Association for Artificial Intelligence* (pp. 461-466), Orlando, FL.

Milenova, B. L., & Campos, M. M. (2003). *Clustering large databases with numeric and nominal values using orthogonal projections.* Paper presented at the 29th VLDB Conference.

Miller, R. A., & Geissbuhler, A. (2007). Diagnostic Decision Support Systems. In E. S. Berner (Ed.), *Clinical Decision Support Systems Theory and Practice* (pp. 99-125). NY: Springer.

Miller, W. C., Ford, C. A., Morris, M., Handcock, M. S., Schmitz, J. L., & Hobbs, M. M. (2004). Prevalence of chlamydial and gonococcal infections among young adults in the United States. *Journal of the American Medical Association, 291*(18), 2229–2236. doi:10.1001/jama.291.18.2229

Miner, M. (2010). Metabolic Syndrome, Testosterone, and Lifestyle Modification: Impact on Erectile Dysfunction, Cardiovascular Disease and All-Cause Mortality. *Urology Times -. Sexual Health*, (Supplement), 16–21.

Mitchell, T. (1997). *Machine Learning.* New York, NY: McGraw Hill.

Mizoguchi, R. (2004). Tutorial on Ontological Engineering: Part 3: Advanced Course of Ontological Engineering. *New Generation Computing, 22*(2).

MMWR. (2007). *Data Source: 2003 Medical Expenditure Panel Survey, 56*(01), 4-7. Available at: http://www.cdc.gov/nchs/nhanes.htm.

Molinara, M., Ricamato, M. T., & Tortorella, F. (2007). *Facing Imbalanced Classes through Aggregation of Classifiers.* IEEE Computer Society Washington, DC, USA.

Morrison, J. L., Breitling, R., Higham, D. J., & Gilbert, D. R. (2005). GeneRank: using search engine technology for the analysis of microarray experiments. *BMC Bioinformatics, 6*, 233. doi:10.1186/1471-2105-6-233

Mortier, P., De Beule, M., Carlier, S. G., Van Impe, R., Verhegghe, B., & Verdonck, P. (2008). Numerical Study of the Uniformity of Balloon-Expandable Stent Deployment. *Journal of Biomechanical Engineering, 130*(2), 021018. doi:10.1115/1.2904467

Mu, T., Nandi, A. K., & Rangayyan, R. M. (2008). Classification of breast masses using selected shape, edge-sharpness, and texture features with linear and kernel-based classifiers. *Journal of Digital Imaging, 21*(2), 153–169. PubMed doi:10.1007/s10278-007-9102-z

Mule, G., Caimi, G., Cottone, S., Nardi, E., Andronico, G., & Piazza, G. (2002). Value of home blood pressures as predictor of target organ damage in mild arterial hypertension. *Journal of Cardiovascular Risk, 9*, 123–129.

Narracott, A. J., Lawford, P. V., Gunn, J. P. G., & Hose, D. R. (2007). Balloon folding affects the symmetry of stent deployment: Experimental and computational evidence. In *Proceedings of the 29th Annual International Conference of IEEE-EMBS, Engineering in Medicine and Biology Society, EMBC'07* (pp. 3069-3073).

Natarajan, A. M., Rajalaxmi, R. R., et al. (2007). A hybrid data transformation approach for privacy preserving clustering of categorical data. *Innovations and Advanced Techniques in Computer and Information Sciences and Engineering*, 403-408, 562.

National Cholesterol Education Program (NCEP). (2002). Expert Panel on Detection, Evaluation, and Treatment of High Blood Cholesterol in Adults (Adult Treatment Panel III). Third Report of the National Cholesterol Education Program (NCEP) Expert Panel on Detection, Evaluation, and Treatment of High Blood Cholesterol in Adults (Adult Treatment Panel III) final report. *Circulation, 106*, 3143–3421.

National Health Service. (2008). *National Health Service Breast Screening Programme* (*Vol. 2008*). U. K.

National Institutes of Health (NIH). (2009). *Metabolic Syndrome.* Retrieved July 13, 2010 from http://www.nlm.nih.gov/medlineplus/metabolicsyndrome.html

Necib, C. B., & Freytag, J. (2003). Ontology Based Query Processing in Database Management Systems. In *Proceedings of the 6th International Conference on Ontologies, Databases and Applications of Semantics for Large Scale Information Systems (ODBASE'2003)* (pp. 37-99).

Neves, J., Alves, V., Nelas, L., Romeu, A., & Basto, S. (1999). An Information System that Supports Knowledge Discovery and Data Mining in Medical Imaging. In *Proceedings of the ECCAI Advanced Course in Artificial Intelligence (ACAI) Workshop (W13) on Machine Learning in Medical Applications,* Chania, Greece.

Newman, L. M., Moran, J. S., & Workowski, K. A. (2007). Update on the management of gonorrhea in adults in the United States. *Clinical Infectious Diseases, 44,* S84–S101. doi:10.1086/511422

Ng, W., & Dash, M. (2006). *An Evaluation of Progressive Sampling for Imbalanced Data Sets.* IEEE Computer Society Washington, DC, USA.

Niccolai, L. M., Livingston, K. A., Teng, F. F., & Pettigrew, M. M. (2008). Behavioral intentions in sexual partnerships following a diagnosis of Chlamydia trachomatis. *American Journal of Preventive Medicine, 46*(2), 170–176. doi:10.1016/j.ypmed.2007.08.013

Noy, N. F., & McGuinness, D. L. (2001). *Ontology Development 101: A Guide to Creating Your First Ontology.* Stanford Knowledge Systems Laboratory & Stanford Medical Informatics Technical Report

Noy, N. F., & Hafner, C. (1997). The State of the Art in Ontology Design: A Survey and Comparative Review. *AI Magazine, 18*(3), 53–74.

Nutrition Health Review. (2009). Menopause and Metabolic Syndrome. *The Consumer's Medical Journal,* 15-15.

Nutrition, A. H. L. (2009)... *Inflammation & Beyond, 36,* 7–7.

O'Connor, M. J., & Das, A. (2006). *A Mechanism to Define and Execute SWRL Built-ins in Protégé-OWL* [Electronic Version]. Retrieved May, 2009 from http://protege.stanford.edu/conference/2006/submissions/abstracts/7.3_Martin_oConnor_BuiltInBridge.pdf.

O'Brien, E., Asmar, R., Beilin, L., Imai, Y., Mallion, J. M., & Mancia, G. (2003). European Society of Hypertension recommendations for conventional, ambulatory and home blood pressure measurement. *Journal of Hypertension, 21,* 821–848.

O'Brien, E., Asmar, R., Beilin, L., Imai, Y., Mancia, G., & Mengden, T. (2005). Practice guidelines of the European Society of Hypertension for clinic, ambulatory and self blood pressure measurement. *Journal of Hypertension, 23,* 697–701.

Obrst, L., Hughes, T., & Steve Ray, S. (2006, May). Prospects and Possibilities for Ontology Evaluation: The View from NCOR. In *Proceedings of the Fourth International Evaluation of Ontologies for the Web Workshop (EON2006),* Edinburgh, UK.

Office of the Privacy Commissioner of Canada. (2000). *Personal Information Protection and Electronic Documents Act (PIPEDA).* Retrieved November 27, 2009 from http://www.priv.gc.ca/legislation/02_06_01_e.cfm

Ohkubo, T., Asayama, K., Kikuya, M., Metoki, H., Hoshi, H., & Hashimoto, J. (2004). How many times should blood pressure be measured at home for better prediction of stroke risk? Ten-year follow-up results from the Ohasama study. *Journal of Hypertension, 22,* 1099–1104.

Ohkubo, T., Imai, Y., Tsuji, I., Nagai, K., & Kato, J., ikuchi, N. K., et al. (1998). Home blood pressure measurement has a stronger predictive power for mortality than does screening blood pressure measurement: a population-based observation in Ohasama, Japan. *Journal of Hypertension, 16,* 971–975.

Ohkubo, T., Kikuya, M., Metoki, H., Asayama, K., Obara, T., & Hashimoto, J. J. (2005). Prognosis of "masked" hypertension and "white-coat" hypertension detected by 24-h ambulatory blood pressure monitoring 10-year follow-up from the Ohasama study. *Journal of the American College of Cardiology, 46,* 508–515.

Ojala, T., Pietikainen, M., & Maenpaa, T. (2002). Multi-resolution gray-scale and rotation invariant texture classification with local binary patterns. *IEEE Transactions on Pattern Analysis and Machine Intelligence, 24*(7), 971–987. doi:10.1109/TPAMI.2002.1017623

O'Keefe, C. M., Yung, M., Gu, L., & Baxter, R. (2004). Privacy-preserving data linkage protocols. In *WPES '04: Proceedings of the 2004 ACM workshop on Privacy in the electronic society* (pp. 94-102). New York: ACM.

Oliveira, S., & Zaiane, O. R. (2002). *Privacy Preserving Frequent Itemset Mining*. Paper presented at the IEEE International Conference on Privacy, Security and Data Mining, Maebashi City, Japan.

Oliveira, S., & Zaiane, O. R. (2003a, July). Algorithms for Balancing Privacy and Knowledge Discovery in Association Rule Mining. In *Proceedings of the 7th International Database Engineering and Applications Symposium (IDEAS)* (pp. 54-63), Hong Kong, China.

Oliveira, S., & Zaiane, O. R. (2003b, November). Protecting Sensitive Knowledge by Data Sanitization. In *Proceedings of the 3rd IEEE International Conference on Data Mining* (pp. 613-616), Melbourne, Florida.

Oliveria, S.A., Felson, D.T., Cirillo, P.A., Reed, J.I., & Walker, A.M. (1999). Body weight, body mass index, and incident symptomatic osteoarthritis of the hand, hip, and knee. *Epidemiology*; *10*, 161e6.

OpenCyc. (2005). *Predicates and Denotational Functions of Cyc* [PowerPoint slides]. Retrieved from Web site: http://www.cyc.com/doc/tut/DnLoad/TheBasicsOfPred-DenoFun.pdf

Osteoarthritis Fact sheet (2008). *News from the Arthritis Foundation*.

Palmer, S. (2009). Putting the Brakes on Inflammation Through Diet and Lifestyle Strategies. *Environmental Nutrition*, *32*, 1–6.

Parati, G., & Stergiou, G. (2004). Self blood pressure measurement at home: how many times? *Journal of Hypertension*, *22*, 1075–1079.

Pear, R. (in press). Warnings over privacy of us health network. *New York Times*.

Pearson, K. (1901). On lines and planes of closest fit to systems of points in space. *Philosophical Magazine*, *2*, 559–572.

Pericevic, I., Lally, C., Toner, D., & Kelly, D. J. (2009). The influence of plaque composition on underlying arterial wall stress during stent expansion: The case for lesion-specific stents. *Medical Engineering & Physics*, *31*(4), 428–433. doi:10.1016/j.medengphy.2008.11.005

Phillips, R. D., Watson, L. T., & Wynne, R. H. (2008). A Shared Memory Parallel Algorithm for Data Reduction Using the Singular Value Decomposition. In H. Rajaei (Ed.), *Proceedings of the 2008 Spring simulation multi-conference* (pp. 459-466). New York: ACM.

Pickering, T. (1996). Recommendations for the use of home (self) and ambulatory blood pressure monitoring, American Society of Hypertension Ad Hoc Panel. *American Journal of Hypertension*, *9*, 1–11.

Pickering, T. G., Hall, J. E., Appel, L. J., Falkner, B. E., Graves, J., & Hill, M. N. (2005). Recommendations for blood pressure measurement in humans and experimental animals: part 1: Blood pressure measurement in humans: a statement for professionals from the Subcommittee of Professional and Public Education of the American Heart Association Council on High Blood Pressure Research. *Circulation*, *111*, 697–716.

Pickering, T. G., James, G. D., Boddie, C., Harshfield, G. A., Blank, S., & Laragh, J. H. (1988). How common is white coat hypertension? *Journal of the American Medical Association*, *259*, 225–228.

Pisanelli, D. M., Gangemi, A., & Steve, G. (1998). An Ontological Analysis of the UMLS Metathesaurus. *Journal of the American Medical Informatics Association*, *5*, 810–814.

Planas, R., Quer, J. C., & Boix, J. (1994). A prospective randomized trial comparing somatostatin and sclerotherapy in the treatment of acute variceal bleeding. *Hepatology (Baltimore, Md.)*, *20*, 370. doi:doi:10.1002/hep.1840200216

Platt, J., Scholkopf, B., Burges, C., & Smola, A. (1999). Fast training of support vector machines using sequential minimal optimization. In Anonymous, (Ed.), *Advances in Kernel Methods - Support Vector Learning*. Cambridge, MA: MIT Press.

Pohlig, S. C., & Hellman, M. E. (1978). An improved algorithm for computing logarithms over GF(p) and its cryptographic significance. *IEEE Transactions on Information Theory*, *24*, 106–110. doi:doi:10.1109/TIT.1978.1055817

Poli, R., Langdon, W. B., & McPhee, N. F. (2010). *A Field Guide to Genetic Programming*. Retrieved from http://www.gp-eld-guide.org.uk

Pollach. (2007). What's wrong with online privacy policies? *Communications of the ACM, 30*(2), 103-108.

Pottie, P., Presle, N., Terlain, B., Netter, P., Mainard, D., & Berenbaum, F. (2006). Obesity and osteoarthritis: more complex than predicted. *Ann Rheum Dis, 65*, 1403e5.

Prapavesis, S. T., Fornage, B. D., Weismann, C. F., Palko, A., & Zoumpoulis, P. (2001). *Breast ultrasound and US-guided interventional techniques.* Thessaloniki, Greece.

Princeton University. (2006). *WordNet 2.1 Database Statistics.* Retrieved from Web site: http://wordnet.princeton.edu/man/wnstats.7WN

Privacy Rights Clearinghouse. (2009). *A chronology of data breaches.* Retrieved November 27, 2009 from http://www.privacyrights.org/ar/ChronDataBreaches.htm

Quinlan, J. R. (1979). Discovering rules by induction from large collections of examples. In Michie, D. (Ed.), *Expert Systems in the Microlectronic age* (pp. 168–201).

Quinlan, J. R. (1993). *C4.5: Programs for machine learning.* San Francisco, CA: Morgan Kaufmann Publishers.

Rajagopala, S. V., Goll, J., Gowda, N. D., Sunil, K. C., Titz, B., & Mukherjee, A. (2008). MPI-LIT: a literature-curated dataset of microbial binary protein--protein interactions. *Bioinformatics (Oxford, England), 24*(22), 2622–2627. doi:10.1093/bioinformatics/btn481

Rajapakse, M., Kanagasabai, R., Ang, W. T. T., Veeramani, A., Schreiber, M. J. J., & Baker, C. J. O. J. (2008). Ontology-centric integration and navigation of the dengue literature *Journal of Biomedical Informatics, 41*(5, October), 806-815.

Raptis, A. E., Spring, M. W., & Viberti, G. (1997). Comparison of blood pressure measurement methods in adult diabetics. *Lancet, 349*, 175–176.

Rauner, M. S., Brailsford, S. C., & Flessa, S. (2005). Use of discrete-event simulation to evaluate strategies for the prevention of mother-to-child transmission of HIV in developing countries. *The Journal of the Operational Research Society, 56*(2), 222. doi:10.1057/palgrave.jors.2601884

Rindfleisch, T. C. (1997). Privacy, information technology, and health care. *Communications of the ACM, 40*(8), 92–100. doi:doi:10.1145/257874.257896

Rizvi, S., & Haritsa, J. R. (2002). *Maintaining Data Privacy in Association Rule Mining.* Paper presented at the VLDB.

Roan, S. (2010). A win-win for breastfeeding. *Fit Pregnancy, 17*, 22–22.

Rosenblatt, F. (1962). *Priciples of Neurodynamics.* New York, NY: Spartan.

Rostad, L., & Edsburg, O. (2006). A study of access control requirements for healthcare systems based on audit trails from access logs. In *proceedings of the Annual Computer Security Applications Conference* (pp. 175-186). Miami Beach, Florida, USA: IEEE Computer Society.

Russell, R. C., Williams, N. S., & Bulstrode, C. J. (Eds.). (2004). *Bailey and Love's Short Practice of Surgery* (24th ed., p. 1030). New York: Arnold.

Russ, J. C. (2007). *The image processing handbook* (5th ed.). Boca Raton, Fla: CRC Press.

Ruzzin, J. (2010). Persistent Organic Pollutant Exposure Leads to Insulin Resistance Syndrome. *Environmental Health Perspectives, 118*, 465–471. doi:10.1289/ehp.0901321

RxHub. (2004). The opportunity and challenge of RxHub meds. RxHub White Paper.

Rybchynski, D. (2005). *Design of an Artificial Neural Network Research Framework to Enhance the Development of Clinical Prediction Models.* Unpublished master's thesis, University of Ottawa, Ottawa, ON, Canada.

Sahai, A., & Waters, B. (2005). Fuzzy identity-based encryption. In R. Cramer (Ed.), *Proceedings of Eurocrypt 2005* (Vol. 3494) (pp. 457-473). New York: Springer Verlag.

Samarati, P., & Sweeney, L. (1998). Protecting privacy when disclosing information: *k*-anonymity and its enforcement through generalization and suppression. In *Proceedings of the IEEE Symposium on Research in Security and Privacy*, Oakland, CA.

Samarati, P. (2001). Protecting Respondents' Identities in Microdata Release. *TKDE, 13*(6), 1010–1027.

Schachter, J., Chow, J. M., Howard, H., Bolan, G., & Moncada, J. (2006). Detection of Chlamydia trachomatis by nucleic acid amplification testing: our evaluation suggests that CDC-recommended approaches for confirmatory testing are ill-advised. *Journal of Clinical Microbiology, 44*(7), 2512–2517. doi:10.1128/JCM.02620-05

Scholkopf, B., & Smola, A. J. (2001). *Learning with Kernels: Support Vector Machines, Regularization, Optimization, and Beyond.* MA, USA: MIT Press Cambridge.

Schunter, M., Herreweghen, E. V., & Waidner, M. (2002). Expressive Privacy Promises how to improve the Platform for Privacy Preferences (P3P). In *Proceedings of the W3C Workshop on Future of P3P.* Dulles, Virginia, USA. Retrieved November 27, 2009 from http://www.w3.org/2002/p3p-ws/pp/ibm-zuerich.pdf

Sega, R., Facchetti, R., Bombelli, M., Cesana, G., Corrao, G., Grassi, G., & Mancia, G. (2005). Prognostic value of ambulatory and home blood pressures compared with office blood pressure in the general population - Follow-up results from the Pressioni Arteriose Monitorate e Loro Associazioni (PAMELA) study. *Circulation, 111,* 1777–1783.

Sega, R., Trocino, G., Lanzarotti, A., Carugo, S., Cesana, G., & Schiavina, R. (2001). Alterations of cardiac structure in patients with isolated office, ambulatory, or home hypertension: Data from the general population (Pressione Arteriose Monitorate E Loro Associazioni [PAMELA] Study). *Circulation, 104,* 1385–1392.

Seino, M. (2006). Classification criteria of epileptic seizures and syndromes. *Epilepsy Research, 70*(2-3 – Supplement), S27-S33.

Sendi, P., & Al, M. J. (2003). Revisiting the decision rule of cost-effectiveness analysis under certainty and uncertainty. *Social Science & Medicine, 57*(6), 969–974. doi:10.1016/S0277-9536(02)00477-X

Seta, K., Ikeda, M., Kakusho, O., & Mizoguchi, R. (1997, June 2-5). Capturing a Conceptual Model for End-User Programming: Task Ontology as a Static User Model. In *Proceedings of the Sixth International Conference on User Modeling* (pp. 203-214). Chia Laguna, Sardinia, Italy.

Shamir, A. (1985). Identity-based cryptosystems and signature schemes. In G. R. Blakely & D. Chaum (Eds.) *Proceedings of Crypto1984 (Vol.* 196 of LNCS) (pp. 47-53). New York: Springer Verlag.

Shaw, P. (2003). *Multivariate statistics for the Environmental Sciences.* London: Hodder-Arnold.

Sherman, F. T. (2009). Baby Boomers court metabolic syndrome. *Geriatrics, 64,* 8–15.

Shoup, V. (2006). Sequences of games: a tool for taming complexity in security proofs. Retrieved October 15, 2009 from http://shoup.net/papers/games.pdf

Shrier, L. A., Harris, S. K., & Beardslee, W. R. (2002). Temporal associations between depressive symptoms and self-reported sexually transmitted disease among adolescents. *Archives of Pediatrics & Adolescent Medicine, 156*(6), 599–606.

Sieg, A., Mobasher, B., & Burke, R. D. (2007). Ontological User Profiles for Representing Context in Web Search. In *Proceedings of Web Intelligence/IAT Workshops* (pp. 91-94).

Sim, I., Gorman, P., Greenes, R., Hayes, R., Kaplan, B., & Lehmann, H. (2001). Clinical decision support systems for the practice of evidence-based medicine. *Journal of the American Medical Informatics Association, 8*(6), 527–534.

Singh, G., Miller, J.D., Lee, F.H., Pettitt, D., & Russell, M.W. (2002). Prevalence of cardiovascular disease risk factors among US adults with self-reported osteoarthritis: data from the Third National Health and Nutrition Examination Survey. *Am J Manag Care, 8*(Suppl 15), S383e91.

Slonim, D., Tamayo, P., Mesirov, J., Golub, T., & Lander, E. (2000). Class prediction and discovery using gene expression data. In *Proceedings of the 4th Annual International Conference on Computational Molecular Biology (RECOMB),* Tokyo, Japan (pp. 263-272). Tokyo, Japan: Universal Academy Press.

Smith, B. C. (1982). *Reflection and Semantics in a Procedural Language.* PhD thesis. Massachusetts Institute of Technology. MIT-LCS-272:154.

Smith, R. A., Saslow, D., Sawyer, K. A., Burke, W., Costanza, M. E., Evans, W. P., et al. (2003). American Cancer Society guidelines for breast cancer screening: update 2003. *CA: a Cancer Journal for Clinicians, 53*(3), 141–169. PubMed doi:10.3322/canjclin.53.3.141

Soghikian, K., Casper, S. M., Fireman, B. H., Hunkeler, E. M., Hurley, L. B., Tekawa, I. S., & Vogt, T. M. (1992). Home blood pressure monitoring, Effect on use of medical services and medical care costs. *Medical Care, 30*, 855–865.

Sourceforge.net. (2007). *OpenCyc* [Computer program]. Retrieved from Web site: http://sourceforge.net/project/showfiles.php?group_id=27274.

Sourceforge.net. (2008). *JWNL – Java WordNet Library* [Computer program]. Retrieved from Web site: http://sourceforge.net/projects/jwordnet.

Staab, S., & Maedche, A. (2000). *Axioms are objects too – Ontology engineering beyond the modeling of concepts and relations.* Research report 399, University of Karlsruhe, Institute AIFB.

Staessen, J. A., Den Hond, E., Celis, H., Fagard, R., Keary, L., Vandenhoven, G., & O'Brien, E. T. (2004). Antihypertensive treatment based on blood pressure measurement at home or in the physician's office: a randomized controlled trial. *Journal of the American Medical Association, 291*, 955–964.

Stephens, S., Morales, A., & Quinlan, M. (2006). Applying semantic Web technologies to drug safety determination. *Intelligent Systems IEEE, 21*(1), 82–88. doi:10.1109/MIS.2006.2

Stergiou, G. S., Argyraki, K. K., Moyssakis, I., Mastorantonakis, S. E., Achimastos, A. D., Karamanos, V. G., & Roussias, L. G. (2007). Home blood pressure is as reliable as ambulatory blood pressure in predicting target-organ damage in hypertension. *American Journal of Hypertension, 20*, 616–621.

Stergiou, G. S., Baibas, N. M., Gantzarou, A. P., Skeva, I. I., Kalkana, C. B., Roussias, L. G., & Mountokalakis, T. D. (2002). Reproducibility of home, ambulatory, and clinic blood pressure: implications for the design of trials for the assessment of antihypertensive drug efficacy. *American Journal of Hypertension, 15*, 101–104.

Stergiou, G. S., Baibas, N. M., & Kalogeropoulos, P. G. (2007). Cardiovascular risk prediction based on home blood pressure measurement: the Didima study. *Journal of Hypertension, 25*, 1590–1596.

Stergiou, G. S., & Parati, G. (2007). The optimal schedule for self-monitoring of blood pressure by patients at home. *Journal of Hypertension, 25*, 1992–1997.

Stergiou, G. S., Salgami, E. V., Tzamouranis, D. G., & Roussias, L. G. (2005). Masked hypertension assessed by ambulatory blood pressure versus home blood pressure monitoring: is it the same phenomenon? *American Journal of Hypertension, 18*, 772–778.

Stergiou, G. S., Skeva, I. I., Zourbaki, A. S., & Mountokalakis, T. D. (1998). Self-monitoring of blood pressure at home: how many measurements are needed? *Journal of Hypertension, 16*, 725–731.

Stergiou, G. S., Zourbaki, A. S., Skeva, I. I., & Mountokalakis, T. D. (1998). White coat effect detected using self-monitoring of blood pressure at home: comparison with ambulatory blood pressure. *American Journal of Hypertension, 11*, 820–827.

Stevens, R., Aranguren, M. E., Wolstencroft, K., Sattler, U., Drummond, N., & Horridge, M. (2007). Using OWL to model biological knowledge. *International Journal of Human-Computer Studies, 65*(65), 583–594. doi:10.1016/j.ijhcs.2007.03.006

Stewart, M. J., Gough, K., & Padfield, P. L. (1995). The accuracy of automated blood pressure measuring devices in patients with controlled atrial fibrillation. *Journal of Hypertension, 13*, 297–300.

Stone, J., Wu, X., & Greenblatt, M. (2004). An Intelligent Digital Library System for Biologists. In *Proceedings of the 2004 IEEE Computational Systems Bioinformatics Conference (CSB 2004)* (pp. 491-492).

Stryker, T., Wilson, M., & Wilson, T. W. (2004). Accuracy of home blood pressure readings: monitors and operators. *Blood Pressure Monitoring, 9*, 143–147.

Sun, M., & Sclabassi, R. J. (1999, October 13-16). *Optimal selection of the sampling rate for efficient EEG data acquisition.* Paper presented at Proceedings of the First Joint BMES/EMBS Conference on Serving Humanity, Advancing Technology, Atlanta, GA.

Supekar, K., Patel, C., & Lee, Y. (2004). Characterizing Quality of Knowledge on Semantic Web. In *Proceedings of the Seventeenth International Florida Artificial Intelligence Research Symposium Conference* (pp. 220-228).

Su, T. C., Jeng, J. S., Chien, K. L., Sung, F. C., Hsu, H. C., & Lee, Y. T. (2001). Hypertension status is the major determinant of carotid atherosclerosis: a community-based study in Taiwan. *Stroke*, *32*, 2265–2271.

Takashima, K., Kitou, T., Mori, K., & Ikeuchi, K. (2007). Simulation and experimental observation of contact conditions between stents and artery models. *Medical Engineering & Physics*, *29*, 326–335. doi:10.1016/j.medengphy.2006.04.003

Tang, P. C., Ash, J. S., Bates, D. W., Overhage, J. M., & Sands, D. Z. (2006). Personal health records: definitions, benefits, and strategies for overcoming barriers to adoption. *Journal of the American Medical Informatics Association*, *13*(2), 121–126. doi:10.1197/jamia.M2025

Tao, G., Abban, B. K., Gift, T. L., Chen, G., & Irwin, K. L. (2004). Applying a mixed-integer program to model re-screening women who test positive for C. trachomatis infection. *Health Care Management Science*, *7*(2), 135–144. doi:10.1023/B:HCMS.0000020653.31862.23

Tao, G., Gift, T. L., Walsh, C. M., Irwin, K. L., & Kassler, W. J. (2002). Optimal resource allocation for curing Chlamydia trachomatis infection among asymptomatic women at clinics operating on a fixed budget. *Sexually Transmitted Diseases*, *29*(11), 703–709. doi:10.1097/00007435-200211000-00014

The personal health working group final report. (2004). *Connecting for health*. Retrieved October 2, 2009 from http://www.connectingforhealth.org/resources/wg_eis_final_report_0704.pdf

The US Department of Health and Human Services. (2003). *Summary of the HIPAA privacy rule*. Retrieved October 2, 2009 from http://www.hhs.gov/ocr/privacy/hipaa/understanding/summary/privacysummary.pdf

Thomasian, A., Castelli, V., & Li, C. (1998). Clustering and Singular Value Decomposition for Approximate Indexing in High Dimensional Spaces. In N. Pissinou, C. Nicholas, J. French, & G. Gardarin (Eds.), *Proceedings of the seventh international conference on Information and knowledge management* (pp. 201-207). New York: ACM.

Thompson, J. R., & Tapia, R. A. (1990). *Nonparametric Function Estimation, Modeling, and Simulation*. Philadelphia: Society for Industrial and Applied Mathematics (SIAM).

Thomson Healthcare. (2008). *Drug Topics Red Book*. Montvale, NJ: Thomson Healthcare.

Timmins, L. H., Moreno, M. R., Meyer, C. A., Criscione, J. C., Rachev, A., & Moore, J. E. (2007). Stented artery biomechanics and device design optimization. *Medical & Biological Engineering & Computing*, *45*, 505–513. doi:10.1007/s11517-007-0180-3

Tsumoto, S. (2003). Automated extraction of hierarchical decision rules from clinical databases using rough set model. *Expert Systems with Applications*, *24*(2), 189–197. doi:10.1016/S0957-4174(02)00142-2

Tyatgat, G. N. J., Classen, M., Waye, J., & Nakazawa, S. (2000). Practical Management of Non-Variceal Upper Gastrointestinal Bleed. In *Practice of Therapeutic Endoscopy* (2nd ed., p. 4).

U. S. National Library of Medicine. (2008). *UMLS Knowledge Sources*. Retrieved from Unified Medical Language System Web site: http://www.nlm.nih.gov/research/umls/umlsdoc.html.

U.S. (2009). Health *Information Technology for Economic and Clinical Health (HITECH) Act*. Retrieved November 27, 2009 from http://waysandmeans.house.gov/media/pdf/110/hit2.pdf

U.S. Department of Health and Human Services. (1996). *Health Insurance Portability and Accountability (HIPAA) Act*. Retrieved November 27, 2009 from http://www.hhs.gov/ocr/privacy/hipaa/administrative/privacyrule/adminsimpregtext.pdf

U.S. President's Information Technology Advisory Committee (PITAC). (2004). *Revolutionizing Health Care Through Information Technology*. Retrieved November 27, 2009 from http://www.nitrd.gov/pitac/reports/index.html

U.S. Preventive Services Task Force. (2005). *Screening for Gonorrhea*. Retrieved from http://www.uspreventiveservicestaskforce.org/uspstf/uspsgono.htm

U.S.A. (2009). *American Recovery and Reinvestment Act (ARRA)*. Retrieved November 27, 2009 from http://frwebgate.access.gpo.gov/cgi-bin/getdoc.cgi?dbname=111_cong_bills&docid=f:h1enr.pdf

Udommanetanakit, K., Rakthanmanon, T., & Waiyamai, K. (2007, August 6-8). *E-Stream: evolution-based technique for stream clustering.* Paper presented at the 3rd International Conference on Advanced Data Mining and Applications (ADMA'07), Harbin, China.

Uemura, H., Arisawa, K., Hiyoshi, M., Kitayama, A., Takami, H., & Sawachika, F. (2009). Prevalence of Metabolic Syndrome Associated with Body Burden Levels of Dioxin and Related Compounds among Japan's General Population. *Environmental Health Perspectives, 117*, 568–573.

Vaidya, J. S., & Clifton, C. (2002). *Privacy preserving association rule mining in vertically partitioned data.* Paper presented at the 8th ACM SIGKDD International Conference on Knowledge Discovery and Data Mining (pp. 639-644).

Vaidya, J., & Clifton, C. (2003). *Leveraging the "multi" in secure multi-party computation.* Paper Presented at the Workshop on Privacy in the Electronic Society held in association with the 10th ACM Conference on Computer and Communications Security.

Vaidya, J., & Clifton, C. (2003). Privacy-preserving k-means clustering over vertically partitioned data. In *Proceedings of the ninth ACM SIGKDD international conference on Knowledge discovery and data mining,* Washington, DC (pp. 206-215). New York: ACM.

Vaidya, J., Clifton, C., & Zhu, Y. (2006). *Privacy Preserving Data Mining.* New York: Springer.

Van Der Pol, B., Ferrero, D. V., Buck-Barrington, L., Hook, E. III, Lenderman, C., & Quinn, T. (2001). Multicenter evaluation of the BDProbeTec ET System for detection of Chlamydia trachomatis and Neisseria gonorrhoeae in urine specimens, female endocervical swabs, and male urethral swabs. *Journal of Clinical Microbiology, 39*(3), 1008–1016. doi:10.1128/JCM.39.3.1008-1016.2001

Van Popele, N. M., Bos, W. J., de Beer, N. A., Van Der Kuip, D. A., Hofman, A., Grobbee, D. E., & Witteman, J. C. (2000). Arterial stiffness as underlying mechanism of disagreement between an oscillometric blood pressure monitor and a sphygmomanometer. *Hypertension, 36*, 484–488.

Vapnik, V. (1995). *The nature of statistical learning theory.* New York: Springer-Verlag.

Verberk, W. J., Kroon, A. A., Lenders, J. W., Kessels, A. G., van Montfrans, G. A., & Smit, A. J. (2007). Self-measurement of blood pressure at home reduces the need for antihypertensive drugs: a randomized, controlled trial. *Hypertension, 50*, 1019–1025.

Verberk, W. J., Thien, T., Kroon, A. A., Lenders, J. W., van Montfrans, G. A., Smit, A. J., & De Leeuw, P. W. (2007). Prevalence and persistence of masked hypertension in treated hypertensive patients. *American Journal of Hypertension, 20*, 1258–1265.

Verdecchia, P., Palatini, P., Schillaci, G., Mormino, P., Porcellati, C. C., & Pessina, A. C. (2001). Independent predictors of isolated clinic ('white-coat') hypertension. *Journal of Hypertension, 19*, 1015–1020.

Verdecchia, P., Porcellati, C., Schillaci, G., Borgioni, C., Ciucci, A., & Battistelli, M. (1994). Ambulatory blood pressure, An independent predictor of prognosis in essential hypertension. *Hypertension, 24*, 793–801.

Verykios, V. S., Elmagarmid, A. K., Elisa, B., Saygin, Y., & Elena, D. (2004). Association Rule Hiding. *IEEE Transactions on Knowledge and Data Engineering, 16*(4), 434–447. doi:10.1109/TKDE.2004.1269668

Visa, S., & Ralescu, A. (2005). *Issues in mining imbalanced data sets-a review paper.*

Visscher, P. M., & Hill, W. G. (2009). The limits of individual identification from sample allele frequencies: theory and statistical analysis. *PLOS Genetics, 5*(10), e1000628. doi:10.1371/journal.pgen.1000628

Wang, R., Li, Y. F., et al. (2009). Learning your identity and disease from research papers: information leaks in genome wide association study. In Proceedings of the 16th ACM conference on Computer and communications security, Chicago (pp. 534-544). New, York: ACM.

Wang, L., Cao, Z., Okamoto, T., Miao, Y., & Okamoto, E. (2006). Authorization-limited transformation-free proxy cryptosystems and their security analyses. *IEICE Transactions on Fundamentals of Electronics, Communications and Computer Science*, (1): 106–114. doi:10.1093/ietfec/e89-a.1.106

Ward, J. H. (1963). Hierarchical Grouping to Optimize an Objective Function. *Journal of the American Statistical Association, 58*(301), 236. doi:10.2307/2282967

Weiss, G. M. (2004). Mining with rarity: a unifying framework. *ACM SIGKDD Explorations Newsletter, 6*(1), 7–19. doi:10.1145/1007730.1007734

Weng, C. G., & Poon, J. (2006). A Data Complexity Analysis on Imbalanced Datasets and an Alternative Imbalance Recovering Strategy. IEEE Computer Society Washington, DC, USA.

Wennber, J., & Cooper, M. M. (1999). *The Dartmouth atlas of medical care in the United States: a report on the medicare program*. Chicago, IL: AHA Press.

Wikipedia (2008). Support vector machine: MediaWiki.

Wikipedia. (2010). *Cluster Analysis*. Retrieved from en.wikipedia.org/wiki/Cluster_analysis

Wikipedia. (2010). *DNA Microarray*. Retrieved from en.wikipedia.org/wiki/DNA_microarray

Wilcox, C. M., Alexander, L. N., & Straub, R. F. (1996). A prospective endoscopic evaluation of the causes of upper gastrointestinal hemorrhage in alcoholics. A focus on alcoholic gastropathy. *The American Journal of Gastroenterology, 91*(7), 1343–1347.

Wilson, R. L., & Rosen, P. A. (2003). Protecting Data Through 'Perturbation' Techniques: The Impact on Knowledge Discovery in Databases. *Journal of Database Management, 14*(2), 14–26.

Witten, I. H., & Frank, E. (2005). *Data mining - Practical machine learning tools and techniques*. United States of America: Morgan Kaufmann, Elsevier.

Wong, R. (2009). *An overview of data protection laws around the world*. Retrieved November 27, 2009 from http://pages.britishlibrary.net/rwong/dpa.html

Wu, C. H., Apweiler, R., Bairoch, A., Natale, D. A., Barker, W. C., & Boeckmann, B. (2006). The Universal Protein Resource (UniProt): an expanding universe of protein information. *Nucleic Acids Research, 34*(Database issue), D187–D191. doi:10.1093/nar/gkj161

Wu, W., Wang, W. Q., Yang, D. Z., & Qi, M. (2007). Stent expansion in curved vessel and their interactions: a finite element analysis. *Journal of Biomechanics, 40*, 2580–2585. doi:10.1016/j.jbiomech.2006.11.009

Xia, Z., Ju, F., & Sasaki, K. (2007). A general finite element analysis method for balloon expandable stents based on repeated unit cell (RUC) model. *Finite Elements in Analysis and Design, 43*, 649–658. doi:10.1016/j.finel.2007.01.001

Xu, G., Niu, Z., Uetz, P., Gao, X., Qin, X., & Liu, H. (2009). Semi-Supervised Learning of Text Classification on Bacterial Protein-Protein Interaction Documents. *International Joint Conference on Bioinformatics, Systems Biology and Intelligent Computing (IJCBS'09)*.

Xu, C., & Prince, J. L. (1998). Generalized gradient vector flow external forces for active contours. *Signal Processing, 71*, 131–139. doi:10.1016/S0165-1684(98)00140-6

Yang, J. (2003). *Dynamic clustering of evolving streams with a single pass*. Paper presented at the 19th International Conference on Data Engineering (ICDE'03).

Yang, Y., & Pedersen, J. O. (1997). A comparative study on feature selection in text categorization. *Fourteenth International Conference on Machine Learning*.

Yao, A. C. (1986). How to generate and exchange secrets. In *Proceedings of the 27th IEEE Symposium on Foundations of Computer Science* (pp. 162-167). Washington, DC: IEEE.

Yao, A. C.-C. (1986). How to generate and exchange secrets. In *Proceedings of the 27th Annual Symposium on Foundations of Computer Science* (pp. 162-167). Washington, DC: IEEE Computer Society.

Yap, M. H., Edirisinghe, E. A., & Bez, B. E. (2007, Feb 2007). *Fully automated lesion boundary detection in ultrasound breast images*. Paper presented at the SPIE Medical Imaging Conference, San Diego, CA.

Yap, M. H., Edirisinghe, E. A., & Bez, H. E. (2009). *A comparative study in ultrasound breast imaging classification*. Paper presented at the SPIE Medical Imaging.

Yap, M. H., Edirisinghe, E. A., & Bez, H. E. (2008). A novel algorithm for initial lesion detection in ultrasound breast images. *Journal of Applied Clinical Medical Physics, 9*(4), 181–199. doi:10.1120/jacmp.v9i4.2741

Yen, S. J., Lee, Y. S., Lin, C. H., & Ying, J. C. (n.d.). *Investigating the Effect of Sampling Methods for Imbalanced Data Distributions.*

Yu, A. (2006). Methods in biomedical ontology. *Journal of Biomedical Informatics, 39*(3), 252–266. doi:10.1016/j.jbi.2005.11.006

Zanchetti, A., Crepaldi, G., Bond, M. G., Gallus, G. V., Veglia, F., & Ventura, A. (2001). Systolic and pulse blood pressures (but not diastolic blood pressure and serum cholesterol) are associated with alterations in carotid intima-media thickness in the moderately hypercholesterolaemic hypertensive patients of the Plaque Hypertension Lipid Lowering Italian Study, PHYLLIS study group. *Journal of Hypertension, 19*, 79–88.

Zanderigo, F., Bertoldo, A., Pillonetto, G., & Cobelli, C. (2009). Nonlinear Stochastic Regularization to Characterize Tissue Residue Function in Bolus-tracking MRI: Assessment and Comparison with SVD, Block-circulant SVD, and Tikhonov. *IEEE Transactions on Bio-Medical Engineering, 56*, 1287–1297. doi:10.1109/TBME.2009.2013820

Zeller, T. (2007). Current state of endovascular treatment of femoro-popliteal artery disease. *Vascular Medicine, 12*, 223–234. doi:10.1177/1358863X07079823

Zeng, Q. T., Tse, T., Crowell, J., Divita, G., Roth, L., & Browne, A. C. (2005) Identifying Consumer-Friendly Display (CFD) Names for Health Concepts. In *Proceedings of the AMIA Annual Symposium* (pp. 859-863).

Zhang, N., Wang, S., & Zhao, W. (2004). *A New Scheme on Privacy Preserving Association Rule Mining.* Berlin Heidelberg: Springer-Verlag.

Zheng, Z., Wu, X., & Srihari, R. (2004). Feature selection for text categorization on imbalanced data. *ACM SIGKDD Explorations Newsletter, 6*(1), 80–89. doi:10.1145/1007730.1007741

About the Contributors

Aryya Gangopadhyay is a professor and the chair of information systems at University of Maryland Baltimore County (UMBC). He is also Associate Chair of Academic Affairs in the Department of Information Systems. Dr. Gangopadhyay has a PhD degree in computer information systems from Rutgers University. He has published peer-reviewed several articles on spatial and spatio-temporal data mining, data mining in medicine, data stream mining and navigating multi-dimensional databases. Dr. Gangopadhyay He has also co-authored and edited three books and he has received funding from NSF, US Department of Education, state and government agencies and private industries.

* * *

Nabil R. Adam is a Professor at Rutgers University and founding Director of the Rutgers CIMIC Research Center. He is currently on an assignment at the Science & Technology Directorate, US Department of Homeland Security. He has directed numerous R&D projects with funding over $18 million from various federal and state agencies including NSF, NSA, NOAA, U.S. EPA, DLA, NLM, NASA, and NJMC. He has published numerous technical papers covering such topics as information management, information security and privacy, data mining, Web services, and modeling & simulation. His papers appeared in referred journals and conference proceedings including, IEEE Transactions on Software Engineering, IEEE Transactions on Knowledge and Data Engineering, ACM Computing Surveys, Communications of the ACM. He co-authored/co-edited ten books. Dr. Adam is the co-founder and the Executive-Editor-in-Chief of the International Journal on Digital Libraries and serves on the editorial board of a number of journals.

Yoo Jung An received M.S. and Ph.D. degrees in Computer Science from New Jersey Institute of Technology (NJIT) in January 2004 and 2008, respectively. During her graduate study years, she received a UPS Foundation Ph.D. Fellowship for Academic Excellence. She also holds an M.S. in Consumer Science from Dongguk Univ., South Korea (1995) and a B.S. in Education from Kookmin Univ., South Korea (1993). She is currently a visiting assistant professor in the Gildart Haase School of Computer Science and Engineering at Fairleigh Dickinson University. Her professional activities include organizing the first ever workshop "The Semantic Web meets the Deep Web" as chair, at the IEEE Joint Conference on E-Commerce Technology and Enterprise Computing, E-Commerce and E-Services 2008, Washington D.C. Her research interests include Semantic Web, Deep Web, Data Warehouses, Artificial Intelligence and Internet Security.

Ajat Shatru Arora was born in Utrakhand, UP, India on April Sept 27, 1969. He received the graduation degree (1990) in Electrical Engineering, post graduation degree (1992) in PAED from University of Roorkee, UP, India and doctorate (2002) in Biomedical Engineering from Indian Institute of Roorkee, UP, India. He has teaching experience of 17 years. He is currently serving Principal of DAV Institute of Engineering & Technology, Jalandhar, Punjab, India. His research interests are in the field of Biomedical Engineering with an emphasis on bio signal analysis, artificial neural networks, support vector machines, statistical analysis and microprocessor based system development. He has published 50 National/ International Journal and Conference papers in these areas.

Darpan Bansal MS is a Senior Resident at SGRD Institute of Medical Sciences, Amritsar, India. Dr. Bansal interest is to study the various risk factors of obstructive jaundice and comparing the role of various investigation procedures in Obstructive Jaundice

Helmut Bez, received a first class honours degree in Mathematics from the University of Wales in 1972, and M.Sc. and D.Phil. degrees from Oxford University in 1973 and 1976 respectively. He joined Rolls Royce Aero Engines in 1976 and in 1980 was appointed to the academic staff of the Department of Computer Science at Loughborough University, where he now holds the title of Reader in Geometric Computation. His doctoral thesis was on applications of group theory to classical and quantum mechanics. His current research interests include: the determination and application of the invariant properties of path and surface functions, rational parametrisation, image processing and parallel computation. He is the author of over 40 journal papers in these topics.

Rafae Bhatti is an information security professional at the Oracle Corporation, Redwood Shores, California. Rafae received his PhD from the Center of Excellence in Information Security at Purdue University. Rafae has experience in Web-based information management systems, in evaluating and analyzing large scale data warehousing workloads, in the design and development of secure database systems and has worked with National Institute of Standards and Technology (NIST) on the development of applications based on the Role Based Access Control (RBAC) standard. Recently, Rafae has published a book on "A Policy Engineering Framework for Federated Access Management".

Pimwadee Chaovalit received her Bachelor of Business Administration degree, majoring in Information Systems, from Chulalongkorn University in Thailand. After working as a consultant at KPMG Advisory (Thailand), she was awarded the Royal Thai Scholarship from the Thai government to pursue her graduate studies. Pimwadee received her Ph.D. in Information Systems from University of Maryland, Baltimore County in 2009. Currently, she is a specialist at the National Science and Technology Development Agency in Thailand, overseeing enterprise IT projects. Her research interests include data mining algorithms, data streams and time series clustering, Thai text mining, and data mining in application domains such as biomedical signal analysis and polarity mining.

Guantao Chen is a professor and Chair of the Mathematics and Statistics Department at Georgia State University. His research focuses on combinatorics, graph theory, operation research and bioinformatics. Research has been supported by the National Security Agency and the National Science Foundation.

Zhiyuan Chen is an assistant professor at information systems department, UMBC. He has a PhD in Computer Science from Cornell University. His research interests include privacy preserving data mining, data navigation and visualization, XML, automatic database tuning, and database compression.

Soon Ae Chun is an assistant professor of Information Systems in CUNY/CSI. Her research and development interests include Dynamic Workflow Composition and Management, Information Security and Privacy, Policy-based Web Service Composition, Ontologies and the Semantic Web, and Geospatial information and satellite image Database systems. Her research projects focus on application areas of e-government, homeland security, environmental and medical informatics, addressing the issues of the process design and personalization, security and privacy, information sharing, interoperability and mobile and geospatial data integration. She received her Ph.D. and M.B.A. in Information Technology from Rutgers University, and M.S. in Computer Science from SUNY Buffalo.

Eran Edirisinghe received B.Sc.Eng. (Hons) degree from Moratuwa University Sri Lanka in 1994, and MSc degree is PhD Degree from Loughborough University in 1996 and 1999 respectively. His doctoral thesis was on Data Compression of Stereoscopic Images and Video. After a short assignment as a Postdoctoral Research Fellow at Glamorgan University, Wales, he was appointed a Lecturer in Computer Science at Loughborough University. He was promoted to a Senior Lecturer in February 2004 and received the title of Reader in Digital Imaging in July 2008. He is a member of the College of Peers of the Engineering & Physical Sciences Research Council, UK and a member of the IASTED committee in image processing. His research interests include, image and signal processing, video coding, texture synthesis and novel mobile applications.

Monique Frize has been a Professor for 20 years, first at University of New Brunswick (1989-1997), then at Carleton University and the University of Ottawa (1997-2010). She currently is Distinguished Professor at Carleton and Professor Emerita at University of Ottawa. Dr. Frize was a biomedical engineer for 18 years in hospitals (1971-1989). She published over 200 papers in journals and conference proceedings on artificial intelligence in medicine, infrared imaging and ethics. She is Senior Member of IEEE, Fellow of the Canadian Academy of Engineering (1992) and of Engineers Canada (2010), Officer of the Order of Canada (1993) and recipient of the 2010 Gold Medal from Professional Engineers Ontario and the Ontario Society of Professional Engineers. She received five honorary doctorates in Canadian universities since 1992. Her book: *The Bold and the Brave: A history of women in science and engineering* was released by University of Ottawa Press in November 2009.

Mariacristina Gagliardi was born in Lamezia Terme in 1983 and graduated in Chemical Engineering in 2006 at the University of Pisa. In 2010 got the Ph.D. degree of Chemical and Materials Engineering at the University of Pisa. From 2008 she delivered lessons on Biomaterials, Bionanotechnologies and Biomedical implantable devices at the Faculty of Engineering of the University of Pisa. From 2009 she is professor assistant of Chemistry. At the present she is a post-doctoral researcher at the Department of Chemical Engineering, Industrial Chemistry and Materials Science of the University of Pisa. Her research activity concerns: synthesis of novel biocompatible polymers and their physicochemical and mechanical characterisation; preparation of polymeric drug-delivery systems; preparation of polymeric scaffolds for cardiac tissue regeneration; Finite Element analysis of the mechanical behaviour of endovascular stents; Mathematical modelling of drug delivery kinetics from drug-eluting stents. She is author of more than 15 scientific papers published in international journals and of more than 15 communications to scientific meetings, both in national and international conferences.

James Geller received an Electrical Engineering Diploma from the Technical University, Vienna, Austria, in 1979, and the MS Degree (1984) and Ph.D. degree (1988) in Computer Science from the State University of New York at Buffalo. Dr. Geller joined the Computer Science Department of the New Jersey Institute of Technology (NJIT) in 1988. He was granted tenure and promoted to associate professor in 1993. Subsequently he was promoted to full professor in 2000. Dr. Geller has authored and co-authored over fifty journal papers and over fifty conference papers. These papers are in a number of areas, including Knowledge Representation, Parallel Reasoning, Semantic Modeling in Object-Oriented Databases, Web Mining, Medical Informatics, Medical Vocabularies, and Auditing of Ontologies and Medical Terminologies.

Bhaswati Ghosh is a graduate student in the Department of Computer and Information Science, Cleveland State University (CSU). She has an MTech degree in Computer and Information Science, University Of Calcutta, India. Prior to joining CSU she served as Lecturer, Computer Science and Engineering Department, Panjab University, India.

Partha Sekhar Ghosh is Child Neurology fellow in Cleveland Clinic Children's Hospital, in Pediatric Neurology and Neurosurgery program. He has completed Pediatrics residency and Neurology fellowship training at Post Graduate Institute of Medical Education and Research, Chandigarh, India. He has published numerous articles and made poster presentations at national and international conferences.

Thomas Gift, PhD is an economist with the Division of STD Prevention, Centers for Disease Control and Prevention. His research focuses on cost-effectiveness analysis and mathematical modeling. Much of his prior and current work has been devoted to the analysis of chlamydia screening and treatment interventions.

Johannes Goll has been a Bioinformatics Engineer at the JCVI since August 2007. He studied bioengineering with an emphasis on software engineering and earned his diploma in bioengineering from the Weihenstephan University of Applied Sciences in Germany. His research focuses on the analysis and visualization of cellular networks and related data. During his thesis with Dr. Peter Uetz, he conducted a bioinformatics analysis of protein interactions of the Syphilis spirochete Treponema pallidum and wrote a book chapter on 'Analyzing Protein Interaction Networks' in 'Bioinformatics-From Genomes to Therapies', edited by Dr. Lengauer. Besides data analysis, Goll has a strong background in object oriented programming (certified Java programmer) and relational database development (certified MySQL Developer). He developed JCVI's Microbial Protein-Protein Interaction Database (MPIDB) for which he has also set up a protein interaction curation interface for Biocurators.

Tyrone Grandison manages the Intelligent Information Systems team in the Computer Science department at the IBM Almaden Research Center, San Jose, CA. Tyrone's research interests are in data disclosure management relevant and applicable to industry verticals. Over the years, Tyrone has worked in data privacy, RFID data management, privacy-preserving mobile data management and text analytics. Tyrone is an ACM Distinguished Engineer, an IEEE senior member and was named Pioneer of the Year by NSBE in 2009. Tyrone received a Ph.D. from Imperial College, London and M.Sc. and B.Sc. degrees from the University of the West Indies, Mona, Jamaica.

Pieter Hartel received his Master degree in Mathematics and Computer Science from the Free University of Amsterdam in 1978 and his PhD degree in Computer Science from the University of Amsterdam in 1989. He has worked at CERN in Geneva (Switzerland), the Universities of Nijmegen, Amsterdam (The Netherlands), and Southampton (UK). He is currently a full Professor of Compter Science at the University of Twente. His research interest is computer security.

Xiaoyun He is a Ph.D. candidate in Information Technology at Rutgers University, Newark, New Jersey. She holds B.S. and M.S. both in Computer Science. Her current research interests include knowledge management and data mining, data privacy issues, and business intelligence. She is a student member of the SIAM and the ACM.

Kuo Chuan Huang is a PhD candidate in Computer Science at New Jersey Institute of Technology, Newark NJ, under the supervision of Prof. Geller and Prof. Halper (at Kean University). His research interests include Semantic Web, Ontologies, and medical informatics. Currently, he is working on some web projects using J2EE with Hibernate and Strut technologies. Before becoming a graduate student at NJIT, Kuo Chuan had many years of software/web developing experience using Java, ASP, Perl/PHP, etc. Kuo Chuan has a Master of Science degree in Computer Science from NJIT and a Bachelor of Science degree in Information Engineering from Tatung University, Taipei Taiwan.

Luan Ibraimi received his Master Degree in Information and Communication Systems Security from the KTH Royal Institute of Technology, Sweden in 2007. He is currently a PhD Candidate at the EEMCS faculty of University of Twente. Recently (2009) he is working at the Information and System Security group in Philips Research in Eindhoven (the Netherlands). His research interests are public key encryption and network security, especially on applying cryptographic techniques to securely manage electronic health records.

Vijender Kumar Jain was born in Sonepat, Haryana, India on Sept 27, 1955. He received the graduation (1977), post graduation (1979) and doctorate degrees (1995) in Electrical Engineering from Kurukshetra University, Haryana. He has teaching experience of 31 years. His area of interest is Biomedical Image and Signal Processing, Reliability Engineering, Control and Energy Systems. He is currently working as Professor and Head of Electrical and Instrumentation Engineering Department at Sant Longowal Institute of Engineering and Technology, Longowal, Sangrur, Punjab, India. His research interests are in the field of Biomedical Image and Signal Processing, Reliability Engineering, Control and Energy Systems. He has published 78 National/ International Journal and Conference papers in these areas.

Willem Jonker studied mathematics and computer science at Groningen University. He then joined Delft University of Technology for his PhD research on knowledge-based systems. He has worked at KPN Research and European Computer industry Research Centre in Munich (ECRC, a joint research laboratory of Bull, ICL and Siemens) . In 1999 he founded the new research department of KPN Research at the campus of Twente University. In September 2001 he joined Philips Research. He started in the PACMan (Processing and Architectures for Content Management) group at Philips Research to work on secure content management in networked environments and to coordinate the cluster activities in this field. In April 2004 he became the department head of the Information & System Security group. In October 2005 he became the sector head of the Digital Lifestyle Technology sector. Finally, he is a part-time full professor of computer science at Twente University. Among his research interest are database systems, multi-media databases, distributed applications, content management, DRM, and security.

Ashish Joshi is a Research Assistant Professor of Department of Information Systems and a Research Director of Consortium for Information Technology and Health Outcomes Research (CITHOR) at UMBC. Dr. Joshi is a trained physician and obtained his Masters in Public Health (majors in Epidemiology and Biostatistics) from Boston University School of Public Health and a certificate in Public Health Informatics from University of Maryland, College Park. Dr. Joshi's research interests includes public health informatics, designing and evaluating tele-health systems for chronic disease management, computer mediated health education and analyses of large clinical, administrative health care databases.

Gurmanik Kaur was received the Diploma (2002) in Electronics and Communication Engineering from Government Polytechnic for Girls, Patiala, Punjab, India, the graduation degree (2005) in Electronics and Instrumentation Engineering from Adesh Institute of Engineering and Technology, Faridkot, Punjab, India, the post graduation degree (2007) with Silver Medal in Instrumentation and Control Engineering from Sant Longowal Institute of Engineering and Technology, Longowal, Sangrur, Punjab, INDIA. During her post graduation degree, she has worked on a project funded by Ministry of Human Resource Development (MHRD), India. She is currently doing regular Ph.D. with scholarship in Electrical and Instrumentation Engineering Department from Sant Longowal Institute of Engineering and Technology, Longowal, Sangrur, Punjab, India. Her research interest is in the field of Biomedical Engineering with an emphasis on bio signal analysis, artificial neural networks, support vector machines, statistical analysis. She has published 13 National/ International Journal and Conference papers in these areas.

Xin Li is currently working as a Bioinformatician at Lombardi Comprehensive Cancer Center in Georgetown University Medical Center, and pursuing his Ph.D. degree in Information Systems at University of Maryland, Baltimore County (UMBC). Mr. Li's research interests include: database and data mining applications on bioinformatics data, heterogeneous data integration, privacy preserving data mining, Web Services, biomedical ontology application, workflow management on biomedical/healthcare, data processing and analysis on genomics, proteomics, and metabolomics, and pathway/gene network analysis. Before joined Georgetown University in 2006, he worked as an associate faculty in UMBC since 2003. Mr. Li received a Bachelor of Engineering in Management Information Systems (1998) and a Master of Management in Management Science (2001) from Beijing University of Aeronautics and Astronautics, and he also received a Master of Science in Information Systems from UMBC in 2003.

Hongfang Liu is currently an Assistant Professor in Department of Biostatistics, Bioinformatics, and Biomathematics (DBBB) of Georgetown University. She has been working in the field of Biomedical Informatics for ten years. Her expertise in clinical informatics includes clinical information system, controlled medical vocabulary, and medical language processing. Her expertise in bioinformatics includes microarray data analysis, biomedical entity nomenclature, molecular biology database curation, ontology, and biological text mining. She received a B.S. degree in Applied Mathematics and Statistics from University of Science and Technology of China in 1994, a M.S. degree in Computer Science from Fordham University in 1998, and a PhD degree in computer science at the Graduate School of City University of New York in 2002.

Simone A. Ludwig joined the Department of Computer Science at North Dakota State University (NDSU) as Associate Professor in Fall 2010. Prior to joining NDSU, she worked at the University of Saskatchewan (Canada), Concordia University (Canada), Cardiff University (UK) and Brunel University (UK). She received her PhD degree and MSc degree with distinction from Brunel University (UK), in 2004 and 2000 respectively. Before starting her academic career Dr. Ludwig worked several years in the software industry. Her research interests include artificial intelligence, evolutionary computation, knowledge engineering, Semantic Grid/Web, and distributed/Grid computing.

Ravinder Singh Malhotra, MBBS, MS, is an Assistant Professor of Surgery at Sri Guru Ram Das Institute of Medical Sciences & Research, Amritsar, Punjab, India. An ardent supporter of public health education and practice, Dr. Singh is well versed with various National Health and Family Welfare Programs. He has been working in close liaison with the Block Development Officers, community leaders, and multiple social welfare agencies in Punjab promoting various health programs in the state.

Shibnath Mukherjee has a BE in Electronics and telecommunication engineering and has done MBA in Systems and Operations. He has also done his PhD in Information Systems specializing in algorithms for privacy preserving data mining. He has worked with IBM India and Deloitte India in consulting and managerial positions in the business intelligence practice. Currently he is working as a research engineer in Yahoo! Research and Development India. His topic of interest lies in the domain of internet advertising and scalable machine learning algorithms over the grid.

Josephine Namayanja is currently pursuing a PhD in Information Systems at the University of Maryland, Baltimore County (UMBC). She received her Master's degree in Information Systems in May, 2010 from the same institution. Her primary research area is data mining and she has a large interest in computational health applications. She is also interested in exploring data mining techniques in previous research studies to understand disease patterns.

Stefanie Roos is currently a graduate student of Darmstadt University, Germany. She started university in Fall 2006, receiving her Bachelor degree in Fall 2009. Stefanie was an exchange student at the University of Saskatchewan, Canada from Fall 2008 to Summer 2009. Her research interests include genetic programming and routing in decentralized networks.

Basit Shafiq is a Research Assistant professor at the Center for Information Management, Integration and Connectivity (CIMIC), Rutgers University. He received his Ph. D. and M.S. in Electrical and Computer Engineering from Purdue University. His research interests include information systems security and privacy, access-control management in distributed systems, semantic Web, Web services composition and verification, and distributed multimedia systems. His research work resulted in several publications in well-renowned journals and conferences.

Iftikhar U. Sikder is an Associate Professor of Computer and Information Science at Cleveland State University. He holds a PhD in Computer Information Systems from the University of Maryland, Baltimore County. His research interests include Semantic data models, spatial databases, spatial data mining and granular computing. He has authored numerous papers in peer-reviewed journals, many book chapters and presented papers in many national and international conferences. He can be reached at i.sikder@csuohio.edu

Kulwinder Singh Ded MS MCh is Professor and Head Department of Surgery at SGRD Institute of Medical Sciences, Amritsar, India. Dr. Ded has MS General Surgery and a MCh in Peidatric Surgery and was earlier Associate Professor of Surgery at Rajindra Hospital, Patiala, India.

Qiang Tang is currently a postdoc researcher at the Distributed and Embedded Security Research Group in the EEMCS faculty of University of Twente. His research interests include cryptography and information security, especially applying cryptographic techniques to solve practical information security problems. Previously, he spent one year as a postdoc researcher at the Crypto Team in Ecole Normale Superieure, France. Even before this, he did his PhD at the Information Security Group of Royal Holloway, University of London, United Kingdom.

Guoyu Tao, PhD. Dr. Tao has worked as health service researcher with the Division of STD Prevention at Centers for Disease Control and Prevention since 1995. He is interested in STD-related health services research, economic evaluation, and policy.

Manabu Torii is a Research Assistant Professor at the Imaging Science and Information Systems (ISIS) Center in Georgetown University Medical Center (GUMC) since December 2007. He is a member of the Division of Integrated Biodefense in the ISIS Center and his current research focuses on information retrieval for Internet-based biosurveillance. His research interests also include natural language processing (NLP), information extraction (IE), machine learning, and their application in the biomedical domain. Before he joined the ISIS Center, he was a postdoctoral fellow at Liu Lab in the Department of Biostatistics, Bioinformatics, and Biomathematics in GUMC. He received his Ph.D. degree in Computer Science from University of Delaware in January 2006.

Jaideep Vaidya received the bachelor's degree from the University of Mumbai and the master's and PhD degrees from Purdue University. He is an assistant professor of computer information systems at Rutgers University, Newark, New Jersey. His research interests include data mining, data management, privacy, and security. He has received two best paper awards from the premier conferences in data mining and databases. He is also the recipient of an NSF Career Award. He is a member of the ACM, and the IEEE Computer Society.

Thomas White is a senior executive within the New York State Office of Mental Health (OMH), and an Associate Professor at Columbia University. He developed the PSYCKES business intelligence + disease management system, which won a national innovation award, and is now using Medicaid claims data to improve prescribing quality throughout New York. His Dialogix system for creating complex, multi-lingual, epidemiological studies has supported over $100 million in NIH-funded research; and extensions to it have become the national standard encoding interoperable assessment instruments. Prior successes included the development of best-of-breed systems for neurophysiology and brain imaging NIMH (CORTEX), and Memorial Sloan Kettering Cancer Center (fMRI); plus a novel content management system for a national insurance regulator (NCCI). Dr. White is now spearheading open-source-based Master Data Management initiatives within OMH and across multiple state agencies, effectively a Health Information Exchange for key government data.

Guixian Xu is a lecturer at College of Information Engineering in Minzu University of China since 2004. She is currently perusing her Ph.D. degree at College of Computer Science in Beijing Institute of Technology. Her research fields include machine learning and artificial intelligence. As a visiting scholar, she worked and studied at Department of Biostatistics, Bioinformatics, and Biomathematics of Georgetown University from March 2008 to March 2009. She cooperated with Dr. Hongfang Liu and conducted research on biological text mining. Her research topics focused on imbalanced text classification as well as semi-supervised learning of text classification on protein-protein interaction documents during the visiting time.

Moi-Hoon Yap received her PhD in Computer Science from Loughborough University in 2009. She received her BSc(hons) in Statistics from Universiti Putra Malaysia (UPM) in 1999, and MSc(IT) in 2001. In 2002 and 2005, she served as a lecturer at the Faculty of Information Technology, Multimedia University (MMU), Malaysia. Currently she is a Postdoctoral Research Assistant in School of Computing, Informatics and Media, University of Bradford, UK. She is actively involving in computer vision research. Her research of interest is facial analysis, medical image analysis, human perception, image and video processing.

Nicole Yu graduated with a Bachelor of Science Double Advanced Major in Chemistry and Biology given by Saint Francis Xavier University (Nova Scotia). With a deep interest for learning and a need for a bigger challenge, she proceeded to obtain her Masters of Applied Science in Biomedical Engineering from the Systems and Computer Engineering Department of Carleton University. When she isn't studying, she loves to play sports, snowboard, learn new hobbies and travel the world.

Kun Zhao is a PhD candidate in the Mathematics and Statistics Department at Georgia State University. He is interested in applying mathematical, statistical and computational techniques to solve disease-related problems in health care services and biomedical research.

Index